P9-CBK-449

Mechanisms of Immunopathology

BASIC AND CLINICAL IMMUNOLOGY

SERIES EDITORS: Stanley Cohen, University of Connecticut Health Center, Farmington. Robert T. McCluskey, Massachusetts General Hospital, Harvard Medical School

Mechanisms of Cell-Mediated Immunity

ROBERT T. MCCLUSKEY AND STANLEY COHEN, *Editors*

Mechanisms of Tumor Immunity

IRA GREEN, STANLEY COHEN, AND ROBERT T. MCCLUSKEY, *Editors*

Immunocytochemistry

LUDWIG A. STERNBERGER

Mechanisms of Immunopathology

STANLEY COHEN, PETER A. WARD, AND ROBERT T. MCCLUSKEY, *Editors*

Mechanisms of Immunopathology

EDITED BY

STANLEY COHEN

University of Connecticut Health Center, Farmington

PETER A. WARD

University of Connecticut Health Center, Farmington

ROBERT T. McCLUSKEY

Massachusetts General Hospital and Harvard Medical School

A WILEY MEDICAL PUBLICATION

JOHN WILEY & SONS New York • Chichester • Brisbane • Toronto

Library of Congress Cataloging in Publication Data:

Main entry under title:

(Basic and clinical immunology) (A Wiley medical
publication)
Includes index.
1. Immunopathology. I. Cohen, Stanley, 1937–
II. Ward, Peter A. III. McCluskey, Robert T.
[DNLM: 1. Immunologic diseases. 2. Immunity.
3. Antigen-antibody reactions. WD300 M486]
RC582.2.M37 616.07'9 78-18290
ISBN 0-471-16429-1

Printed in the United States of America

10 9 8 7 6 5 4 3 2 1

Contributors

Chester A. Alper, M.D.
Scientific Director, Center for Blood Research
Professor of Pediatrics
Children's Hospital Medical Center
Harvard Medical School
Boston, Massachusetts 02115

Pierluigi E. Bigazzi, M.D.
Associate Professor of Pathology
University of Connecticut Health Center
Farmington, Connecticut 06032

Charles G. Cochrane, M.D.
Member
Department of Immunopathology
Scripps Clinic and Research Foundation
La Jolla, California 92037

Stanley Cohen, M.D.
Professor and Associate Chairman
Department of Pathology
University of Connecticut Health Center
Farmington, Connecticut 06032

Robert B. Colvin, M.D.
Assistant Professor of Pathology
Harvard Medical School
Assistant in Pathology
Massachusetts General Hospital
Boston, Massachusetts 02114

Michael V. Doyle, Ph.D.
Research Fellow
Department of Immunopathology
Scripps Clinic and Research Foundation
La Jolla, California 92037

Harold F. Dvorak, M.D.
Professor of Pathology
Harvard University
Associate Pathologist
Massachusetts General Hospital
Boston, Massachusetts 02114

Gabriel Fernandes, Ph.D.
Visiting Investigator
Memorial Sloan-Kettering Cancer Center
New York, New York 10021

Robert A. Good, Ph.D., M.D.
President and Director
Sloan-Kettering Institute for Cancer Research
New York, New York 10021

Philip D. Greenberg, M.D.
Instructor
Department of Medicine
University of California
San Diego, California 92103

Clive L. Hall, M.D.
Associate Professor
Department of Pathology
Massachusetts General Hospital
Boston, Massachusetts 02114

Helen M. Hallgren, M.S.
Associate Professor
Department of Laboratory Medicine
University of Minnesota
Minneapolis, Minnesota 55455

Barry S. Handwerger, M.D.
Assistant Professor
Department of Medicine
University of Minnesota
Minneapolis, Minnesota 55455

Lawrence M. Lichtenstein, M.D.
Professor of Medicine
Clinical Immunology Division
Department of Medicine
The Johns Hopkins University
School of Medicine
Good Samaritan Hospital
Baltimore, Maryland 21239

Richard Lindquist, M.D.
Associate Professor
Department of Pathology
University of Connecticut Health
Center
Farmington, Connecticut 06032

Robert T. McCluskey, M.D.
Professor of Pathology
Harvard Medical School
Chief Pathologist
Massachusetts General Hospital
Boston, Massachusetts 02114

D. Elliot Parks, Ph.D.
Assistant Member
Department of Immunopathology
Scripps Clinic and Research
Foundation
La Jolla, California 92037

Carole G. Romball, M.S.
Senior Technologist
Department of Immunopathology
Scripps Clinic and Research
Foundation
La Jolla, California 92037

Noel R. Rose, M.D., Ph.D.
Professor and Chairman
Department of Immunology and
Microbiology
Wayne State University
Detroit, Michigan 48201

Fred S. Rosen, M.D.
Chief, Immunology Division
Children's Hospital Medical Center
James L. Gamble Professor of
Pediatrics
Harvard Medical School
Boston, Massachusetts 02115

Thomas P. Stossel, M.D.
Associate Professor
Department of Pediatrics
Harvard Medical School
Massachusetts General Hospital
Boston, Massachusetts 02114

Peter A. Ward, M.D.
Professor and Chairman
Department of Pathology
University of Connecticut Health
Center
Farmington, Connecticut 06032

William O. Weigle, Ph.D.
Member and Acting Chairman
Department of Immunopathology
Scripps Clinic and Research
Foundation
La Jolla, California 92037

Curtis B. Wilson, M.D.
Member
Department of Immunopathology
Scripps Clinic and Research
Foundation
La Jolla, California 92037

Takeshi Yoshida, M.D.
Associate Professor
Department of Pathology
University of Connecticut Health
Center
Farmington, Connecticut 06032

Edmond J. Yunis, M.D.
Professor of Pathology
Harvard Medical School
Chief Physician of Immunogenetics
Sidney Farber Cancer Institute
Boston, Massachusetts 02115

Nathan J. Zvaifler, M.D.
Professor of Medicine
University of California
San Diego, California 92103

Preface

The field of immunopathology encompasses a variety of phenomena. Perhaps most obviously, it deals with the various derangements of biologic processes that arise as a consequence of immunologic reactions. Aberrant, excessive, or inappropriate immunologic responses can lead to pathologic changes. Some examples are allergies, autoimmunity, and various kinds of immune complex-induced damage. Even when the immunologic response is initiated as a part of a normal defense reaction, pathologic alterations can result. In analogy, one can think of the reaction between the immune system and pathogen as a battle, and note that in a war, even if the right side wins, the battlefield can remain scarred.

Another aspect of immunopathology involves intrinsic defects in the immune system, and the consequence to the host of such defects. Finally, immunopathology includes a number of fields that are different from the categories mentioned above, but that involve similar kinds of mechanisms. Two examples are transplantation and the role of the immune system in aging.

From the above, it is obvious that aside from intrinsic defects of immunologic function, immunopathology involves the activation of various effector mechanisms that result in pathologic consequences. These mechanisms, for the most part, represent an interface between the immune system and the inflammatory system. To a very large extent, immunopathology depends upon immunologically induced inflammation.

Rather than attempt the usual encyclopedic cataloging of every disease entity thought to involve immunopathologic mechanisms, this book focuses on the themes outlined above. It begins with an overview of the major inflammatory mediators that can be generated via the workings of the immune system. Following are chapters that deal with our current understanding of the mechanisms of anaphylactic reactions, immune complex-induced reactions, and cell-mediated immunity. In the latter, special attention is given to the lymphocyte-derived mediators, their in vivo significance, and basic principles involving desensitization and regulation that may relate to defects of cellular immunity in disease. In these chapters, an attempt is made to explore interrelationships of the various systems, since the immune system has a great deal of built-in, fail-safe redundancy. One chapter is devoted to the role of granulocytes in cell-mediated immunity, since it is still widely and erroneously held that the unique effector cell in this class of reaction is the macrophage.

These topics plus a discussion of the relation between aging and immunity, followed by an extensive review of tolerance, provide the introduction for the subsequent chapters dealing with various aspects of autoimmune and immune-complex disease. The chapters on tolerance and autoimmunity deal with similar topics and concepts, but examine them from different perspectives in order to provide a well-balanced view. From there we turn to defects of the immune system, not only with respect to classic immunologic deficiency states but with respect to certain kinds of mediator dysfunction and effector cell dysfunction. The book concludes with an account of some of the mechanisms involved in transplantation immunity.

Although methodology is not stressed, considerable information regarding clinically useful assay procedures is provided throughout the book. Examples include discussions on ways of detecting circulating complexes and descriptions of various in vitro and in vivo manifestations of lymphokine activity.

With this mechanism-oriented approach, we hope that the book will prove useful not only to clinicians and investigators in various fields involving immunopathologic processes but to students who wish a more in-depth exposure to these concepts than is generally available in introductory texts.

October 1978

Stanley Cohen
Peter A. Ward
Robert T. McCluskey

Contents

Chapter 1:	**Mediators of Inflammatory Responses** PETER A. WARD	**1**
Chapter 2:	**Anaphylactic Reactions** LAWRENCE M. LICHTENSTEIN	**13**
Chapter 3:	**Immune Complex-Mediated Tissue Injury** CHARLES G. COCHRANE	**29**
Chapter 4:	**Lymphokine-Mediated Reactions** STANLEY COHEN AND TAKESHI YOSHIDA	**49**
Chapter 5:	**Role of Granulocytes in Cell-Mediated Immunity** ROBERT B. COLVIN AND HAROLD F. DVORAK	**69**
Chapter 6:	**Aging and Immunity** EDMOND J. YUNIS, BARRY S. HANDWERGER, HELEN M. HALLGREN, ROBERT A. GOOD, AND GABRIEL FERNANDES	**91**
Chapter 7:	**Immunoregulation in Tolerance and Autoimmunity** MICHAEL V. DOYLE, D. ELLIOT PARKS, CAROLE G. ROMBALL, AND WILLIAM O. WEIGLE	**107**
Chapter 8:	**General Aspects of Autoimmune Disease** NOEL R. ROSE	**143**

Chapter 9: Thyroiditis as a Model of Autoimmune Disorders in Man 157
PIERLUIGI E. BIGAZZI

Chapter 10: Immunopathology of Anti-Basement Membrane Antibodies 181
CURTIS B. WILSON

Chapter 11: Human Immune Complex Diseases 203
CLIVE L. HALL, ROBERT B. COLVIN, AND ROBERT T. MCCLUSKEY

Chapter 12: Immunopathology of Rheumatoid Arthritis 247
NATHAN J. ZVAIFLER AND PHILIP D. GREENBERG

Chapter 13: Disorders of Phagocytic Effector Cells 271
THOMAS P. STOSSEL

Chapter 14: Human Complement Deficiencies 289
CHESTER A. ALPER AND FRED S. ROSEN

Chapter 15: Immunodeficiency Diseases 307
FRED S. ROSEN

Chapter 16: Mechanisms of Transplantation Immunity 323
RICHARD LINDQUIST

Index 355

Chapter One

Mediators of Inflammatory Responses

PETER A. WARD

Department of Pathology, University of Connecticut Health Center, Farmington, Connecticut

Except for those few immunopathologic reactions in which the inflammatory response and the tissue injury are attributable to direct cell-cell contact between sensitized lymphocytes and target cells, most reactions that result in tissue damage do so secondary to the induction of an inflammatory reaction. In essence, the immune response triggers a highly focused elaboration of phlogistic mediators, the outcome of which is a localized accumulation of inflammatory cells and plasma constituents. It is the presence of these blood-derived elements that is most directly associated with the tissue damage. This is true not only for antibody-mediated reactions but also for various manifestations of cell-mediated immunity, as will be discussed in subsequent chapters.

Inflammatory reactions can be looked upon in terms of the two key elements that characterize an inflammatory reaction: vasopermeability changes and the arrival of leukocytes from the circulation (1). Secondary changes include the activation of fibroblasts leading to production of collagen, and the proliferation of endothelial cells resulting in formation of new capillaries. Mediators have been described that can account for each of these changes. The increased vasopermeability is due to the transient opening of endothelial junctions, permitting egress of soluble substances such as plasma proteins, electrolytes, and water. It is of interest that virtually all the vasopermeability mediators were originally found to be capable of causing smooth muscle contraction. The mechanism by which these mediators are currently presumed to work is through their ability to induce contraction of the actin-myosin elements in endothelial cells. This causes them to become "wrinkled" and shrunken, leaving gaps in the junctional zones between endothelial cells (2). This hypothesis, which explains the mechanism of

Table 1. Some Effects of Chemotactic Factors on Leukocytes

Transmembrane fluxes of Na^{+}, K^{+}, Ca^{++}
Membrane depolarization
Cell swelling
Cell aggregation
Proesterase activation
Activation of hexose monophosphatase shunt activity
Increased glycolysis and superoxide anion production
Enhanced random migration ("chemokinesis")
Directed (unidirectional) migration
Secretion of lysosomal enzymes

vasopermeability, accounts also for the muscle-contracting activities of vasopermeability mediators, as well as their ephemeral and reversible nature.

The leukotactic mediators appear to be, in general, separate and distinct factors from the vasopermeability mediators. As a general rule, the leukotactic mediators do not contract smooth muscle, and injection of vasopermeability mediators does not result in accumulation of inflammatory cells.

Leukotactic factors have a variety of effects on leukocytes, as described in Table 1. The changes described in the table occur after contact of neutrophils with any of many chemotactic factors (C3 and C5 factors, bacterial factors, and synthetic peptides). Although studies have not been done in as great detail, it seems likely that monocytes and macrophages behave similarly after contact with these chemotactic mediators. The changes listed in the table may not all be directly related to the chemotactic movement of the leukocyte, but they cannot be dissociated; the loss of one implies the loss of all others (3). Some of the cell responses, such as cell aggregation, may relate to what has been seen in vivo (4). For instance, after infusion of chemotactic factor into a peripheral ear vein of rabbits, leukocytes accumulate along endothelial surfaces (perhaps by adherence), and they sequester as intravascular aggregates in the first capillary bed contacted, which in this example would be the pulmonary capillary network (5). These phenomena suggest that increased adherence or "stickiness" of white cells may be part of the outcome of contact of leukocytes with chemotactic factors.

In the following paragraphs I will try to highlight the current knowledge about important inflammatory mediators and will point out instances in which some of the mediators have been demonstrated in ongoing inflammatory reactions.

THE MEDIATORS

The Prostaglandin (PG) System

Details of the chemistry and function of the prostaglandin (PG) system are still emerging (6). PGs presumably arise from arachidonic acid, which is derived by the action of membrane-associated phospholipase A2 of cells. Several years ago aspirin and indomethacin, which are well known to have anti-inflammatory effects, were demonstrated to block cyclo-oxygenase, which converts archidonic

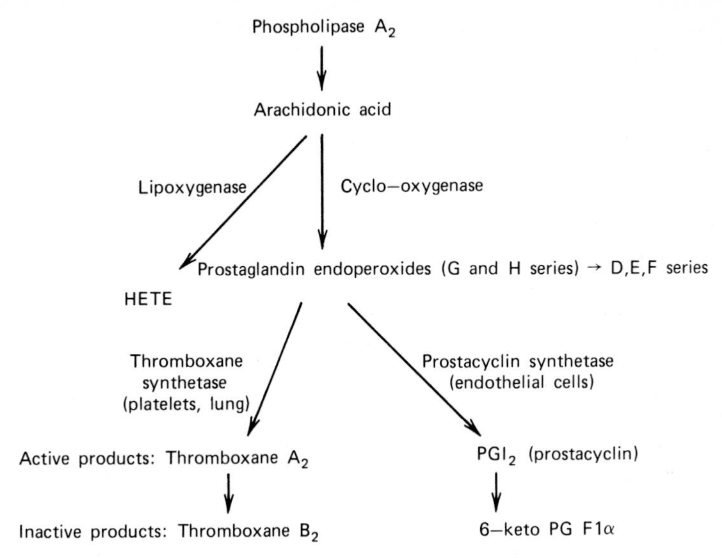

Figure 1. The prostaglandin system.

acid into the PG G and H series (Fig. 1). It was widely assumed that the blocking of PG synthesis by these drugs was proof that PGs are direct mediators of the inflammatory response (7). Since that time, as the relatively stable PGE and PGF series have been studied, it has become apparent that other PGs are probably endowed with much more biologic activity, that many highly active PGs are exceedingly unstable, and that PGs have a wide spectrum of activities that may be proinflammatory or anti-inflammatory, depending on the PG in question and the organ or tissue bed under study. This is well demonstrated by the finding that platelets and lung tissue, through their thromboxane synthetase, produce thromboxanes A_2 and B_2, the former being highly active in causing platelet clumping and arterial constriction. In contrast, endothelial cells contain a prostacyclin synthetase that leads to formation of PGI_2, an antagonist of the actions of PGA_2. Thus, the PG system is highly complex and far from being completely understood.

As is described in Chapter 2, PGs have the ability to modify profoundly the functional responses of leukocytes. The release of vasoactive amines from mast cells and/or basophils can be modulated by PGs as well as other drugs. The ultimate effect of these manipulations is, presumably, a change in intracellular levels of cyclic AMP or cyclic GMP, which subsequently depresses or enhances cell responsiveness.

The Kinin-Forming System

Generation of kinins (bradykinin, lysyl-bradykinin, and methionyl-lysyl-bradykinin) from plasma substrates occurs by an indirect activation step that involves activation of factor XII (Hageman factor) of the intrinsic clotting system (Fig. 2). These events are described in greater detail in Chapter 3. This activation, which can be initiated by bacterial lipopolysaccharide, plasmin,

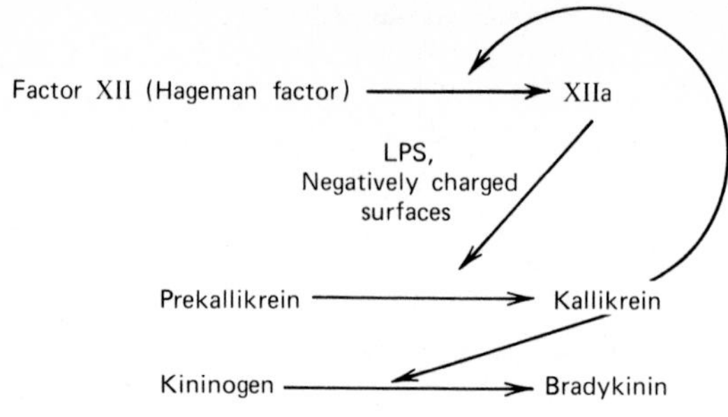

Figure 2. The kinin-forming system.

by contact of plasma with negatively changed surfaces, or by kallikrein itself, involves either a conformational change in factor XII or its fragmentation, or both. The active form of Hageman factor, or XIIa, is now known to be identical with the "permeability factor of dilution" (PF/dil.) first described by Miles and Wilhelm (8). It was noted that this permeability factor was acting as if a latent period was required for expression of activity. This can now be explained by the fact that it is an enzyme and that its effects are ultimately mediated through its role in the generation of bradykinin. The result is conversion of factor XII to its active form (XIIa), which, in turn, leads to conversion of plasma prekallikrein into the active form, kallikrein. By cleavage of an arginyl bond in a plasma substrate, kallikrein causes production of bradykinin, or the two other derivatives of bradykinin, which are listed above.

Bradykinin has long been thought to play an important biologic role, although there is no direct evidence for this contention. The biologic effects of the nonapeptide include bradycardia, hypotension, contraction of isolated strips of smooth muscle, and increased vasopermeability. Part of the difficulty in delineating a role for this peptide is the fact that it is rapidly inactivated by a plasma kininase (described in a later section). Thus, it is virtually impossible to find bradykinin in active form in biologic fluids, and this has complicated the search for its biologic significance.

The Leukokinin-Forming System

In contrast to bradykinin and its derivatives, which are very cationic peptides with molecular weights of approximately 1,000, the leukokinins represent a chemically different class of active peptides with vasopermeability effects (9). The leukokinins are acidic peptides with molecular weights of approximately 3,500. They were originally described in experiments employing extracts of lysosomal granules. These extracts, when incubated with plasma, produced a smooth-muscle-contracting and vasopermeability factor that was recognized to differ from bradykinin. It was later found that the term "leukokinin" was a misnomer, since the leukokinin-generating enzyme could be extracted not only from leukocytic lysosomal granules but also from a variety of other cell types, including tumor cells. The latter observation has led to the interesting finding that in mice with malignant tumors, which produce abundant ascitic fluid, the tumor cells release a leukokinin-generating enzyme that acts on a substrate (present in plasma) in the peritoneal cavity (9). The generation of leukokinins appears to lead to the production of ascites, a manifestation of the increased vasopermeability. The leukokinin-generating enzyme can be blocked with pepstatin, which interferes with the formation of ascites. There is no information available on the role of the leukokinin-forming system in non-neoplastic diseases.

The Basophil (and Mast Cell) Factors

Increasingly, as emphasized in Chapter 5, basophils are known to have a prominent role in both cell-mediated immune reactions and humoral immune reactions. To date, there appears to be little difference in the release mechanisms and the products released from basophils and from mast cells. Although the mediator substances relevant to the participation of basophils in cellular immune reactions have not been identified, the mechanisms of the participation of basophils in humorally mediated reactions are reasonably clear. These can be attributed to the active secretory release of vasoactive amines (histamine and/or serotonin), the release of other anaphylactic mediators (see below), and the release of platelet activating factor (PAF), which, in turn, can lead to aggregation of platelets, inducing the release of serotonin from platelet granules (10).

The role of vasoactive amines, especially histamine, is strongly incriminated in the deposition of circulating immune complexes in renal glomerular basement membrane (see Chapter 3). The anaphylactic mediators of the basophil, described in Chapter 2, include the slow-reacting substance of anaphylaxis (SRS-A), the eosinophil chemotactic factor of anaphylaxis, and histamine. The platelet activating factor (PAF) is also released under conditions in which other "anaphylactic mediators" are also released. PAF is not yet structurally defined. It seems to be some type of acidic lipid, perhaps a prostaglandin. Its action ties together the functional responses of both basophils and platelets. It should also be emphasized that many of the products of basophil secretion, in addition to being released under anaphylactic conditions (as described above), can be released by contact of basophils with the complement-derived anaphylotoxins (C3a and C5a). (See the section on complement, below.) Thus, there are at least two separate and distinct biologic reactions that can lead to basophil secretion. It should be stressed that virtually all these products will cause smooth muscle contraction and increased vasopermeability.

Another secretory product of the basophil, the plasminogen activator, has been very recently described. This substance may, through its purported leukotactic activity and its ability to activate plasmin, have secondary effects on other mediator systems.

Factors Affecting Vascular and Stromal Elements

Two different factors affecting stromal elements have been described. These include the tumor angiogenesis factor (TAF) and the fibroblast activating factor (11,12). Since these involve soluble factors and since they affect vascular and fibrous connective tissue elements, their effects on the outcome of an inflammatory response may be exceedingly important. TAF is a protein-like, diffusible substance with an estimated molecular weight of 10^5 daltons. This factor causes neovascular growth at the rate of 0.2 to 0.8 mm/day. The factor was originally found in extracts of malignant tumors and in culture filtrates of tumor cells maintained in vitro. A major problem in the demonstration of TAF has been the requirement for an in vivo assay, using either the chorioallantoic membrane of hen eggs or the cornea of a variety of animals. In the latter model, limbal vessels can be seen growing toward the corneal implant. Unless there is a continuing presence of TAF for at least the first 16 hours, rapid regression of the newly formed vessels occurs. Very recently, a nontumor cell source of angiogenesis factor has been found in cultures of macrophages activated by phagocytosis (11). These latter observations are of particular interest because of the profusion of newly formed vessels in reactions that are rich in mononuclear cells, such as the chronic inflammatory reactions of viral hepatitis, tuberculosis, chronic viral infections, etc.

Fibroblast activating factors, which lead either to proliferation of fibroblasts or to increased secretion of collagen, or both, have been described in fractions of serum, in platelets, and in culture supernatant fluids of antigen- or mitogen-stimulated lymphoid cells. These latter represent, by definition, lymphokines. None of these factors has yet been characterized in physical-chemical terms, but their recognition implies discrete control of collagen production by nonfibroblast factors.

The Complement Mediators

With few exceptions, the complement-derived phlogistic mediators are derived from the middle portion of the complement system (Fig. 3). An exception to this is the putative "C142 kinin," which was first described in association with permeability change induced in the skin of persons injected with C1 esterase (C1s) (13). This vasopermeability reaction occurred in C3-deficient but not in C2-deficient individuals. It was later demonstrated that in vitro mixtures of C1, C4, and C2 resulted in the formation of a kinin-like activity that would cause contraction of smooth muscle. This activity has not been chemically characterized, and it is not seen predictably in incubation mixtures of purified complement compo-

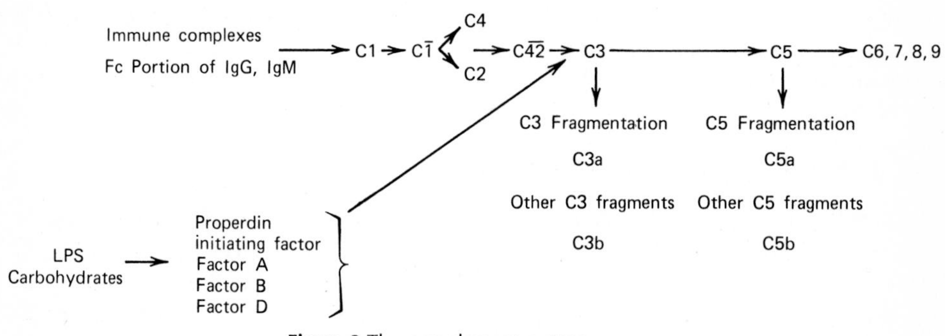

Figure 3. The complement system.

Table 2. Phlogistic Mediators from the Complement System

Source	Designation	Biological Activity
C1,4,2	"C1,4,2 kinin"	Contracts smooth muscle
C3	C3a (anaphylatoxin)	Contracts smooth muscle Releases histamine from mast cells and basophils
	C3 fragment (not C3a)	Leukotactic for neutrophils, eosinophils, and monocytes
	C3b fragment	Opsonic factor
C5	C5a (anaphylatoxin)	Contracts smooth muscle; leukotactic for monocytes, neutrophils, basophils, and eosinophils Releases histamine from mast cells and basophils Leukotactic for neutrophils, eosinophils, and monocytes
	C5 fragments (not C5a)	Leukotactic for neutrophils, eosinophils, and monocytes
C567	$\overline{C567}$	"Membrane attack" factor, leukotactic for neutrophils

nents. Interest in the pathophysiologic role of this factor has arisen in studies of patients with deficiency of the inhibitor that controls C1s (discussed below).

The biologic activities emanating from the complement system are reviewed in Table 2. Fragmentation products of C3 include the classical C3a anaphylatoxin that contracts smooth muscle and also causes histamine release from mast cells and basophils (14,15). Histamine release may be the mechanism of smooth muscle contraction by C3 anaphylatoxin, since its effects can be blocked with antihistaminic drugs. Depending on the circumstances of fragmentation, C3 fragments that do not have anaphylatoxin activity, but that are leukotactically active, have also been described (16). Although the C3a fragment, which has an estimated molecular weight of 8,500, is presumed to arise from a cleavage point near the amino terminal end of the alpha chain of C3, no structural information is available on the other biologically active fragments. However, the non-C3a biologically active fragments can be produced by the actions of a variety of neutral proteases, including trypsin, thrombin, and a tissue protease (16). Under the usual conditions of complement activation in normal human serum, no biologically active C3 fragments are found. This may be due either to lack of generation of C3 fragments or, more likely, inactivation of biologically active fragments by serum inhibitors.

The C3b fragment is the large, residual portion of the C3 molecule remaining after the splitting off of C3a (14). The residual molecule thus has two peptide chains that are held together by disulfide bonds, minus the alpha chain amino terminal segment. With a molecular weight of around 180,000, C3b is hydrophobic and, therefore, tends to affix to cell membranes. As such, C3b is the major opsonic factor of the complement system for which there are receptors both on neutrophils and on monocytes. Accordingly, particles, cells, or complexes with C3b will be phagocytically removed either by the blood leukocytes or by the reticuloendothelial system. Although C5b has not been studied to the same extent, similar statements about its biologic activity can be made. The additional biologic activities of C3b include activation of the alternative complement pathway and activation of B lymphocytes, causing these cells to produce and release lymphokines (see Chapter 4).

The lower-molecular-weight C5-related products with biologic activity include fragments (circa 15,000 to 20,000 molecular weight) produced either by activation of the complement system or by direct enzymatic cleavage of C5 (17). C5a is the product of complement activation via the alternative or the classical pathway, or the result of limited trypsin cleavage of the molecule. The C5a molecule is a basic peptide of molecular weight 15,000, about 25% of which is due to the presence of sugars. This molecule is active in both anaphylatoxin and chemotactic assays at concentrations of approximately 10^{-9}M. Because C5a is rapidly destroyed in normal serum by the anaphylatoxin inactivator, and because chemotactic activity exists under the same conditions, the relationship, if any, between the anaphylatoxin peptide and the chemotactic factor is not established. It has been recently proposed that the inactivation of C5a results in C5a des arg, a peptide with limited chemotactic activity and no anaphylatoxin activity (18). Whether this explains the origin of the chemotactic factor in activated serum, or whether a second, unrelated C5 peptide with chemotactic activity is produced in serum, cannot presently be resolved.

In addition to leukotactic activity, C5a anaphylatoxin induces contraction of smooth muscle and causes histamine release from mast cells and basophils. There is evidence that the receptors in smooth muscle for C3a and C5a are different, since tachyphylaxis is specific for the anaphylatoxin peptide causing loss of muscle-contracting activity (14). Althouth C5b is an opsonic factor, much as C3b (see above), there is as yet no indication that C5b can activate the alternative complement pathway; nor has there been any evidence that a natural inactivator for C5b exists in serum.

The macromolecular $\overline{C567}$ complex was the first complement-derived chemotactic factor to be described; the available evidence indicates that it is chemotactic only for neutrophils (19). $\overline{C567}$ is also described as having the a "membrane attack" activity. By this is meant that cell membranes are first altered by $\overline{C567}$ and "prepared" for interaction with C8 and C9, which results in cytoly-

Table 3. Presence of Inflammatory Mediators in Ongoing Inflammatory Reactions

Reaction	Mediator(s) Identified
Immunologic vasculitis	C5 chemotactic fragment and $\overline{C567}$
Synovial fluids from patients with inflammatory nonrheumatoid arthritis	C5 chemotactic fragment and $\overline{C567}$
Peritoneal challenge of animals with lipopolysaccharide	C5 chemotactic fragments
Synovial fluids from patients with inflammatory nonrheumatoid arthritis	C3 chemotactic fragments
Antigen challenge of animals sensitized for anaphylaxis	SRS-A, ECF-A, histamine, platelet activating factors, protaglandins

tic damage to the cell. The most recent, available evidence suggests that the damage is due to the formation of an ion "channel" in the membrane, perhaps because of a detergent-like effect of the terminal complement components. The highly publicized "holes" found in cytolytically damaged membranes have not been correlated with the terminal complement component action (20). There is reasonably conclusive evidence that the cytotoxin events are not related to an activation of a phospholipase.

EVIDENCE FOR IN VIVO ACTIVITY OF THE INFLAMMATORY MEDIATORS

Inflammatory mediators have been demonstrated in vivo in a variety of conditions, which are summarized in Table 3. One of the difficulties in securing evidence that the mediators listed above are in fact being found in vivo (a prerequisite to proof that they in fact are important mediators for in vivo reactions) relates to the rapid destruction of these mediators by factors present in plasma. Thus, bradykinin cannot be demonstrated in human plasma or in synovial or other biologic fluids. However, it can be demonstrated that in certain circumstances the serum substrate (kininogen) for bradykinin is depressed in amount, suggesting but not proving that kinin production has occurred. The same problem relates to the anaphylatoxins, which are rapidly inactivated by plasma. In the case of anaphylactic reactions, however, a series of mediators has been found in vivo or in perfused tissues after antigen challenge. These mediators include histamine, SRS-A, ECF-A, and platelet activating factors, as well as prostaglandins and kallikrein, all of which will be discussed in greater detail in subsequent chapters. Perhaps the most convincing data for the role of complement mediators have come from studies of experimental vasculitis and from humans with arthritis (21,22).

It has been demonstrated that complement depletion in vivo precludes development of inflammatory reactions and vascular injury in reversed passive Arthus reactions (23). It was subsequently shown that developing Arthus reactions are associated with the presence of C5 chemotactic products (namely C5 fragment and $\overline{C567}$) in extracts of the developing vasculitis reactions (24). In another experimental approach, the injection of bacterial lipopolysaccharide (a potent activator of the alternative complement pathway) into the peritoneal cavities of experimental animals also results in the production of C5 chemotactic fragment and the induction of a prompt, acute neutrophil-rich inflammatory response (25). In patients with active rheumatoid arthritis, the synovial fluids of inflamed joints contain both C5 chemotactic fragment, as well as $\overline{C567}$. In patients with inflammatory nonrheumatoid arthritis (such as Reiter's syndrome), the inflamed joint fluids contain C3 chemotactic fragments (22). Thus, there is good evidence that the complement-derived chemotactic factors exist in vivo. Their presence closely correlates with development of inflammatory reactions. The availability of immunochemical reagents for the various mediators described above would probably permit the detection of several of these mediators, even if the mediators do not persist in a functionally active state in plasma or in other tissue fluids.

CONTROL OF INFLAMMATORY MEDIATORS

The mediators described in this chapter are active at very low concentrations. Obviously, activation of pathways leading to mediator production must be under some type of regulatory control, or else the inflammation would quickly escalate out of control. Control of bradykinin has been referred to above. Its inactivation occurs by a plasma-associated carboxypeptidase, which also inactivates the complement-derived anaphylatoxins. The best understanding of this concept comes from studies of the complement system.

There are two types of controls built into activation mechanisms for the complement system: inhibition of activation of complement-associated enzymes and inactivation of the products of the complement system. The first is best known by the presence in serum of the " $C\bar{1}$ esterase inhibitor" ($C\bar{1}$ INH) (26). $C\bar{1}$ INH blocks the ability of C1 esterase to cleave C4 and C2, resulting in a bimolecular complex (C42) that is enzymatically active and is directed against C3. $C\bar{1}$ INH also blocks the ability of C1 esterase to hydrolyze the synthetic substrate tosylarginine methyl ester (TAMe). Although complement activation can obviously override this inhibitor, the presence of $C\bar{1}$ INH modulates the intensity of the activation process. Although it was at first thought that these facts provided a reasonable explanation for the findings in hereditary angioedema, which occurs in individuals who lack inhibitor activity in their serum, the story quickly became complicated when it was found that $C\bar{1}$ INH also inhibits kallikrein and plasmin. In view of the fact that plasmin can activate both C1s and also directly cleave C3 into chemotactic peptides, and with the potential of kinin generation of kallikrein, the pathogenesis of $C\bar{1}$ INH deficiency syndrome cannot be easily explained (27). It is known that intradermal injection of C1 esterase causes local increases in vasopermeability in C3-deficient (but not in C2-deficient) persons. This explanation, that C1 esterase-associated permeability changes can indeed be directly ascribed to complement products, as suggested by the initial reports of the "$C\overline{142}$ kinin" (described above), awaits confirmation. At the present time, no other inhibitors of complement components containing enzymatic activities (such as $C\overline{42}$) have been definitively described.

Several inhibitors of the products of complement activation have been described, including the C3b inactivator, the anaphylatoxin inactivator, and the chemotactic factor inactivator (Table 4). The C3b inactivator appears to be a critical element in controlling levels of C3b and, thereby, regulating activation by C3b of the alternative complement pathway (28). This is most dramatically demonstrated by a patient who, lacking C3b inactivator, has unfettered activation of this pathway, leading to consumptive depletion of C3. The biologic consequence of this is the loss of control of complement activation and the inability to withstand bacterial infections as a result of the depleted levels of C3.

The C3b inactivator is thought to have enzymatic properties, since the inactive C3b preparation shows evidence of fragmentation. However, no definitive evidence for the enzymatic nature of C3b inactivation has been provided. There appears to be a co-factor in human plasma that enhances the rate of inactivation of C3b by the C3b inactivator. This co-factor is termed the β1H globulin (a designation of its electrophoretic behavior) and was first found as a contaminant in C5 preparations. There is no evidence that β1H globulin has any direct interaction with C3b.

Table 4. Regulators of Complement-Derived Inflammatory Mediators

1. Inhibitors of activated enzymes—$C\bar{1}$ esterase inhibitor ($C\bar{1}$ INH)
2. Inactivators of biologically active products—
a. C3b inactivator (and β1H co-factor)
b. Anaphylatoxin inactivator (also has kininase activity)
c. Chemotactic factor inactivators

The anaphylatoxin inactivator (AI) is an alpha globulin present in normal human serum; it irreversibly inactivates both C3a and C5a by a cleavage of the C terminal arginyl residue (29). AI is the same carboxypeptidase that inactivates bradykinin, a peptide that also ends in the same C terminal residue. Because of the presence of this inhibitor, neither C3a nor C5a activity can be demonstrated in normal human serum that has been treated with complement activating agents such as immune complexes, zymosan, cobra venom factor, etc. At present, no abnormalities in levels of AI have been described.

The chemotactic factor inactivator (CFI) is a system of at least two inhibitors in normal human serum (30). It is known that one CFI irreversibly inactivates the C5 (and the C3) chemotactic peptide, while an entirely different serum CFI inactivates the bacterial chemotactic factor produced from *Escherichia coli.* Although CFI is presumed to be an enzyme, it is not known how it inactivates the C5 chemotactic peptide. CFI is not inhibited by the serum protease inhibitors; nor is it blocked by di-isopropylfluorophosphate. Purified human CFI is a potent inhibitor of C5-dependent inflammatory reactions, such as immune complex-induced vasculitis and pulmonary alveolitis (31).

Clinical interest in CFI has arisen with the finding that patients with sarcoidosis, Hodgkin's disease, hepatic cirrhosis, and lepromatous leprosy have elevations in the levels of CFI (32). Clinically, they usually appear to be anergic. The leprosy patients, as would be expected with high levels of CFI, demonstrated about a half-normal mobilization of both neutrophils and monocytes into skin windows. Thus, a good correlation exists between abnormal levels of CFI and defective inflammatory reactions. These studies raise the possibility that eventually it might be possible to manipulate plasma levels of CFI in ways that would alter inflammatory responses.

COMPLEXITIES OF THE MEDIATOR SYSTEMS

Considerable knowledge is now available about the inflammatory mediator systems. Because of the intricate relationships between the various mediator systems, dissection of each in the context of one ongoing inflammatory reaction is difficult and is even more difficult in the context of specific deficiency states. Examples of the interrelationships between the mediator systems include the multiple effects of inhibitors (e.g., $C\bar{1}$ INH and its ability to react with C1 esterase, kallikrein, and plasmin); the multiple effects of activators (e.g., bacterial lipopolysaccharide can activate the alternative complement pathway and generate the complement-derived factors; lipopolysaccharide can also activate factor XII of the intrinsic clotting system, leading to the production of kinins and plasmin, which has effects on the clotting system and, also, on the complement system); also the multiple effects of inactivators (see above) can induce an amplification or marked dampening of a stimulus, depending on the interplay of the various parts. Finally, many of the effects of the mediators described in this chapter can be duplicated by the lymphokines. Understanding these complex relationships is one of the most formidable challenges today in the field of inflammation.

REFERENCES

1. Ryan, G. B., and Majno, G., *Am. J. Pathol.* **86,** 183 (1977).
2. Majno, G., Shea, S. M., and Leventhal, M., *J. Cell Biol.* **42,** 647 (1969).
3. Kreutzer, D. L., O'Flaherty, J. T., Orr, W., Showell, H. J., Ward, P. A., and Becker, E. L., submitted.
4. O'Flaherty, J. T., Kreutzer, D. L., and Ward, P. A., *J. Immunol.* **119**, 232 (1977).
5. O'Flaherty, J. T., Showell, H. J., and Ward, P. A., *J. Immunol.* **118**, 1586 (1977).
6. Pike, J. E., *Sci. Am.* **225** (5), 84 (1971).
7. Piper, P. J., and Vane, J. R., *Ann. N.Y. Acad. Sci.* **180**, 363 (1971).
8. Miles, A. A., and Wilhelm, D. L., *Br. J. Exp. Pathol.* **36,** 71 (1955).
9. Greenbaum, L. M., *Am. J. Pathol.* **68**, 613 (1972).
10. Henson, P. M., and Benveniste, J., Blackwell Scientific Publications, Oxford, 1971, p. 243.
11. Folkman, J., and Cotran, R., *Int. Rev. Exp. Pathol.* **16**, 207 (1976).
12. Ross, R., Glomset, J., and Harker, L., *Am. J. Pathol.* **86**, 675 (1977).
13. Ratnoff, O. D., *Thromb. Diath. Haemorrh.* Suppl. **45**, 109 (1971).
14. Müller-Eberhard, H. J., *Complement. Ann. Rev. Biochem.* **38,** 389 (1969).
15. Hugli, T. E., in *Proteases and Biological Control* (E. Reich, D. B. Rifkin, and E. Shaw, eds.), Cold Spring Harbor Laboratory, Long Island, N.Y., 1975.
16. Hill, J. H., and Ward, P. A., *J. Exp. Med.* **130**, 505 (1969).
17. Ward, P. A., and Newman, L. J., *J. Immunol.* **102**, 93 (1969).
18. Fernandez, S., and Hugli, T. E., *J. Immunol.* (in press).
19. Ward, P. A., Cochrane, C. G., and Müller-Eberhard, H. J., *J. Exp. Med.* **122**, 327 (1965).
20. Polley, M. J., Müller-Eberhard, H. J., and Feldman, J. D., *J. Exp. Med.* **133**, 53 (1971).
21. Ward, P. A., and Hill, J. H., *J. Immunol.* **108**, 1137 (1972).
22. Ward, P. A., and Zvaifler, N. J., *J. Clin. Invest.* **50**, 606 (1971).
23. Ward, P. A., and Cochrane, C. G., *J. Exp. Med.* **121**, 215 (1965).
24. Ward, P. A., and Hill, J. H., in *Chemical Biology of Inflammation* (B. K. Forscher and J. C. Houck, eds.), *Excerpta Medica,* 1971, p. 52.
25. Snyderman, R., Phillips, J., and Mergenhagen, S. E., *J. Expl. Med.* **134**, 1131 (1971).
26. Donaldson, V. H., and Evans, R. R., *Am. J. Med.* **35**, 37 (1963).
27. Ward, P. A., *J. Exp. Med.* **126**, 189 (1967).
28. Alper, C. A., Rosen, F. S., and Lachmann, P. J., *Proc. Natl. Acad. Sci.* (U.S.A.) **69**, 2910 (1972).
29. Müller-Eberhard, H. J., Bokisch, V. A., and Budzko, D. B., in *Immunopathology,* Sixth Int. Symp. (P. A. Miescher, ed.), Schwabe, Basel, 1971, p. 191.
30. Berenberg, J. L., and Ward, P. A., *J. Clin. Invest.* **52**, 1200 (1973).
31. Zigmond, S. H., and Hirsch, J. G., *J. Exp. Med.* **137**, 387 (1973).
32. Ward, P. A., Johnson, K. J., and Kreutzer, D. L., *Am. J. Pathol.* **88**, 701 (1977).

Chapter Two

Anaphylactic Reactions

LAWRENCE M. LICHTENSTEIN

Clinical Immunology Division, Department of Medicine, The Johns Hopkins University School of Medicine at The Good Samaritan Hospital, Baltimore, Maryland

The study of human allergic disease and the mechanism of reactions of immediate hypersensitivity may be considered as a field of research whose time has come. Although investigation in this area has been continuous since the demonstration by Prausnitz and Küstner that allergic diseases are due to a special class of "reaginic" antibodies, the diversity of the clinical problems and pragmatic approaches to therapy has, until recently, tended to obscure the nature of the immunopathologic events that cause anaphylaxis (1). In the last 20 years, however, rapid strides have been made. This progress is the result of (1) a series of controlled clinical evaluations of various modalities of treatment, (2) the development of sophisticated immunochemical, serologic, and biochemical techniques, and (3) appropriate in vitro models of the allergic response.

The diseases considered to be "allergic" range from the relatively benign, such as ragweed, tree, or grass pollinosis, affecting 10 to 15% of the entire population, through the less common, more obscure, and serious disorders, such as urticaria and asthma, to rare and life-threatening episodes of anaphylaxis. In this latter instance, such as the case illustrated in Fig. 1, we are studying immediate hypersensitivity in its purest form; the response here is clearly due to the release of mediators from mast cells and basophils, which then cause the dramatic and immediate effects noted. The pathophysiology of anaphylaxis can be understood in some detail, and therapeutic maneuvers, such as the administration of the adenylate cyclase stimulating drug, epinephrine, can be understood in terms of mechanism. In the other disease processes, such as allergic rhinitis or asthma,

Supported by Grants AI 08270 and AI 07290 from The National Institute of Allergy and Infectious Diseases, The National Institutes of Health. Publication No. 312 from The O'Neill Research Laboratories, The Good Samaritan Hospital.

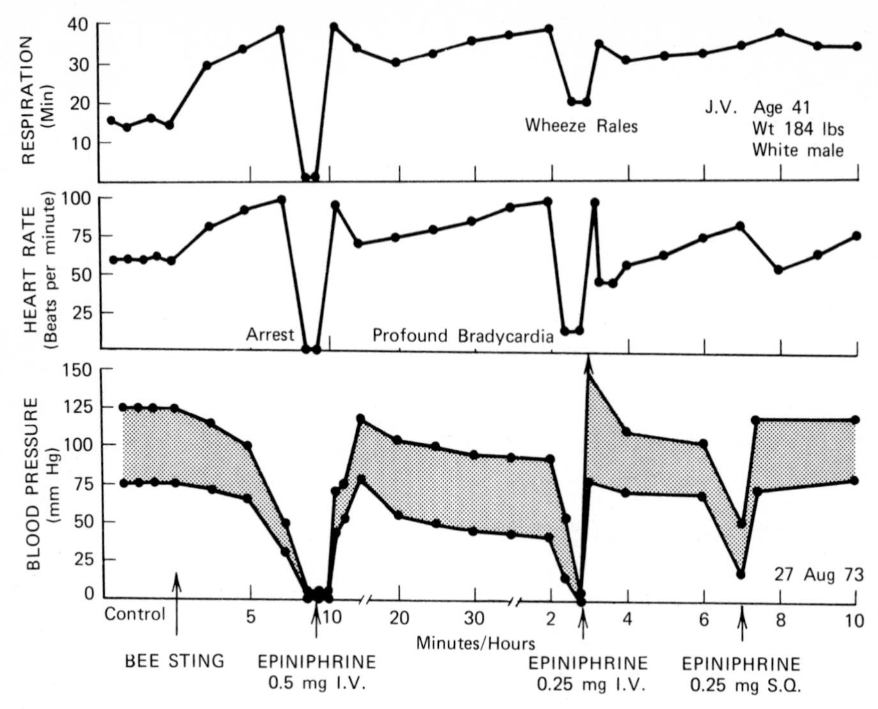

Figure 1. The course of anaphylaxis in an individual sensitive to honeybee venom.

"pure" immediate hypersensitivity reactions initiate the episode, but it appears that more prolonged inflammatory responses also play a role. This is illustrated, in clinical terms, by the fact that corticosteroids, which have little or no effect on immediate anaphylaxis or mediator release, have profound effects on the symptomatology of rhinitis and asthma.

One of the purposes of this chapter will be to place immediate hypersensitivity in the context of research on the inflammatory response in general, so that the whole spectrum of disease processes that result from or are involved in IgE-mediated events may be considered. The various parameters involved in allergic reactions will be discussed seriatim.

IgE ANTIBODIES

Perhaps the most significant element in the research that provided the impetus for the increased tempo of investigations of immediate hypersensitivity was the demonstration, by the Ishizakas, that the reaginic antibodies that cause allergic disease constitute a special class of immunoglobulins, which they designated as IgE (2). Actually, investigators had known for many decades that reagins are unusual antibodies: their titer did not correlate with the antibody titer measured by precipitation or hemagglutination methods, and they were known to be labile to heat and sulfhydryl reagents. Their most unique characteristic, however, was the ability to "fix" to skin and remain in situ for days to weeks. The work of the Ishizakas demonstrated that IgE immunoglobulins shared the light chains of other immunoglobulin classes but had a distinct heavy chain, the epsilon chain.

Their painstaking isolation and characterization of IgE, which exists in nanogram-per-milliliter concentrations in human serum, was aided considerably by the discovery of an IgE myeloma by Johansson and Bennich (3). This myeloma protein and the half-dozen other IgE myelomas that have subsequently been uncovered have provided enough material for structural studies and, from a clinical point of view, have allowed large-scale production of specific anti-IgE antibodies. With these reagents there developed a new diagnostic technology that is becoming increasingly important. (For a review of this technology see ref. 4).

A number of techniques have been used to measure total serum levels of IgE; these measurements have been carried out in groups of people from a large variety of ethnic and racial and disease categories (5,6). IgE is unique in that the serum level, which averages a few hundred nanograms per milliliter, has an extraordinary variability. Persons who are normal by all criteria may have undetectable levels of IgE (less than 1 nanogram per milliliter) or levels as high as several thousand nanograms per milliliter. The highest levels of IgE are seen in parasitized individuals, in whom concentrations of 10 to 20 μg per ml have been reported (7). Studies by the Ishizakas have demonstrated that the IgE-producing lymphocytes are predominantly in transmucosal locations, so that antigenic stimulation through the respiratory or gastrointestinal tract tends to produce the highest IgE levels; this explains the high levels seen in individuals who carry parasites (8). In Western, nonparasitized populations, it has been clearly demonstrated that persons with an allergic diathesis, such as atopic rhinitis or asthma, have, on the average, higher levels of total IgE than controls. There is, however, considerable overlap, and it is possible that a highly allergic individual may have little IgE, and an apparently nonatopic individual, high IgE levels. Recent improvements in IgE measurements have considerably reduced this apparent overlap, and although exceptions still occur, atopic and normal populations can be clearly defined by total IgE level (7).

In addition to being highly variable, in terms of the serum concentration, the IgE immunoglobulin system is unique in that a large percentage of the total IgE may be directed against a single antigen or antigenic determinant. Studies from the laboratories of Gleich and Adkinson, using independent techniques, have demonstrated that the IgE directed against one of the ragweed antigens, antigen E, may account for as much as 40% of the total circulating IgE (9,10). Although this is the exception, the majority of patients with simple grass or ragweed hay fever as their only atopic disease have 5 to 15% of the total IgE directed against one allergen. In penicillin-allergic persons, as much as 20% of the total IgE may be directed against a single haptenic determinant, the penicilloyl group (9).

The measurement of specific IgE antibody against an antigen (allergen) is of greater clinical importance than the total level of the immunoglobulin. The technology in use today, designated the radioallergosorbent test (RAST), was first described in Sweden by Wide and his colleagues (11). It is a relatively straightforward procedure, which is depicted in Fig. 2. It was, however, of limited value until recently, because the IgE titers were relative rather than absolute and, with no standards in general use, titers varied from one laboratory to another and there was no basis for comparison. As indicated above, work by Adkinson and Gleich has, in theory, solved this problem, allowing for measurements of IgE antibody in absolute, nanogram-per-milliliter terms. These mea-

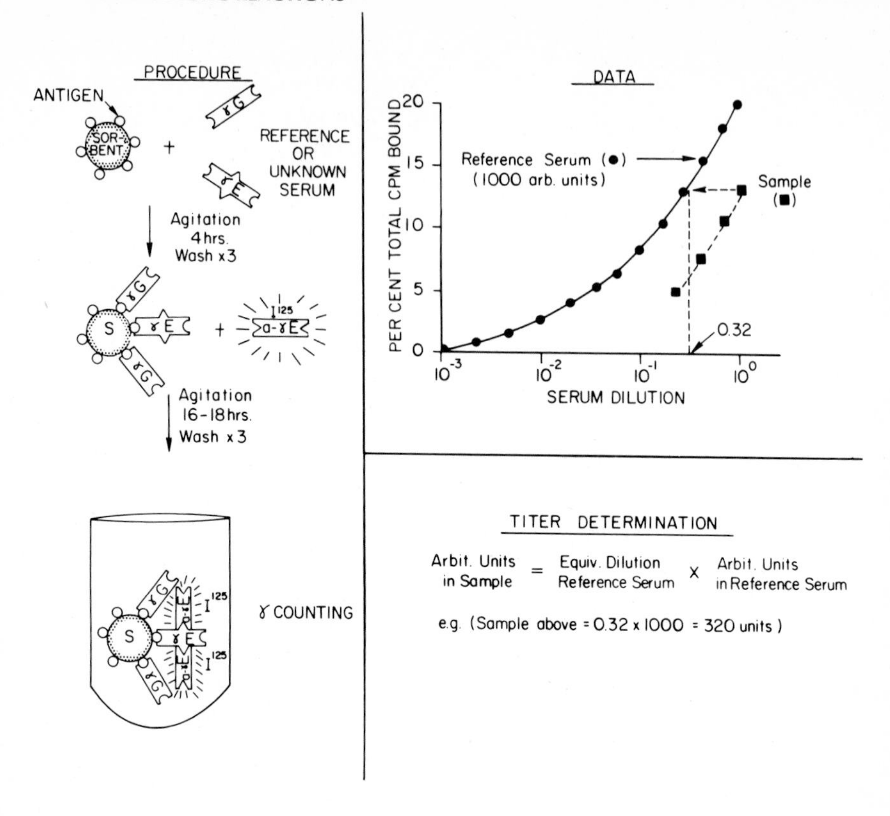

Figure 2A. The technique of the radioallergosorbent test (RAST).

surements are made using a procedure called the RAST elution technique, which is depicted in Fig. 2B. Once a standard serum has been established, it can be used to calibrate the usual RAST assays. Although this capability has not yet been translated into practice, full application of the procedure should be accomplished shortly.

The diagnostic value of RAST technology has been examined in a number of studies (12,13). These have explored the relationship between RAST titers and clinical history and contrasted the RAST with other diagnostic techniques, such as skin testing, basophil-induced histamine release, and various types of provocation tests, in which the lungs, nose, or eyes are challenged with the appropriate antigen. In general, there has been a good correlation among these various measurements of the allergic condition, at least in a statistical sense. Since the RAST procedure is entirely serologic, it does not assess a number of other important parameters, such as the ease of releasability of mediators from person to person (which is subject to marked variation) or individual sensitivity to released mediators. Moreover, the serum IgE level need not reflect the concentration of these molecules on the target mast cells or basophils. It is, therefore, common to find patients who show wide discrepancies between serum IgE antibody levels and biologic measurements; the final opinion on which test provides

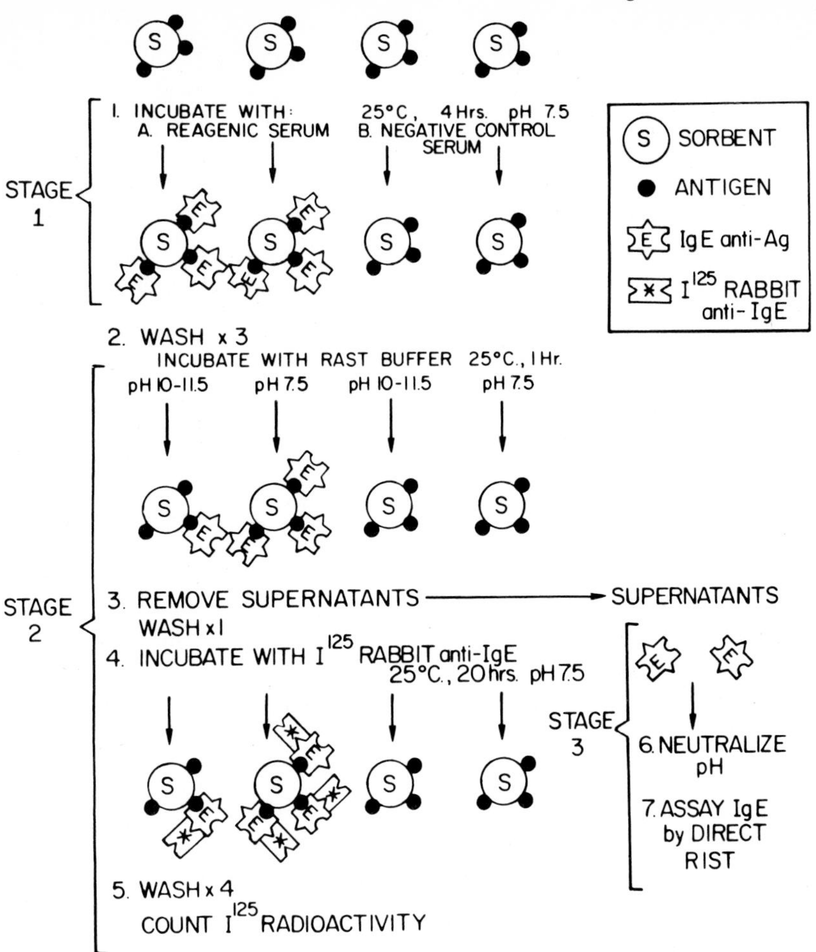

Figure 2B. The RAST elution technique, which allows absolute quantitation of IgE antibody against an allergen.

the best diagnostic information has not yet been established (7). The skin test, which provides an index of sensitivity that encompasses all the various components of the allergic response, probably gives the most information but, as carried out in this country, is usually inappropriately executed with nonstandardized allergens and, at best, semiquantitative technique.

It has been appreciated for as long as allergic diseases have been studied in an organized fashion that the propensity toward atopic conditions is familial. No defined genetic mechanism of inheritance has as yet been described, but a number of laboratories have recently begun to explore this problem. It would appear that, subject to marked environmental influence, the total IgE level is genetically controlled, with the population showing a non-Gaussian distribution (14). From this it follows that persons with genetically high levels of IgE are more likely to respond to multiple antigens than persons with low levels of IgE. As in other immunoglobulin systems, it is today generally believed that the ability to respond to a particular antigen with IgE antibody is dependent upon Ir genes that may be linked to the HLA cell surface antigens. Marsh, for example, has demonstrated that sensitivity to particular grass or ragweed allergens occurs more commonly in persons with certain HLA types, and this association is more marked if one considers only those individuals with low total IgE levels (15). On the other hand, Levine, in family studies, has noted an association between various different HLA haplotypes and sensitivity to ragweed antigen (16). Although it is apparent that further study of immunogenetics as related to allergy is needed, several techniques promise to be powerful tools in achieving a better understanding of these disorders.

There have been sporadic but repeated reports that immunoglobulins other than IgE can mediate human allergic reactions (17, 18). This is likely to be true, since most mammalian species have not only an IgE-like molecule but also a "fast" gamma immunoglobulin which, though it is not heat-labile and does not "fix" as avidly to mast cells as does IgE, can initiate the same cascade of reactions leading to mediator release. A recent report suggests that IgG may play an important role in cromolyn-resistant asthma (19). It is too early to be certain of this observation, but even if it is established that one or another subclass of IgG can induce reactions similar in type to those induced by IgE, its role in human disease will probably be quantitatively quite small.

IgG ANTIBODY

Whereas IgG antibodies probably play little or no role in the induction of anaphylactic reactions in primates, blocking antibodies, as they are usually referred to in this context, are widely believed to protect against the antigenic insult that leads to anaphylaxis. Indeed, this is the basis for "hyposensitization," a misnomer for the immunotherapeutic regimens used to treat allergic individuals. It has been clearly demonstrated that immunotherapy as commonly used clinically leads to an increase in IgG antibody. In spite of a reasonable theoretical basis, however, evidence supporting a protective role for IgG in human disease has not been overly convincing. This problem has been primarily studied in diseases such as ragweed pollinosis. A definite association between the increase in IgG antibody induced by immunotherapy and clinical protection can be noted, but this relationship is statistical, and the correlation coefficient ($\approx .70$) suggests that, at best, this is but one parameter in the clinical response (20).

It is more likely that IgG blocking antibodies can be shown to play a protective role in anaphylactic reactions to allergens encountered parenterally. We recently had occasion to study this question in patients who were sensitive to insect stings. Immunization with the venom proteins led to an increase in IgG antivenom antibody and clinical protection. Again, however, this might have been merely a temporal, rather than a causal, association. To pursue this, we initiated a protocol in which patients who were hypersensitive to honeybee venom were challenged with that venom to the point of a mild systemic reaction. They were then infused with a hyperimmune preparation of IgG from beekeepers and rapidly rechallenged. In five of five instances this led to clinical protection in that subsequent challenge with the same, or higher, doses of antigen caused no systemic reaction (21). This is perhaps the best evidence yet generated that IgG antibody can be protective clinically.

No quantitative study of the levels of IgG blocking antibody in man has been reported. It should be recognized, however, that these antibodies are present at much lower levels than immunologists are accustomed to work with in their hyperimmune animals. A typical "high-dose" immunotherapeutic regimen in man, which increases the IgG antibody tenfold to one hundredfold above the untreated state, may involve the administration of 0.1 to 1 mg of antigen over the course of a year. The IgG antibodies are present in concentrations too low to precipitate in solutions or gels, so that other methods of measurement are necessary (22). To study absolute levels of IgG in man, we used a "plateau" binding method involving radiolabeled antigen precipitated by goat anti-IgG in the presence of carrier IgG. We found that untreated patients allergic to honeybee venom have about 100 to 300 ng of IgG antibody per ml; this was increased by venom immunotherapy to tenfold or, sometimes, to one hundredfold these levels. It is worth repeating that these quantities of antibody are too low to precipitate in vivo and therefore to cause the type of reaction described by Arthus. Although it has been suggested that human IgG antibody causes so-called type III reactions, critical analysis suggests that there is not enough antibody to produce these lesions.

The studies described above also yielded an estimate of the average equilibrium constant of the IgG antibody, which, surprisingly, was quite high and rather homogeneous from person to person, ranging from approximately 1 to 4 $\times 10^{10}$ moles per liter.

IN VITRO MODELS FOR THE STUDY OF IMMEDIATE HYPERSENSITIVITY

Our understanding of the mediators that are involved in immediate hypersensitivity, and progress in studying the mechanism by which these mediators are released following an immunologic event, have depended primarily on the use of a variety of in vitro models. These models are based on the recognition that IgE antibody is fixed to receptors that exist only on mast cells and basophils, and the observation that histamine, the major mediator in question, is likewise stored in these cells. Tissues or cell suspensions that contain mast cells or basophils have therefore been used. The earliest quantitative work employed rat peritoneal cells, which include a relatively high percentage of mast cells. More recently, techniques have been devised for the purification of rat mast cells in which they approach 98% of the total cell number (23). This provides a very considerable advantage in carrying out biochemical studies. Chopped tissues, such as guinea pig or primate lung or skin, have also provided useful models, as have human peripheral leukocytes, which contain approximately 1% basophils.

Although a thorough description of these model systems is beyond the scope of this review, a number of points can be made. Primate anaphylaxis differs considerably from that in other mammalian species in the type of mediators that are released, the mechanism of their release, and the sensitivity of the tissues to different mediators. Rodents, for example, are unreactive to concentrations of histamine that would cause serious systemic reactions in the guinea pig or man. The rodent species also have mast cells that contain both histamine and serotonin, the latter not being found in the mast cells of any other species; the rat and mouse are more sensitive to serotonin than they are to histamine. In most other species, serotonin is contained in the platelets, but in the rabbit the platelets also contain histamine. Because of these differences, much recent work has used systems in which the cells or tissues are derived from primate sources, although the rat mast cell system remains the only model in which highly purified preparations of cells can be obtained, and, therefore, this model is of critical interest to the field.

In general, the in vitro models are rather similar, employing simple buffers in which the isolated cells or tissue minces are suspended. These preparations are challenged with the appropriate antigens in actively sensitized tissues, or the cells are passively sensitized with reaginic serum, washed and treated with antigen. The reaction is allowed to proceed for a period of minutes, and the supernatant is then examined for the mediator(s) that is of interest. These fluid phase systems are readily amenable to studies of drug activity, influence of cations, temperature, and the like, and their use has clarified the mechanism of mediator release considerably.

THE MEDIATORS OF ANAPHYLACTIC REACTIONS

The mediators of anaphylactic reactions have been dealt with in Chapter 1, but this subject can be reviewed quite briefly here. A review is, perhaps, useful in two sections of this book because this is a rapidly moving field and one's appreciation of the role of the various mediators varies according to one's research vantage point.

Histamine

Since its discovery by Sir Henry Dale, histamine has been considered the main mediator of allergic reactions. The biologic activities of histamine are well known. A recent development, which was anticipated by the work of Schild over a decade ago, has been the synthesis and characterization, by Black, of histamine-2 antagonists (24,25). Schild had found that histamine interacted with two types of receptors. The histamine-1 receptors were those with which we are familiar, i.e., those that cause smooth muscle contraction, vasodilatation, pruritis, etc., and that are antagonized by the standard antihistamines. A number of actions of histamine, however, such as gastric acid secretion, contraction of the uterus, and certain effects on cardiac function were not blocked by histamine-1 antagonists. The development of the new histamine antagonists has led to the clear definition of these receptors as histamine-2. It is also beginning to be appreciated that there are histamine-2 receptors that are important in influencing the contraction of vascular and bronchial smooth muscle as well as in mediating the effects of histamine on cardiac contractibility. More significant, perhaps, the introduction of the histamine-2 antagonists has allowed understanding of the marked anti-inflammatory activities of histamine.

Both in vitro and in vivo, it has been shown that histamine, acting through histamine-2 receptors, can negatively modulate histamine and other mediator release from mast cells and basophils (26). It also depresses T lymphocyte killing, lymphokine production, and the manifestations, in vivo, of delayed hypersensitivity (27–29). Both phagocytic and chemotactic events are also strongly modulated by histamine-2 receptors. Thus, the role of histamine released after an anaphylactic reaction is quite complex, and a considerable period of study will be required before it is fully understood. The multiple functions of histamine as they are currently understood are outlined in Table 1.

SRS-A

SRS-A, the slow-reacting substance of anaphylaxis, was first described by Brockelhurst and others over 20 years ago (30). Exhaustive work by Orange et al. has failed to provide precise chemical definition of this molecule, although it is known to be a low-molecular-weight, sulfate-containing lipid (31). Unlike histamine, which is a preformed mediator, SRS-A is generated only after the immune event. Its measurement remains by bioassay, that is, the prolonged contraction of guinea pig ileum in a Schultz-Dale apparatus. This has considerably hampered progress towards its characterization. SRS-A is known to contract human bronchial muscle and is thought to play a role in asthma, but this has not been fully documented. Although there are drugs that provide partial SRS-A antagonism, a highly selective antagonist has not been developed. It was thought that in primates SRS-A was generated only from mast cells and basophils, but recent experiments using a calcium ionophore, which mimics an immunologic stimulus, demonstrated that it was possible to release SRS-A from human

Table 1. Effects of Histamine on Inflammatory Processes

	H_2 *Receptor*
Histamine inhibits:	
Mediator release from basophils (human)	+
Mediator release, lung and skin (monkey)	+
PCA reaction (rabbit)	+
Neutrophil phagocytosis (human)	+
Neutrophil chemotaxis (human)	+
Neutrophil lysosomal enzyme release (human)	?
Eosinophil chemotaxis (high dose) (human)	+
T cell cytotoxicity (murine)	+
MIF production (guinea pig)	+
Delayed skin reactivity (guinea pig)	+
Ab production or secretion (murine)	?
Histamine permits:	
Immune glomerulonephritis (rabbit)	H1
Footpad swelling (murine)	?

granulocytes as well (32). The pathogenetic significance of this mediator arising from an inflammatory cell remains to be established.

ECF-A

Eosinophils tend to accumulate at the site of lesions of immediate hypersensitivity as a result of the release from mast cells, on appropriate immunologic stimulus, of the eosinophil chemotactic factor of anaphylaxis (ECF-A) (33). ECF-A is assayed by its ability selectively to cause eosinophils to migrate through millipore filters mounted in Boyden chambers; it selectively desensitizes these cells to subsequent ECF-A stimuli if they are exposed under nongradient conditions. ECF-A has been characterized by Austen's group as two preformed acidic peptides (Val-Gly-Ser-Glu; Ala-Gly-Ser-Glu) (34). ECF-A can also be released from human basophils by antigen, anti-IgE, or ionophore stimulation. As with SRS-A, an eosinophil chemotactic factor of a size similar to ECF-A (molecular weight $\approx$ 500 daltons) is released from human polymorphonuclear cells, either by the ionophore or by phagocytic stimulation (35,36). The demonstration that a mediator that was previously associated only with immediate hypersensitivity reactions can be released during phagocytosis has wide-ranging implications that will be considered below.

Other Factors

A considerable number of other potential mediators have been described. These include a neutrophil-immobilizing factor, a material with kallikrein activity that can produce bradykinin on interaction with serum kininogen, and others (37,38). In general, the pathogenetic significance of these mediators is less well defined than with those discussed above, and they are considered beyond the scope of this section.

THE MECHANISM OF MEDIATOR RELEASE

In the last several years, the work of Sutherland and his colleagues, demonstrating the control of secretory reactions by changes in the cyclic AMP level, has been extended to reactions of immediate hypersensitivity and, subsequently, to other aspects of the inflammatory response. It was first observed that β-adrenergic agonists such as epinephrine and isoproterenol, which are known stimulators of adenylate cyclase, inhibit histamine release from basophils (39). It was also demonstrated that theophylline, which inhibits the phosphodiesterase that destroys cyclic AMP, was inhibitory and that the two together had an additive or synergistic effect. This work was extended to studies using primate or human lung and has been coupled with direct measurement of cyclic AMP levels in both these tissues and leukocyte preparations (40, 41). The observation that increased cyclic AMP levels inhibited mediator release had a logical corollary, i.e., that one of the early stages following the antigen-IgE interaction on a mast cell or basophil surface was a fall in the cyclic AMP level and that this served to initiate the series of events that lead to mediator release. For technical reasons, this change cannot be demonstrated in the mixed cell preparations that are available when using primate or human tissues. In the rat mast cell system, however, it has been demonstrated that there is a fall in cyclic AMP following antigen-IgE interaction (42).

It thus appears that the target cells of the allergic reaction contain on their surface β-adrenergic receptors which, if stimulated, block the antigen-induced fall in cyclic AMP and are thus of critical importance in modulating the release of mediators. This work has been extended to show that there are other receptors on the cells. These include receptors for the prostaglandin series and, as referred to above, a histamine-2 receptor that also causes an increase in cyclic AMP levels. These studies, together with those using cholera enterotoxin, a highly specific and potent adenylate cyclase activator, have demonstrated that both the dose response and kinetic changes induced by these agonists, in terms of cyclic AMP, are paralleled by the resulting inhibition of mediator release (43,44). Appropriate studies with antagonists, such as propranolol or the antihistamines for type 2 receptors, have shown that abrogation of the cyclic nucleotide response also blocks the inhibition of mediator release (43–45). Since the target cells are bathed in a fluid that can contain variable quantities of β-adrenergic agonists, prostaglandins, and histamine, these hormone-receptor interactions would seem to be of primary importance in determining the eventual results of an antigenic challenge. As indicated above, with respect to histamine, similar hormone receptor interactions have been shown to control virtually all aspects of the inflammatory response from T lymphocyte function to phagocytosis and lysosomal enzyme release. In each instance, increased cyclic AMP levels lead to diminution of the response.

There are discrepancies in the data reported with regard to other hormone-receptor interactions. It appears from work in human lung, for example, that α-adrenergic stimulation, postulated to lead to a fall in cyclic AMP levels, potentiates mediator release; this cannot be demonstrated in the basophil system (46). Similarly, acetylcholine, or its analogues, potentiates the release process. This is thought to be due to an increase in the cyclic GMP level, and studies with cyclic GMP and its analogues revealed potentiation of the release process (46). The cyclic GMP-related phenomena also cannot be demonstrated in the basophils, suggesting a basic difference in the control mechanism in these two cell types. Cyclic GMP is, however, reported to potentiate lysosomal enzyme release during phagocytosis in a manner entirely similar to its effect on mast cells (47,48). There is dispute about the role of cholinergic agonists on T lymphocyte function: it has been reported that such treatment potentiates killing of tumor cells by rat lymphocytes, while in what appears to be a similar system, using mouse lymphocytes, no effect was demonstrable (49).

In pursuing the mechanism of mediator release, investigators have made efforts to divide the acute allergic response into stages. There is general agreement that at least two stages can be generated. The first is an antigen-dependent, calcium-independent process in which the cells are rapidly activated and if allowed to incubate at 37°C in the absence of calcium, are rapidly and nonspecifically desensitized (50). If the cells are separated from antigen early in the

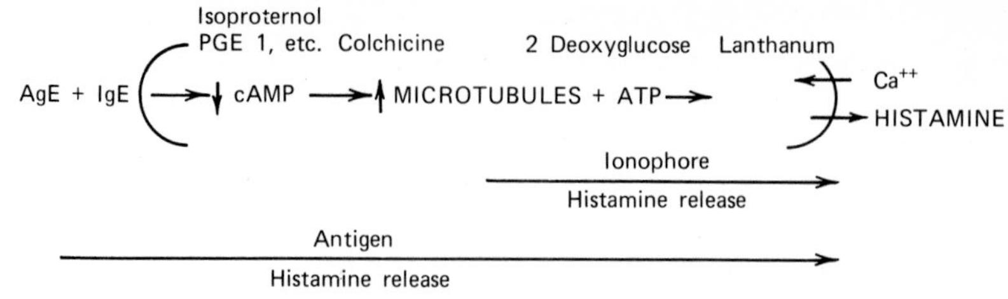

Figure 3. The stages of histamine release as delineated by studies with drugs and the calcium ionophore A23187.

activation phase, washed and resuspended in a calcium-containing medium, mediator release proceeds during a second stage. Studies with the various agonists described above have indicated that cyclic nucleotide-related events occur only in the first stage (51). Second-stage release involves microtubule-associated events as indicated by its sensitivity to heavy water, which potentiates microtubule aggregation and promotes release, and to colchicine, which causes the disaggregation of microtubules, and inhibits the release process (52). The second stage is also energy-dependent, since 2-deoxyglucose, a metabolic inhibitor that has no effect in the first stage, completely blocks the second-stage release process. The stages of histamine release have been further studied with the calcium ionophore A23187, which, as indicated, mimics the secretory stimulus in many tissues (53). This is a noncytotoxic, completely calcium-dependent process that seems to mimic second-stage events. The stages of mediator release that have been elucidated by use of the various agonists and inhibitors are summarized in Fig. 3.

These biochemical studies of mediator release are in their infancy, but have provided some insight into the process. The point to stress is that they have revealed that mediator release from basophils, mast cells, and neutrophils, and to some extent from lymphocytes, is a secretory process that is controlled in a fashion similar to that in other secretory events. The major difference, which seems to apply to each of the cell types involved in inflammation, is that an increase in cyclic AMP *decreases* the response, whereas in almost all other secretory responses the reverse is true.

IMMEDIATE HYPERSENSITIVITY AS ONE ASPECT OF THE INFLAMMATORY PROCESS

The marked similarities between immediate hypersensitivity and other inflammatory reactions have been referred to above (see review in ref. 54). One parallel between mediator release from mast cells/basophils, lysosomal enzyme release from phagocytosing polymorphonuclear cells, and lymphokine release from lymphocytes is that each may be considered an active, energy-requiring, secretory process. Some aspects of these responses, which cannot be strictly viewed in this manner, are, nonetheless, examples of stimulation-secretion coupling in which the stimulus, together with calcium, leads to a response that in broad terms contributes to the mounting of an inflammatory response.

Another parallelism is seen in the stereotyped fashion in which the control of the inflammatory events in basophils, mast cells, lymphocytes, and polymorphonuclear cells is regulated by changes in cyclic nucleotide levels induced by hormones present in the body. Further to this point are the experiments describing the direct effects of histamine release on the development of delayed hypersensitivity reactions and our beginning appreciation of cutaneous basophil hypersensitivity, in which a traditional delayed reaction is fundamentally related to the infiltration of basophils (55). The increasing inability to segregate various types of inflammatory responses also indicates their interrelationships. The most recent observation in this context is that mediators that have heretofore been associated only with immediate hypersensitivity, such as SRS-A and eosinophil chemotactic factors, can be released by polymorphonuclear cells, the latter as the result of phagocytosis.

Schemes that define immunopathogenetic (allergic) mechanisms into types I, II, III, and IV may be useful for classification (56). They may, on the other hand, obscure and hold back progress by causing investigators to look narrowly, rather than broadly, into the field of inflammation. It was by adherence to this scheme, for example, that late reactions to allergens were designated as type III or Arthus reactions. A simple definition of Arthus reactions reveals, however, that they involve amounts of antibody that very rarely can be found in man. Only recently has it been shown by the work of Gleich and Dolovitch that late reactions to allergens can be passively transferred solely by IgE antibody (57,58). Rather than attempting to fit these reactions into a scheme similar to the Arthus reaction in animals, we must attempt to understand the mechanism by which IgE-mediated events can cause a long-delayed response.

Perhaps there is a time in the development of a scientific field when rigid classification is necessary for progress; it would appear, however, that this time in the study of the immunopathogenesis of inflammatory lesions is long past, and that a more general view that stresses the known interactions and the large areas of ignorance is a more viable model for progress.

CLINICAL CONSIDERATIONS

Approaches to the therapy of allergic disorders in man have proceeded mainly in two directions. One has been to employ immunotherapy ("shots," desensitization, or hyposensitization). This approach was introduced by Noon in 1911, long before the nature of allergic disorders was understood; Noon actually thought he was producing an antitoxic immunity (59). The administration of the antigens to which the patient is sensitive is, by far, the most widespread form of therapy and is used in all disease processes that can be broadly called "allergic." It is clearly overused in that its efficacy has not been demonstrated in the majority of clinical situations in which it is prescribed; this is particularly true in asthma. Controlled studies yielding clear-cut results have been carried out only with respect to grass and ragweed pollinosis (hay fever). In these diseases, appropriately designed, blinded, and controlled protocols produced data indicating that immunotherapy leads to a significant amelioration of symptoms (60). This regimen, however, certainly does not ablate the disease.

Immunotherapy is accompanied by a number of readily measurable immunologic changes. As noted, the IgG blocking antibody increases dramatically; the relationship between blocking antibody levels and clinical symptoms has been discussed above. IgE antibody is also increased early in the course of therapy, and in rapid ("rush") immunotherapy the total and specific IgE level may rise five- to tenfold in the first few weeks of treatment. With time, however, the IgG antibody continues to rise, but the IgE antibody levels off and then begins to fall (61). It can be shown that there is a rough correlation between the magnitude of the rise in IgG and the fall in IgE antibody, but the mechanism by which the IgE response is diminished is not clear. This is a very active area of current research. In the absence of immunotherapy, the IgE antibody tends to fall to its lowest level before the appropriate pollen season and is, then, boosted, perhaps twofold. In patients who are receiving immunotherapy, this seasonal increase is not noted (61). Other studies of immunotherapy have revealed changes in the response of circulating basophils to allergen challenge; these changes, a decrease in sensitivity or reactivity, have in general correlated with reduction in clinical symptoms (62). Although immunotherapy leads to a modest rise in secretory IgA antibody (which is much less marked, and not correlated with the blocking antibody response in serum), it has been impossible to demonstrate any relationship between the IgA antibody and the clinical results of immunotherapy (63).

The other major approach to therapy, and the one that holds out the most significant hope for the future, is the pharmacologic approach. The major modalities of therapy have to date used agents that affect the cyclic AMP system. Epinephrine and theophylline are, for example, the mainstays of treatment in asthmatic conditions. These drugs were used before their pharmacology in allergic conditions was fully understood, and it is still a question as to how much their effect is due to the suppression of mediator release and how much it relates to their effects on smooth muscle. Other, more novel pharmacologic modalities can now be studied in the in vitro models referred to above. There are literally dozens of compounds receiving testing in various pharmaceutical and university laboratories which have the ability to turn off mediator release and which operate through a mechanism that is not dependent upon the cyclic AMP system. Some of these have been used in preliminary clinical trials, but it is too early to assess their utility. It seems highly likely, however, that the next major step in the treatment of allergic diseases will be in the pharmacologic control of mediator release.

CONCLUSIONS

My aim has been to review our rapidly developing understanding of the allergic response in man, a process that has brought these reactions into a position in which they are indistinguishable from inflammation in general and in which they in fact constitute only a part of cell biology. The strictly immunologic developments, such as IgE measurements and a beginning of the understanding of the role of IgG antibody, together with an ability to quantitate these parameters, has clearly improved the diagnosis and approaches to the immunotherapeutic management of immediate hypersensitivity conditions. Although this aspect is important, our knowledge of the biochemistry of the acute allergic response is, in the long run, of more therapeutic potential. The last decade has seen a marked increase in the development of drugs that have a broadly antiallergic effect. The numerous model systems and the various stages upon which these drugs can operate are beginning to produce an armamentarium of pharmaceutical tools that seem likely to have, in the immediate future, dramatic therapeutic consequences.

REFERENCES

1. Prausnitz, C., and Küstner, H., in *Clinical Aspects of Immunology* (P. G. H. Gell and R. R. A. Coombs, eds.), F. A. Davis, Philadelphia, 1963, p. 808.
2. Ishizaka, K., and Ishizaka. T., *J. Immunol.* **99**, 1187 (1967).
3. Johansson, S. G. O., and Bennich, H., *Immunology* **13**, 381 (1967).
4. Adkinson, N. F., Jr., in *Manual of Clinical Immunology* (N. R. Rose and H. Friedman, eds.), American Society for Microbiology, Washington, D.C., 1976, p. 590.
5. Johansson, S. G. O., *Lancet* **2**, 951 (1967).
6. Yunginger, J. W., and Gleich, G. J., *Pediatr. Clin. North Am.* **22**, 3 (1975).
7. Lichtenstein, L. M., and Hamburger, R. N., in *Immunological Diseases* (M. Samter, ed.), Little, Brown, Boston (in press).
8. Tada, T., and Ishizaka, K., *J. Immunol.* **104**, 377 (1970).
9. Schellenberg, R. R., and Adkinson, N. F., Jr., *J. Immunol.* **115**, 1577 (1975).
10. Gleich, G. J., and Jacob, G. L., *Science* **190**, 1106 (1975).
11. Wide, L., Bennich, H., and Johansson, S. G. O., *Lancet* **2**, 1105 (1967).
12. Berg, T., Bennich, H., and Johansson, S. G. O., *Int. Arch. Allergy Appl. Immunol.* **40**, 770 (1971).
13. Berg, T. L. O., and Johansson, S. G. O., *J. Allergy Clin. Immunol.* **54**, 209 (1974).
14. Hamburger, R. N., Orgel, H. A., and Bazaral, M., in *Mechanisms in Allergy: Reagin-Mediated Hypersensitivity* (L. Goodfriend, A. Sehon, and R. Orange, eds.), Marcel Dekker, New York, 1973, p. 131.
15. Marsh, D. G., Bias, W. B., and Ishizaka, K., *Proc. Natl. Acad. Sci. (U.S.A.)* **71**, 3588 (1974).
16. Levine, B. B., Stember, R. H., and Fotuno, M., *Science* **178**, 1201 (1972).
17. Reid, T. R., *J. Immunol.* **104**, 935 (1970).
18. Parish, W. E., *Clin. Allergy* **1**, 369 (1971).
19. Bryant, D. H., Burns, M. W., and Lazarus, L., *J. Allergy Clin. Immunol.,* **56**, 417 (1975).
20. Lichtenstein, L. M., Norman, P. S., and Winkenwerder, W. L., *Am. J. Med.* **44**, 514 (1968).
21. Lessof, M. H., Sobotka, A. K., and Lichtenstein, L. M., *Johns Hopkins Med. J.* **142,** 1, (1978).
22. Sobotka, A., Valentine, M. D., Ishizaka, K., et al., *J. Immunol.* **117**, 84 (1976).
23. Bach, M., Bloch, K. J., and Austen, K. F., *J. Exp. Med.* **133**, 752 (1971).
24. Ash, A. S. F., and Schild, H. O., *Br. J. Pharmacol. Chemother.* **27**, 427 (1966).
25. Black, J. W., Duncan, W. A. M., Durant, C. J., et al., *Nature* **236**, 385 (1972).
26. Bourne, H. R., Melmon, K. L., and Lichtenstein, L. M., *Science* **173**, 743 (1971).
27. Plaut, M., Lichtenstein, L. M., Gillespie, E., et al., *J. Immunol.* **111**, 389 (1973).
28. Plaut, M., Lichtenstein, L. M., and Henney, C. S., *J. Clin. Invest.* **55** , 856 (1975).
29. Rocklin, R. E., *J. Clin. Invest.* **57**, 1051 (1976).
30. Brocklehurst, W. E., *J. Physiol.* (London) **151**, 416 (1960).
31. Orange, R. P., Murphy, R. C., Karnovsky, M. L., et al., *J. Immunol.* **110**, 760 (1973).
32. Conroy, M. C., Orange, R. P., and Lichtenstein, L. M., *J. Immunol.* **116**, 1677 (1976).
33. Kay, A. B., Stechschulte, D. J., and Austen, K. F., *J. Exp. Med.* **133**, 602 (1971).
34. Goetzl, E. F., and Austen, K. F., *Proc. Natl. Acad. Sci.* **72**, 4123 (1975).
35. Czarnetzki, B. M., König, W., and Lichtenstein, L. M., *J. Immunol.* **117**, 229 (1976).
36. König, W., Czarnetzki, B. M., and Lichtenstein, L. M., *J. Immunol.* **117**, 235 (1976).
37. Goetzl, E. J., Gigli, I., Wasserman, S., et al., *J. Immunol.* **111**, 938 (1973).
38. Newball, H. H., Talamo, R. C., and Lichtenstein, L. M., *Nature* **254**, 635 (1975).
39. Lichtenstein, L. M., and Margolis, S., *Science* **161**, 902 (1968).
40. Bourne, H. R., Lichtenstein, L. M., and Melmon, K. L., *J. Immunol.* **108**, 695 (1972).
41. Orange, R. P., Austen, W. G., and Austen, K. F., *J. Exp. Med.* **134**, 1365 (1971).

42. Kaliner, M., and Austen, K. F., *J. Immunol.* **112**, 664 (1974).
43. Lichtenstein, L. M., Henney, C. S., Bourne, H. R., et al., *J. Clin. Invest.* **52,** 691 (1973).
44. Bourne, H. R., Lehrer, R. I., Lichtenstein, L. M., et al., *J. Clin. Invest.* **52**, 698 (1973).
45. Lichtenstein, L. M., and Gillespie, E., *J. Pharmacol. Exp. Ther.* **192**, 441 (1975).
46. Kaliner, M., Orange, R. P., and Austen, K. F., *J. Exp. Med.* **136**, 556 (1972).
47. Henson, P. M., in *Progress in Immunology* II, *Biological Aspects* I (L. Brent and J. Holborow, eds.), Proc. Second Int. Cong. of Immunol., Brighton, England, **2**, 95 (1974).
48. Zurier, R. B., Weissmann, G., Hoffstein, S., et al., *J. Clin. Invest.* **53**, 297 (1974).
49. Strom, T. B., Diesseroth, A., Morganroth, J., et al., *Proc. Natl. Acad. Sci.* **69**, 2995 (1972).
50. Lichtenstein, L. M., *J. Immunol.* **107**, 1122 (1971).
51. Lichtenstein, L. M., and DeBernardo, R., *J. Immunol.* **107**, 1131 (1971).
52. Gillespie, E., and Lichtenstein, L. M., *J. Clin. Invest.* **51,** 2941 (1972).
53. Lichtenstein, L. M., *J. Immunol.* **114**, 1692 (1975).
54. Bourne, H. R., Lichtenstein, L. M., Henney, C. S., et al., *Science* **184**, 19 (1974).
55. Richerson, H. B., Dvorak, H. B., and Leskowitz, S., *J. Exp. Med.* **132**, 546 (1970).
56. Gell, P. G. H., and Coombs, R. R. A., in *Clinical Aspects of Immunology* (P. G. H. Gell and R. R. A. Coombs, eds.), Philadelphia, F. A. Davis, 1968, p. 575.
57. Dolovitch, J., Hargreave, F. E., Chalmers, R., et al., *J. Allergy Clin. Immunol.* **52**, 38 (1973).
58. Solley, G. O., Larson, J. B., Jordon, R. E., et al., *J. Allergy Clin. Immunol.* **55**, 112 (1975).
59. Noon, L., *Lancet* **1**, 1572 (1911).
60. Lichtenstein, L. M., Norman, P. S., and Winkenwerder, W. L., *Ann Intern. Med.* **75,** 663 (1971).
61. Lichtenstein, L. M., Ishizaka, K., Norman, P. S., et al., *J. Clin. Invest.* **52**, 472 (1973).
62. Sadan, N., Rhyne, M. B., Mellits, D., et al., *N. Engl. J. Med.* **280**, 623 (1969).
63. Platts-Mills, T. A. E., von Maur, R. K., Ishizaka, K., et al., *J. Clin. Invest.* **57**, 1041 (1976).

Chapter Three

Immune Complex-Mediated Tissue Injury

CHARLES G. COCHRANE

Department of Immunopathology, Scripps Clinic and Research Foundation, La Jolla, California

In the past 15 years, much information has accumulated establishing the role of antigen-antibody complexes per se as pathogenetic agents capable of inducing in particular anatomic sites a variety of injuries, ranging from acute through chronic inflammation to hyaline degeneration. Apparently, the interaction of antigen with antibody forms a macromolecular complex which, if soluble, can circulate in the host and, upon further reaction with serum factors or cells, can injure any tissue in which it is deposited. Similar reactions appear in situations where the complex forms in the tissues.

Experimental demonstration of the pathogenic qualities of antigen-antibody complexes began with the studies of Freidmann (1) and Frieberger (2) of the anaphylactogenic properties of mixtures of immune serum and antigen. Later, it was established that the lesions of serum sickness developed at the time of antigen-antibody interaction in the circulation (3,4). Independent and quite different lines of investigation in several laboratories all pointed to the actual antigen-antibody complex as a pathogenetic agent. The earlier studies of anaphylaxis were extended to demonstrate that purified, soluble antigen-antibody complexes could, by themselves, induce systemic anaphylaxis (5). The study of experimental serum sickness employing isotopically labeled antigens and the fluorescent antibody technique made it possible to demonstrate soluble, circulating antigen-antibody complexes during the development of the disease (6), and further to demonstrate localization of antigen, host Ig, and host complement, presumably as immunologic complexes, in the lesions simultaneously

The work was supported by USPHS Grants A107007, the NHLBI 16411, and the Council for Tobacco Research.

with their development (7,8). It was shown that soluble antigen-antibody complexes would induce smooth muscle contraction in vitro (9,10), produce cutaneous reactions of increased vascular permeability (11), and even actual vascular necrosis (12).

Following these observations, a partial definition of those properties of complexes responsible for their pathogenicity was achieved. Complexes formed in moderate antigen excess, that is, complexes that were large enough to be capable of reacting with complement, were found most active in producing systemic anaphylaxis (5). A series of subsequent studies demonstrated some of the molecular characteristics of pathogenic complexes (13,14). Using increased vascular permeability in a local cutaneous reaction as a test system, it was shown that the activity of a complex depended upon the properties of the antibody, not the antigen, and that the abilities of complexes to fix to tissues and to react with C resided in the Fc portion of the antibody molecule—a portion devoid of antibody-combining sites but rich in carbohydrate; and the activity of soluble complexes was associated with a change in the property of optic rotation of the complex. These findings led to the proposal that the configuration of antibody molecules was altered when brought into close apposition in an immunologic complex, and that this altered configuration was responsible for the complexes' changed optic rotation and their ability to fix C and to induce a phlogogenic stimulus.

If all that was needed to produce biologically active complexes was to bring antibody molecules into close apposition and thereby alter their configuration, means of causing apposition of antibody molecules other than antigen-antibody reactions should have a similar effect. It was demonstrated that human gamma globulin and rabbit gamma globulin aggregated by chemical means or by heat developed the ability to fix C (15). Some of these aggregates also had an affinity for tissues, and these showed pathologic activity, i.e., they increased vascular permeability in cutaneous reactions. In the fixation of C and induction of skin reactions, these heat-aggregated and chemically aggregated gamma globulins were qualitatively and quantitatively quite similar to the immune complexes. This supported the suggestion that the biologic activity of the antigen-antibody complex was related to the interactions of adjacent gamma globulin molecules, with resultant alterations causing a phlogogenic stimulus. The fact that gamma globulins aggregated nonimmunologically in vitro may have biologic activity suggests the possibility that aggregation of a nonimmunologic basis might occur in vivo, perhaps among partially denatured, or in other ways altered, gamma globulins, with formation of pathogenic complexes.

The nature of the disease caused by soluble antigen-antibody (AgAb) complexes is determined by the distribution and extent of their localization in tissues. Thus, the size of the complexes, their concentration, and the duration of their presence in the circulation are of great importance. Since these complexes appear to localize in tissues for anatomic and physiologic reasons and not as a result of immunologic specificity, their physical properties are the determining factors. Small complexes (Ag_2Ab) may remain in the circulation for long periods without depositing in tissues and producing injury, whereas larger complexes seem to be trapped in structures that ordinarily either exclude or are permeable to serum proteins. Large concentrations of pathogenic complexes in the circulation for brief periods, as seen in conventional serum sickness, usually cause exudative polymorphonuclear leukocytic and proliferative endothelial lesions with necrosis of tissue, whereas lower levels of similar complexes in the circulation for periods of weeks or months cause chronic lesions with hyaline degeneration of vessel walls (16). Once the complexes are deposited in the tissues, their interaction with humoral and cellular elements of the host induces biochemical, pharmacologic, and morphologic events quite similar to those caused by other kinds of antigen-antibody reactions, such as the reactions of antitissue antibodies with their target tissues.

EXPERIMENTAL LESIONS INDUCED BY IMMUNOLOGIC COMPLEXES

The Arthus Phenomenon

Pathogenetically, the simplest complex-induced lesion is the Arthus reaction, a localized, acute necrotizing vasculitis (17,18). Essential to the full development of this lesion is the formation of relatively large amounts of antigen and antibody precipitates in the vessel walls (12). In order to so localize the reaction, one of the reactants, either antigen or antibody, must be in the circulation and the other injected locally. Early in the reaction, antigen and antibody diffuse toward each other, meeting and precipitating in the vessel walls (Fig. 1). This antigen-antibody precipitate or complex, after its reaction with C, is chemotactic for polymorphonuclear leukocytes (PMNs), and within a few hours these cells

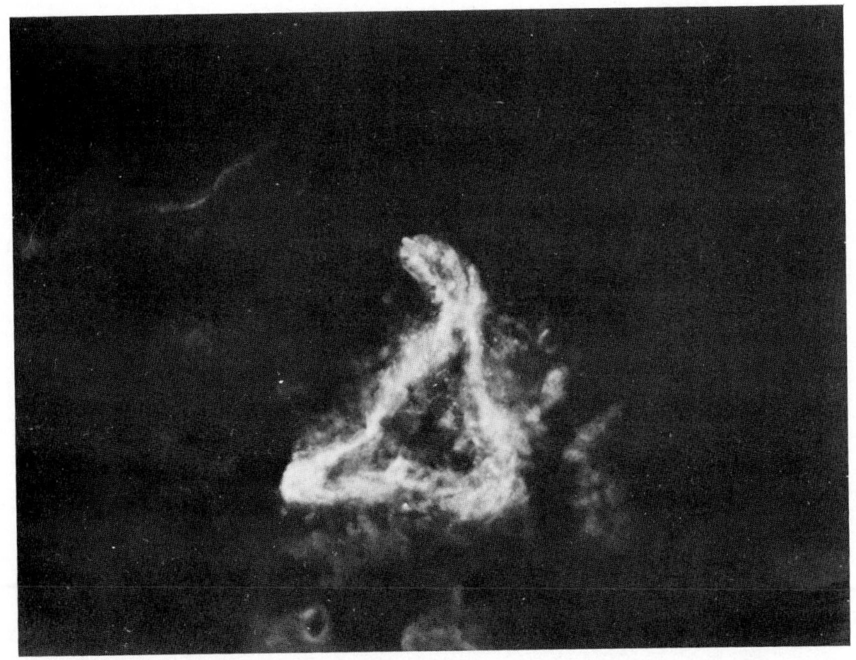

Figure 1. Fluorescent photomicrograph of an inflamed venule as seen in Fig. 2. The section was treated to indicate the position of the antigen. Antibody and complement (C'3) were similarly localized. (Magnification × 250.)

infiltrate the involved vessels, which by now are undergoing necrosis (Fig. 2). The PMNs phagocytose the antigen-antibody complex and appear to carry it away from the site of the reaction. Not only do the PMNs take up the complexes, but they are capable of degrading them rapidly, as shown by in vitro studies (19).

Serum Sickness

Serum sickness, either in experimental animals or in humans, is induced by the intravenous infusion of a single large dose of foreign serum or purified serum protein. Fig. 3 illustrates the relationship of most of the events that occur in this disease (7). The antigen level in the serum, in this case determined by following an isotopic label, can be seen to decline in three distinct phases. The first sharp fall results from equilibration of the intravenously injected foreign protein between intra- and extravascular serum protein pools. Next, there is a period of relatively slow loss caused by nonimmune catabolism of circulating free antigen at a rate characteristic for the particular protein injected and the recipient species. Finally, there is a phase of rapid loss just preceding the appearance of free circulating antibody. The antibody as it forms combines with the antigen in the circulation, at first in an extreme antigen excess environment predisposing to the formation of small complexes capable of remaining in the circulation as indicated by the first part of the complex line. As the amount of antibody formed increases, the antigen-antibody complexes become larger and are finally rapidly removed.

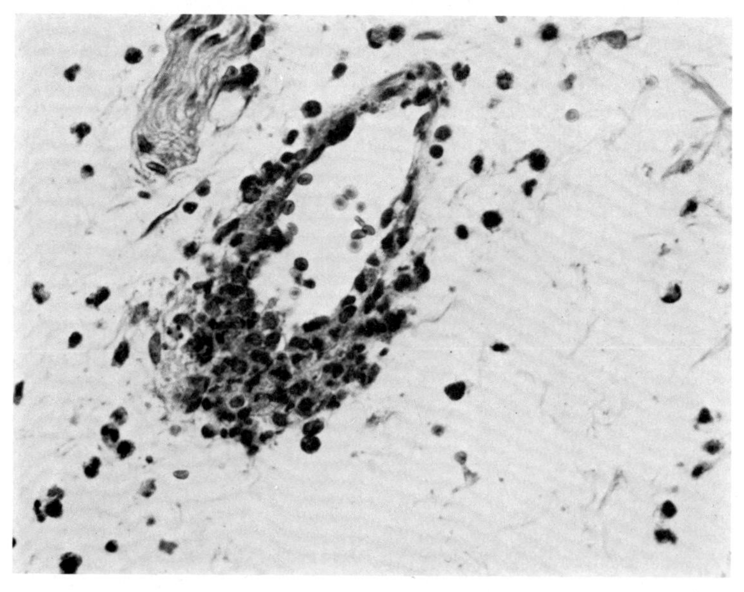

Figure 2. Photomicrograph of a venule taken from a reversed passive Arthus reaction in a rabbit. Large numbers of neutrophils have accumulated in the vessel wall. Extravasated red cells and edema were present in the surrounding tissues.

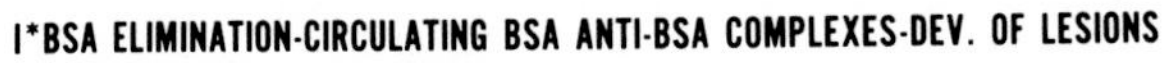

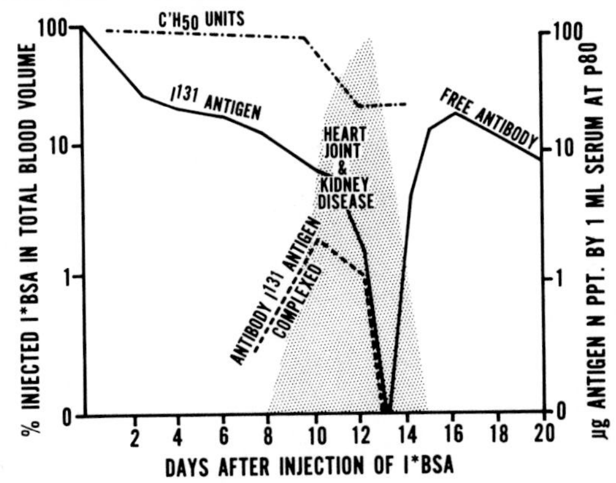

Figure 3. Sequence of events following injection of 250 mg of I*BSA/kg body weight in rabbits Elimination of ^{131}I antigen (by *solid line*) and antigen-antibody complexes plotted as percent of total I*BSA injected (*broken line*) relate to log scale at left. Amount of free antibody in the circulation, level of total complement (C'H_{50} units) plotted as percent of normal, and incidence of cardiovascular, joint, and kidney disease (*shaded area* reaching 100% on day 13) relate to log scale at right.

Coincidental with the presence of antigen-antibody complexes in the circulation, there is a fall in the serum C level and the appearance of acute inflammatory lesions in the kidneys (Fig. 4), heart, arteries (Fig. 5), and joints, strongly reminiscent of lesions of acute glomerulonephritis, rheumatic fever, lupus erythematosus, polyarteritis nodosa, and rheumatoid arthritis in human beings. These lesions vary in the degree to which the different cellular responses to antigen-antibody complexes participate, but prominent in most are endothelial proliferation, increased vascular permeability, and a variable PMN infiltration.

Presumptive evidence for the presence of immune complexes in the lesions has been obtained by fluorescent antibody staining of antigen, host gamma globulin (Fig. 6), apparently specific antibody, and host C in the cardiovascular and renal lesions. The substances were specifically concentrated in the lesions and appeared to be deposited coincidentally with their development. Additional support for the etiologic role of complexes in the cardiovascular and renal lesions was provided by Benacerraf and associates (20) and McCluskey and associates (21), who infused complexes into normal animals and produced arteritis, endocarditis, and glomerulitis. Although it cannot be determined whether the initial, local phlogogenic stimulus in serum sickness lesions results from systemic liberation of active humoral agents that act locally, or from the fortuitous focal deposition of small amounts of complexes, it is likely that the accumulation of complexes from the circulation in the developing lesions, as a result of increasing vascular permeability, and so forth, causes the snowballing inflammatory reaction. With the combination of all antigen into complexes and its subsequent elimination from the circulation, the inflammatory lesions in all sites rapidly resolve, and only occasional microscopic scars remain.

If antigen-antibody complexes are involved in the chronic clinical entities such as glomerulonephritis and rheumatic fever, it seems likely that experimental conditions designed to keep small amounts of such complexes present in the circulation for long periods of time should produce chronic progressive disease.

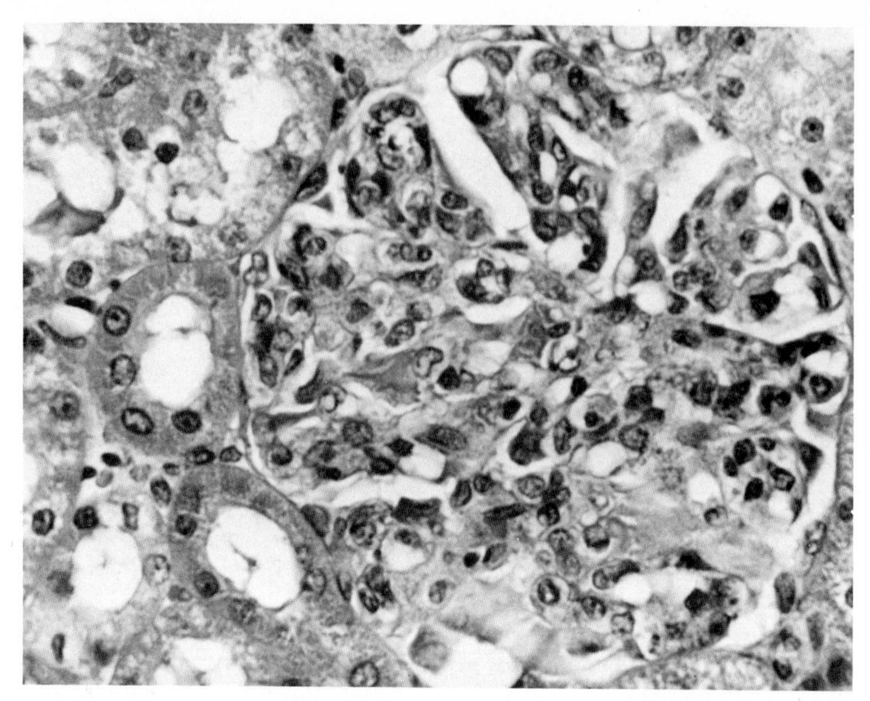

Figure 4. Hematoxylin-eosin-stained section of glomerulus of a rabbit with serum sickness on day of antigen elimination. Glomerulus is swollen, avascular, and filled with an increased number of endothelial and, to a lesser extent, epithelial cells.

These conditions were met a number of years ago in a model (22) in which small amounts of heterologous serum proteins were injected daily into rabbits (16). As shown in Table 1, bovine serum albumin (BSA), human serum albumin (HSA), bovine gamma globulin (BGG), and human gamma globulin (HGG) all served as satisfactory antigens. The antibody responses to daily injection of these antigens were of three types: (1) *Very large,* the animal having a large excess of antibody in the circulation at all times and no circulating soluble complexes; (2) *nonexistent,* in which case antigen in considerable amounts without antigen-antibody complexes was found in the circulation; and (3) *intermediate,* in which case the antibody that was formed combined with the injected antigen excess environment and formed soluble antigen-antibody complexes—these complexes persisting in the circulation for much of the interval between the daily antigen injections.

The diseases that resulted from the daily antigen-antibody reaction depended primarily on the relative amounts of antigen and antibody in the subject and relatively little upon the absolute amounts of antibody or upon the immunologic characteristics of the antigen. The rabbits making a vigorous response passed from an antigen excess environment to an antibody excess environment during the second week of injections and had at this time for a period of several days sizable amounts of antigen-antibody complexes in the circulation. As might be expected, while these complexes were circulating, typical serum sickness with acute inflammatory lesions of the heart, blood vessels, and kidney developed. As with "one-shot" serum sickness, the complexes were identifiable in the lesions. As soon as the rabbit had made sufficient antibody to achieve permanent antibody

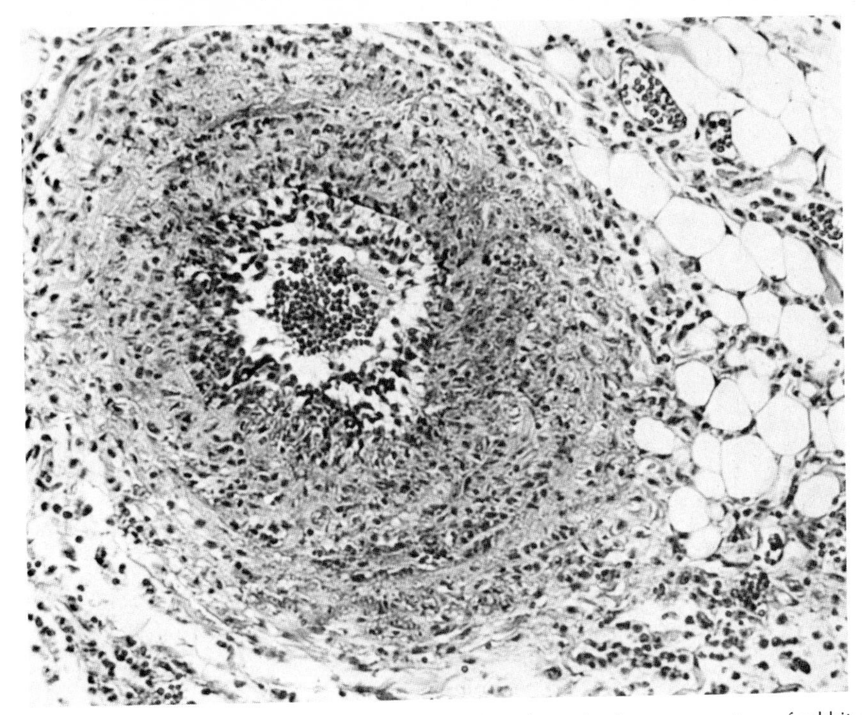

Figure 5. Hematoxylin-eosin-stained paraffin section of medium-sized coronary artery of rabbit with serum sickness on day of antigen elimination. There is considerable proliferation and infiltration of endothelium. Muscular media is almost entirely replaced by fibrinoid. There is moderate infiltration by polymorphonuclear leukocytes and mononuclear cells in the media and adventitia.

excess, each injection of antigen was incorporated immediately into soluble antigen-antibody aggregates and quickly removed from the circulation. This was sometimes accompanied by symptoms of anaphylaxis but without progression of the tissue lesions of serum sickness. The rabbits making no antibody response had considerable amounts of antigen in the circulation at all times without any evidence of disease, a result indicating the lack of toxicity of antigen alone.

It was among the animals making antibody responses too small to cause elimination of antigen but sufficient to result in the formation of circulating complexes that chronic progressive disease developed (Table 1). This pathogenic immunologic balance was achieved in some animals making little antibody and given only 0.5 mg of antigen per day and in some animals making much antibody and given 100 to 200 mg of antigen per day. After one or more months of injections and periods of one to several weeks during which antigen-antibody complexes were circulating a large part of each day, the animals developed a progressive glomerulonephritis. In most rabbits, disease could be turned off or on by changing the dose of antigen. If the dose was either lowered to allow a continual antibody excess or raised to give a very large antigen excess, progression of disease stopped. If the dose was again returned to a level giving rise to soluble complexes, the disease progressed.

The chronic glomerulonephritis was detectable clinically by proteinuria, in some instances hematuria, hypoproteinemia, and elevated serum cholesterol and urea levels. The most common and probably the earliest anatomic form of this

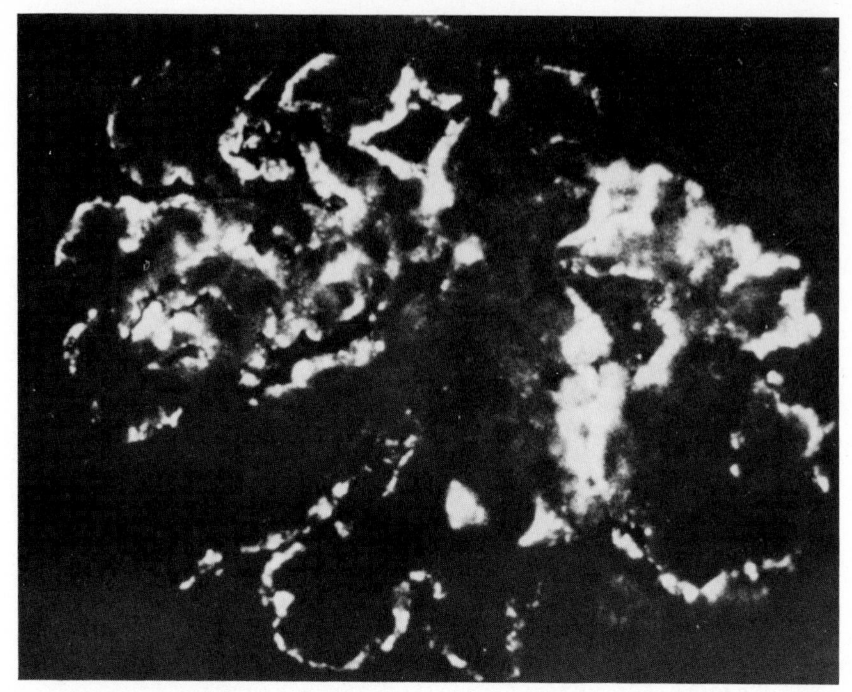

Figure 6. Fluorescent photomicrograph of glomerulus of a rabbit with acute serum sickness taken at day 12 after injection of antigen. The gamma globulin of the antibody is demonstrated complexed with antigen, giving a granular pattern when the complex becomes entrapped along the basement membrane.

disease was a membranous glomerulonephritis characterized by thickened glomerular capillary basement membranes with little or no endothelial proliferation. This lesion was much less inflammatory than degenerative by morphologic criteria. As the disease progressed, proliferative and scarring reactions became more evident (Figs. 7 and 8). Again, as would be expected if the complexes were causing this renal lesion, antigen, host gamma globulin, and host C were found concentrated in the thickened basement membranes (Fig. 9). By electron microscopy, a lumpy, dense deposit was seen along the outer aspect of the basement membranes corresponding to the antigen, gamma globulin, and C-rich deposits visualized with the fluorescent antibody technique (Fig. 10). Subsequent electron-microscopic studies with ferritin-labeled antibody have confirmed this

Table 1. Glomerulonephritis—Daily Injections

Antigen	Dose Range (mg/day)	No. of Rabbits Injected	Antibody Response		
			Ab Excess	Equiv.	Ag Excess
BSA	0.5–200	85	46 (2)[a]	26 (22)[a]	10
HSA	10 – 25	11	10	1 (1)	0
BGG	10 – 50	36	8	15 (15)	13
HGG	10 – 50	31	10	7 (5)	14
TOTALS		160	74 (2)	49 (43)	37

[a]Numbers in parentheses indicate rabbits with chronic glomerulonephritis.

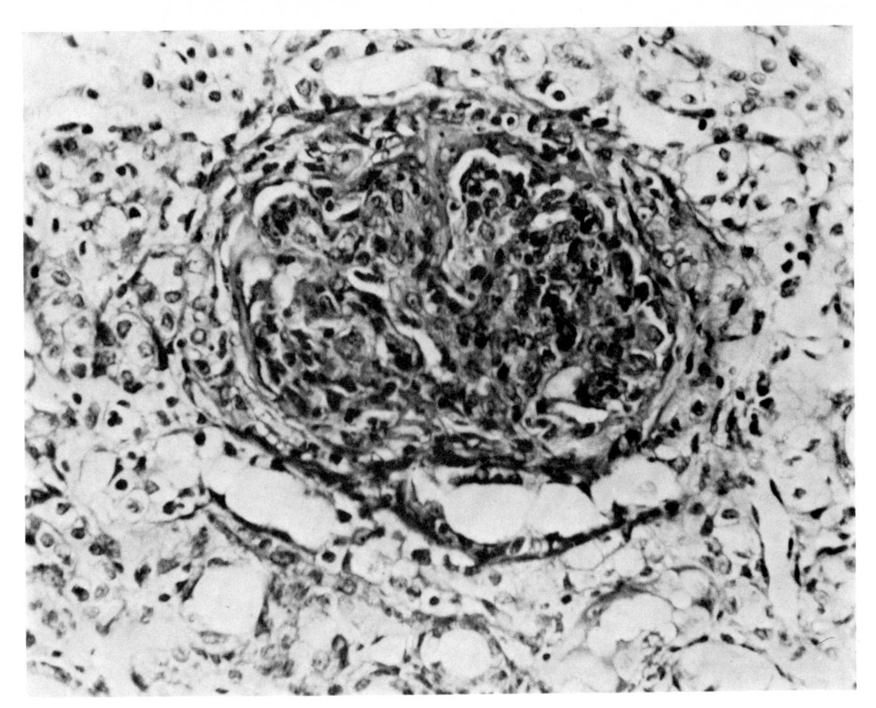

Figure 7. Hematoxylin-eosin-stained section of glomerulus of a rabbit given daily injections of BSA. This glomerulus has undergone prolonged inflammation and is now virtually obliterated by scarring. Capillary lumens are occluded, and the normal glomerular capillary tufts are no longer visible. Some nuclear fragments and other cell debris are visible.

correspondence. Once in this site, the immunologic reactants and the morphologically demonstrated deposits persisted for long periods—as much as one year after cessation of antigen injections—with persistence of associated renal malfunction.

Since the circulating complexes in either "one-shot" or "daily-injection" serum sickness bear no known immunologic relationship to the tissues that are injured, the factors predisposing certain parts of certain organs to injury by the complexes are apparently nonimmunologic. In the prolonged daily exposure to low levels of circulating complexes, the kidneys were the only organs injured, whereas in "one-shot" serum sickness with larger amounts of complexes present, heart, vessels, and joints also suffered lesions. This vulnerability of the kidneys in the presence of low levels of complexes may be related to the extensive renal blood flow and the normal filtering function of this organ.

The considerable concentration of complexes along the outer aspect of the basement membranes of the renal glomeruli is also probably determined by anatomic and physiologic peculiarities of the kidney. Some complexes apparently traverse the basement membrane but then are retained at its outer aspect or between the basement membrane and epithelial cells. It may be that as the complexes progress through the basement membrane, they tend to aggregate and become less soluble as a result of a reduction of excess antigen in the environment. Once here, the complexes appear to be sequestered from circulating cells or tissue cells capable of degrading them. Fresh complexes are also

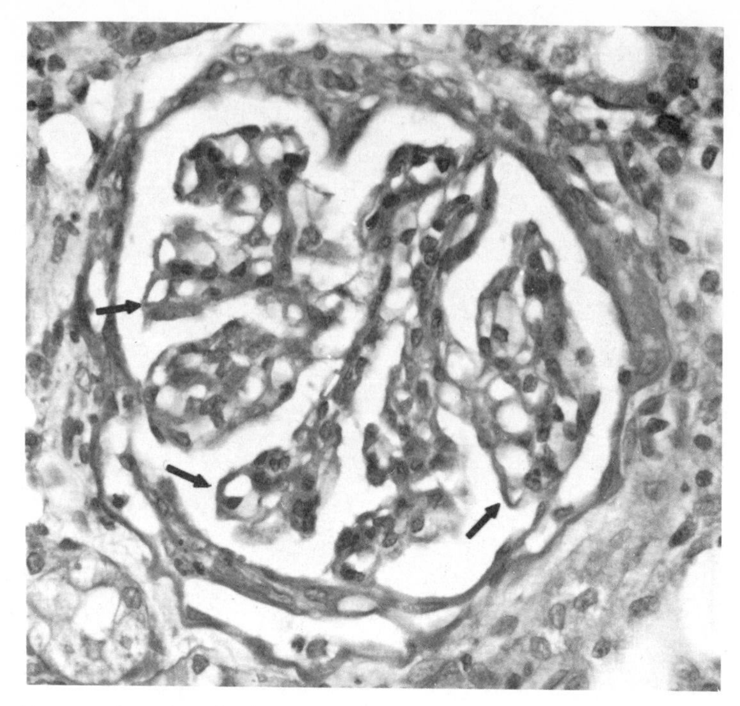

Figure 8. Hematoxylin-eosin-stained section of glomerulus of a rabbit with chronic membranous glomerulonephritis following daily injections of BSA. Capillary lumens are widely patent, but the capillary walls show hyaline thickening. Number of fixed glomerular cells is normal or only slightly increased. Figure obtained from Dr. Curtis Wilson.

deposited on the inner aspects of glomerular capillaries or vessels elsewhere. These newly deposited complexes may form the major injurious complex even in chronic disease where they are in contact with host mediation systems of the circulation.

In the prolonged daily exposure to circulating complexes, the kidneys were the only organs injured. When large amounts of antigen were administered to rabbits producing considerable antibody, deposits of immune complexes appeared in the alveolar walls and interstitium of the lung. Pneumonitis resulted, marked by fibrin deposition, inflammatory cell accumulation, and fibrosis.

MEDIATION OF IMMUNE COMPLEX LESIONS

Immune complexes injure tissues through their ability to activate humoral and cellular mediation systems. Rather than list all the mediator systems shown by in vitro methods to be associated, either directly or indirectly, with the antigen-antibody reaction, the mediation systems known to participate in experimental immune complex injury will be presented. The mediators involved are both humoral and cellular. They include plasma complement and as yet poorly defined serum permeability substances, along with proteolytic enzymes and other

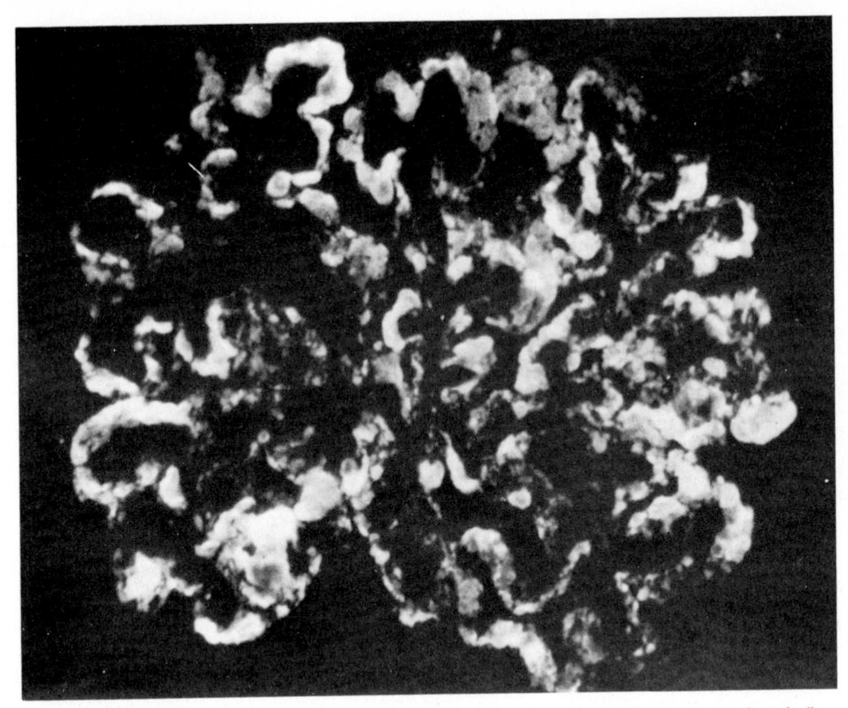

Figure 9. Fluorescent photomicrograph of glomerulus similar to that in Fig. 8. Stained with fluorescent anti-BSA. A lumpy fluorescent deposit is scattered along the glomerular capillary walls. Fluorescent staining for host gamma globulin gave comparable results. The gray tubular autofluorescence is barely visible around the glomerulus.

permeability factors contained within cells. Mediators involved in the release of histamine by immunologic reactants will not be discussed.

Polymorphonuclear Leukocytes: Their Essential Role in Immune Complex-Induced Tissue Injury

The Arthus vasculitis was the first antigen-antibody-induced lesion to be found dependent upon PMNs. Specific removal of PMNs by treatment with nitrogen mustard or heterologous anti-PMN sera has been shown to lead to striking inhibition of the reaction in several species (24–26,19). In depleted animals little or no evidence of injury is apparent microscopically at eight hours, when normal reactions are at their maximum. Microscopically, there is no evidence of injury found in the vessel walls, even though deposits of immunologic reactants and complement may be readily demonstrated. By using dye-marked albumin (Evans' blue), however, it is apparent that a small amount of edema occurs in these reaction sites, suggesting some increase in vascular permeability despite the absence of PMNs. This is most readily demonstrated when large amounts of antibody and antigen are employed in passive reactions.

In a different immunologic disease, serum sickness of rabbits, when PMNs are removed just prior to development of the lesions, the usual necrotizing arteritis does not appear. Intimal proliferation is markedly inhibited or absent, PMN

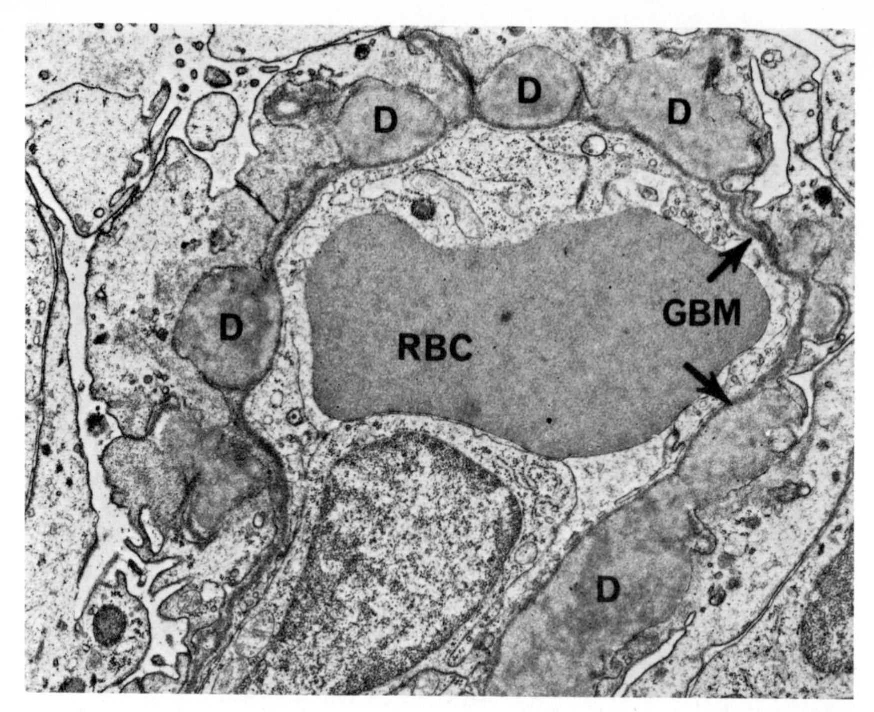

Figure 10. Electron photomicrograph of glomerulus of a rabbit with chronic serum sickness. The basement membrane can be seen as a lightly staining band covered for the most part on its inner aspect by endothelial cell cytoplasm. Studded along the outer part of the basement membrane (GBM) are the dense deposits (D) which in some places appear to be discrete and in other places appear to fuse with the basement membrane. The epithelial cell visible here has lost all its foot processes but contains a complex multistructured cytoplasm.

infiltration does not occur, and there is no destruction of the internal elastic lamina or fibrinoid necrosis in the arterial walls (27). The glomerulitis, normally seen in serum sickness, is not affected by PMN removal, which is not surprising in view of the paucity of PMNs in glomeruli in acute immune complex disease of rabbits.

Another immunologic disease of glomeruli is that of acute nephrotoxic nephritis. In this lesion, which is based on the reaction of injected antibody with the glomerular basement membrane, a clear role of PMNs also is apparent in the development of injury. Within two hours after the injection of antibody, a large accumulation of PMNs may be observed in the glomeruli (Figs. 11 and 12) (28). This accumulation lasts for about six hours, and the numbers of PMNs found thereafter in the glomeruli diminish. Proteinuria is first detected when PMNs accumulate and the numbers of PMNs in the glomeruli correlate reasonably well with the amount of protein in the urine. Removal of the PMNs by using either purified anti-PMN antibody or nitrogen mustard markedly or completely inhibits the occurrence of proteinuria (Table 2). As in the Arthus reaction, when large amounts of antibody are used, glomerular permeability increased in spite of the absence of PMNs. This indicates that factors other than those in PMNs can take part in the development of injury to the glomerulus. Both PMN-dependent and PMN-independent reactions can be elicited in several species.

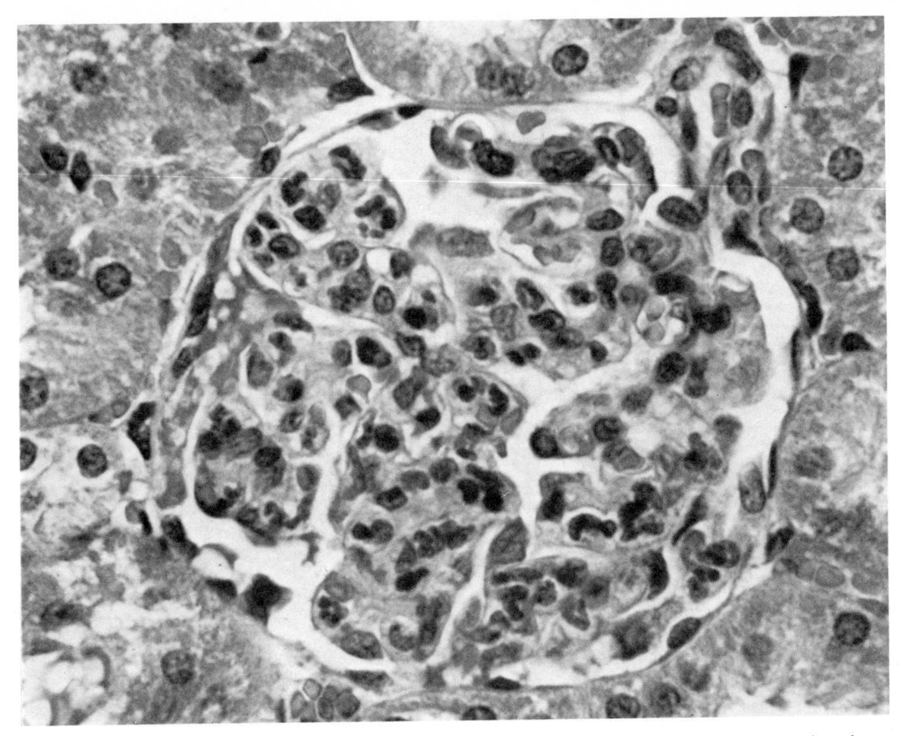

Figure 11. Microscopic section of glomerulus taken from a rat 2.5 hours after the injection of nephrotoxic globulin. Note the influx of polymorphonuclear leukocytes. Fluorescent antibody studies revealed the presence of nephrotoxic globulin and rat C along the basement membranes in similar sections of the same kidney.

MECHANISMS OF ACCUMULATION OF POLYMORPHONUCLEAR LEUKOCYTES

Early concepts as to the mechanisms of accumulation of PMNs were based solely on multitudinous studies of this process in general inflammation. These studies demonstrated several important concepts, among which are the following: (1) A humoral factor may well exist in areas of inflammation capable of attracting PMNs into the site of injury. Although early evidence was inconsistent with this (29), studies by Buckley employing microfoci of injury were most indicative (30). (2) From in vitro studies there was some evidence suggesting a serum factor that could be important in the attraction of PMNs toward a site of tissue injury (31,32). From in vitro studies employing a wide variety of substances that were chemotactic, from washed bacteria to extracts of burned tissue and serum, it appeared that there was more than one substance capable of attracting PMNs chemotactically.

Studies on the attraction of PMNs to immunologic reactants in tissues have strongly implicated plasma complement as being essential for the generation of the chemotactic factor. Four reactions have been studied in detail: the Arthus phenomenon (33), acute nephrotoxic nephritis (28), arteritis associated with

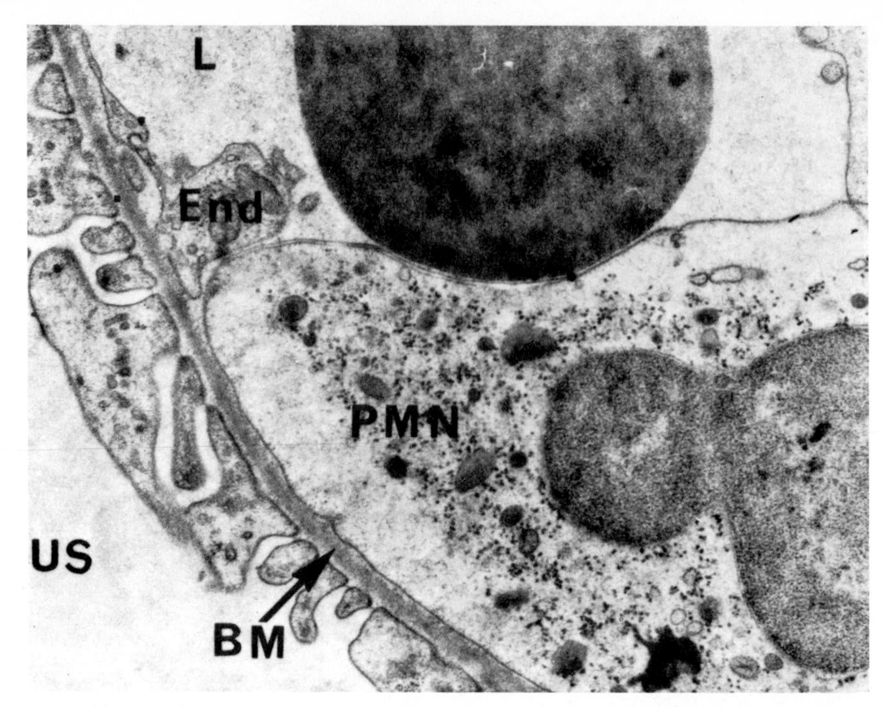

Figure 12. Electron photomicrograph of a capillary loop taken from a rat 2.5 hours after an intravenous injection of nephrotoxic globulin. The endothelial cell (End) has been swept aside by the neutrophil (PMN), leaving the basement membrane (BM) exposed only to the surface of the PMN. The neutrophil has thus gained intimate contact with the basement membrane. L = lumen.

immune complex deposition (34), and synovitis resulting from antigen-antibody combination in small vessels in joint tissues (35). Two approaches were taken, the first consisting of depleting animals of plasma complement (C) prior to induction of reactions, and the second using antibodies to induce reactions (in normal animals) that were incapable of fixing C. Under both circumstances, PMN infiltration was absent, even though antigen and antibody deposits were detected in the vessel walls with fluorescent antibody techniques. In each case, however, little or no C3 could be found in the vascular structure. Thus, in both C-depleted and normal animals, a correlation existed between the ability of the antibody to fix C and the accumulation of PMNs at the antigen-antibody site (Table 3). These findings are in keeping with those of Block et al. (36), who analyzed the biologic properties of guinea pig γ_1 and γ_2 7S antibody to a single antigen. The γ_1 fixed complement poorly and failed to induce full Arthus reactions in homologous guinea pigs. The γ_2 antibody did fix complement and cause severe Arthus reactions.

Table 2. Proteinuria in First 24 Hours After Injection of Nephrotoxic Serum

	Normal		PMN-Depleted	
	No.	mg/24 hours	No.	mg/24 hours
Rats	8	246	5	59
	6	50	7	6
Rabbits	5	1,843	5	0.2

Table 3. Effect of Complement Depletion on PMN Accumulation in Arthus Reaction and Early Nephrotoxic Nephritis

	No. of Rats	PMN Accumulation	Fluorescent Results		$C'H_{50}$	PMN (per mm^3)	Platelets
			C′	AgAb			
Nephrotoxic nephritis							
C-depleted	7	−	±	4+	<7.5	10,960	—
Controls	6	+	3+	4+	38	4,200	—
Arthus reaction							
C-depleted	10	−	±	4	<8	7,300	591,000
Controls	5	+	3+	4+	49	4,300	610,000

Complement might bring about the accumulation of neutrophils in two ways: (1) through immune adherence; and (2) by releasing chemotactic agents that cause a directional migration of neutrophils toward the point of greatest concentration, i.e., the antigen-antibody complex where complement components are being activated.

Immune adherence is a phenomenon by which neutrophils and macrophages from most species, platelets from some species, and erythrocytes only of primates bind to an immune aggregate. In a few species the IgG antibody together with antigen is sufficient to induce adherence of the cells, but in all species the fixation of complement, especially the third component, greatly augments the adherence. Presumably, when immune complexes deposit or form in blood vessel walls, and complement through the third component is bound, neutrophils in the circulation would bind. This would be eliminated by depletion of C3, as was accomplished in the experiments noted in Table 3.

Until recently, chemotaxis has been a phenomenon observed exclusively in vitro. The directional migration of neutrophils to a source of a humoral stimulating agent has been successfully examined in chambers separated into two compartments by a micropore filter. Cells such as neutrophils, placed in the upper chamber, migrate through the filter to a source of chemotactic material in the bottom compartment. By this method, antigen-antibody complexes were observed to generate chemotactic activity from fresh serum with an intact complement system (37,38). Subsequently, three chemotactic agents have been derived from activated components of complement, C5–6–7 (38,39), C3a (40,41), and C5a (42,43). Recently, a role of chemotaxis has been observed in vivo. In synovial tissues, PMNs were observed to migrate over 200 μ to a point where complement components were activated by an immunologic reaction (44). Blocking activation of the complement system inhibited migration of the PMNs.

Thus, complement appears to play an important role in the accumulation of PMNs at the site of immunologic reactions.

Vascular Structures Injured by PMNs in Immunologic Reactions

In attempting to analyze the various components of PMNs responsible for the damage of blood vessel walls during immunologic reactions, it was necessary to gain first an understanding of the specific structures within vessel walls that were damaged. In the arteritis of serum sickness, the internal elastic lamina was disrupted.

In other PMN-dependent reactions, the vascular basement membrane apparently was a critical target structure. In the Arthus reaction, studies of the vessel wall during the influx of PMNs revealed marked disruption of the basement membrane of the vessel wall (45). In addition, in glomeruli, especially in acute nephrotoxic nephritis, morphologic evidence has suggested that the glomerular basement membrane is the site of primary injury (28). As noted in Fig. 12, PMNs forced aside the endothelial cells to gain intimate contact with the underlying basement membrane. It was during this time that proteinuria commenced. Analysis of the urine during this acute phase has revealed basement membrane fragments that were released during the PMN attack (46).

The Role of PMN Constituents in the Alteration of Vascular Integrity

In further considerations of the apparent attack of PMNs on basement membranes, it was found that lysates of PMNs or of the PMN cytoplasmic granules were capable of attacking semipurified glomerular basement membrane in vitro (45). These studies showed that peptides were released from the basement membrane by the PMN lysates. The agents responsible were found to be cathepsins D and E of rabbit PMNs (45).

In human PMNs, a neutral protease hydrolyzes isolated basement membrane much in the same way as the acid cathepsins of rabbit PMNs (47). PMNs also contain a collagenase that hydrolyzes collagen as well as basement membranes (48,49). In addition, an elastase has been isolated that cleaves porcine elastin (49) and may be responsible for breakdown of the internal elastic lamina of arteries observed in serum sickness (27).

Fibrinolytic activity is also observed in extracts of PMNs (50). The enzymes appear in both active and activatable form (51,52).

Protein polysaccharide of cartilage (53,54) also serves as substrate of PMN granule enzymes. PMN proteases also degrade nuclear histones (55,56).

Neutrophils in addition bear on their surfaces an extrinsic membrane protein possessing protease activity. When exposed to plasma, the protease liberates a neutral peptide with a molecular weight of about 1,000 that contracts smooth muscle and enhances vascular permeability (57).

At least four basic proteins have been isolated fom the lysosomes of neutrophils that are capable of increasing vascular permeability. The effect of one of these follows its action on mast cells and the consequent release of histamine (58). The other three act independently by means as yet unclear (59).

Another potentially injurious series of substances given off by granulocytes are the free radicals derived from oxygen. These include superoxide ($\cdot O_2^-$), hydrogen peroxide, hydroxyl radicals, and singlet oxygen. The potent oxidants bear microbicidal activity and could possibly produce injury of tissues.

A composite of the numerous potential agents by which neutrophils can mediate injury of vessels is shown in Table 4.

Table 4. Biologically Active Constituents of Neutrophils

Constituent	Activity
Proteases	Hydrolysis of basement membrane, histone, proteoglycan
Fibrinolysis	Degradation of fibrin
Collagenase	Hydrolysis of collagen basement membrane
Elastase	Hydrolysis of internal elastic lamina
Basic proteins	
Bands 1,3,4	Increase in vascular permeability
Band 2	Activation of mast cells
Thrombin-activating material	Thromboplastin
Slow-reacting substance	Vascular permeability and smooth muscle contraction
Kininogenase	Release of kinin from kininogen
Free radicals of oxygen	?
Surface protease	Kinin release from plasma alpha globulin

IMMUNOLOGIC INJURY THAT OCCURS INDEPENDENTLY OF THE PRESENCE OF NEUTROPHILS AND COMPLEMENT

Immunologic injury has been shown to develop independently of the presence of neutrophils and complement. This has been observed in both immune complex (60) and anti-glomerular basement membrane (GBM) (nephrotoxic) nephritis (61), both of which are reactions of vascular permeability. The mediation of the PMN-complement-independent injury is not yet understood, and that mediators are at all involved is not certain. Nevertheless, evidence suggests that mediation systems are required for the injury: (1) anti-GBM antibody is known to react along the endothelial surface of the GBM, and the position of injury of the neutrophil-independent nephritis apparently lies on the epithelial side of the GBM where the filtration of smaller proteins of the plasma occurs. This is over 1,000 A away from the position where the antigen-antibody reaction takes place; (2) Fab anti-GBM can be reacted with the GBM in large amount, i.e., over ten times the amount of whole IgG antibody, and yet it fails to produce injury as detected by proteinuria and histologic examination; (3) an IgG_2 has been isolated in the author's laboratory from sheep antirabbit GBM that binds in vivo to the rabbit GBM, but fails to cause injury. These final observations have been confirmed in Dr. Keith Peters' laboratory.

Whereas the proteinuria of neutrophil-dependent immunologic injury is nonselective, the proteinuria of neutrophil-independent injury is selective, being almost exclusively albuminuria. GBM fragments and neutrophilic enzymes and basic peptides do not appear in the urine (61).

Additional experimental evidence of complement-neutrophil-independent injury has been gained recently. Guinea pigs injected with human GBM develop an autoallergic glomerulonephritis in which antibody to the heterologous GBM cross-reacts with the guinea pig GBM. Few neutrophils were observed, and deposition of complement was not associated with development of injury (62). In addition, rats injected with γ_1 guinea pig antirat GBM developed proteinuria with antibody that activated little, if any, rat complement (63).

Antibody Responsible for Each Mediator Pathway in Glomerulonephritis

Using heterologous sheep antirabbit GBM to induce glomerulonephritis in rabbits, a distinction has been observed in the type of mediation system responsible for the injury. γ_2 anti-GBM induced glomerular injury that was unaffected by depletion of neutrophils, whereas a γ_1 antibody induced injury that was in large part dependent upon neutrophils. The γ_2 antibody failed to activate complement in vitro when exposed to isolated GBM, whereas the γ_1 antibody did (64,65). The sheep γ_2 antibody therefore resembles avian antibody that behaves similarly in that it injures the GBM in the absence of PMNs and complement.

Thus, evidence exists for the participation of separate antibody classes responsible for activation of distinct mediation pathways. This finding may be of great assistance in detecting members of the second mediator pathway.

IgE antibody has been reported in glomeruli of human idiopathic glomerulonephritis (66), although this finding has lacked confirmation (67). Otherwise, IgG, IgM, and, in special cases, IgA are commonly found in human acute and chronic glomerulonephritis, offering the potential activation of complement-neutrophil-dependent and complement-neutrophil-independent pathways.

SUMMARY

Tissue injury of many types may be caused by deposited complexes of antigen and antibody. The circumstances under which the complexes form and deposit often determine the location and type of injury observed: if the complex forms in the circulation, deposition may occur in arterial walls and glomeruli, initiating lesions in those tissues. If the complex forms in the synovial tissues or spaces, then the reaction will develop at that point, etc. Any local source of antigen will initiate these lesions once antibody is formed. If the source of antigen persists, antibody-forming cells will soon establish themselves locally as they do in the active Arthus reaction, and injury will become chronic.

When the antibody formed is capable of activating complement, polymorphonuclear leukocytes (PMNs, neutrophils) will accumulate, leading to release of injurious constituents. Such is the case in acute glomerulonephritis, arteritis, synovitis, and vasculitis, as is illustrated herein. The ability of complement to attract the PMNs has been demonstrated as an in vitro phenomenon and as a clear possibility in vivo. The requirement of PMNs in the development of the lesions has been demonstrated.

The constituents of PMNs capable of injuring tissue in various ways are described, from peptides capable of increasing vascular permeability, to enzymes that indirectly bring more PMNs and other cells into the lesion, to proteolytic enzymes that hydrolyze vital structures in the tissues. These agents were most likely designed to rid the host of invaders; but at times they unfortunately are directed against the host's own tissues.

The process by which PMNs and other cells (platelets, mast cells, basophils, and macrophages) release injurious constituents is of great interest currently. The exocytosis of their cytoplasmic granules constitutes the major mechanism of release and involves a complicated series of events as outlined in this chapter.

REFERENCES

1. Friedman, U., *Z. Immunitätsforsch.* **2**, 591 (1909).
2. Frieberger, E., *Z. Immunitätsforsch.* **3**, 692 (1909).
3. Hawn, C. V. Z., and Janeway, C. A., *J. Exp. Med.* **85**, 571 (1947).
4. Germuth, F. G., *J. Exp. Med.* **97**, 257 (1953).
5. Germuth, F. G., and McKinnon, G. E., *Bull. Johns Hopkins Hosp.* **101**, 13 (1957).
6. Dixon, F. J., *J. Cell. Comp. Physiol.* **50**, 27 (1957).
7. Dixon, F. J., Vazquez, J. J., Weigle, W. O., and Cochrane, C. G., *Arch. Pathol.* **65**, 18 (1958).
8. Dixon, F. J., Vazquez, J. J., Weigle, W. O., and Cochrane, C. G., in *Symposium on Cellular and Humoral Aspects of the Hypersensitive States* (H. S. Lawrence, ed.), Hoeber Div., Harper and Row, New York, 1959, p. 354.
9. Kulka, A. M., *J. Immunol.* **43,** 273 (1942).
10. Trapani, I. L., Garvey, J. S., and Campbell, D., *Science* **127**, 700 (1958).
11. Ishizaka, K., and Campbell, D., *Proc. Soc. Exp. Biol. Med.* **97**, 635 (1958).
12. Cochrane, C. G., and Weigle, W. O., *J. Exp. Med.* **108**, 591 (1958).
13. Ishizaka, K., and Campbell, D., *J. Immunol.* **83**, 116 (1959).
14. Ishizaka, T., Ishizaka, K., and Borsos, T., *J. Immunol.* **87**, 433 (1961).
15. Christian, C. L., *J. Immunol.* **84**, 117 (1960).
16. Dixon, F. J., Feldman, J. D., and Vazquez, J. J., *J. Exp. Med.* **113**, 899 (1961).
17. Arthus, M. C. R., *Soc. Biol.* (Paris) **55**, 817 (1903).
18. Arthus, and Breton, M. C. R., *Soc. Biol.* (Paris) **55**, 1478 (1903).
19. Cochrane, C. G., Weigle, W. O., and Dixon, F J., *J. Exp. Med.* **110**, 481 (1959).
20. Benacerraf, B., Potter, J. L., McCluskey, R. T., and Miller, F., *J. Exp. Med.* **111**, 195 (1960).
21. McCluskey, R. T., Benacerraf, B., Potter, J. L., and Miller, F., *J. Exp. Med.* **111**, 181 (1960).
22. McLean, C. R., Fitzgerald, J. D. L., Younghusband, O. Z., and Hamilton, J. D., *Arch. Pathol.* **51**, 1 (1951).
23. Kniker, W. T., and Cochrane, C. G., *J. Exp. Med.* **127**, 119 (1968).
23a. Bentjens, J. R., O'Connell, D. W., Pawlowski, J. B., Hsu, K. C., and Andres, G. A. *J. Exp. Med.* **140**, 104 (1974).
24. Stetson, C. A., *J. Exp. Med.* **94**, 347 (1951).
25. Humphrey, J. H., *Br. J. Exp. Pathol.* **36,** 268 (1955).
26. Humphrey, J. H., *Br. J. Exp. Pathol.* **36**, 283 (1955).
27. Kniker, W. T., and Cochrane, C. G., *J. Exp. Med.* **122**, 83 (1965).
28. Cochrane, C. G., Unanue, E. R., and Dixon, F. J., *J. Exp. Med.* **122**, 99 (1965).
29. Harris, H., *Physiol. Rev.* **34**, 529 (1954).
30. Buckley, I. K., *Exp. Mol. Pathol.* **2**, 402 (1963).
31. Hurley, J. V., and Spector, W. G., *J. Pathol. Bacteriol.* **82**, 403 (1961).
32. Hurley, J. V., in *The Acute Inflammatory Process,* N.Y. Acad. Sci. **116**, 918 (1964).
33. Ward, P. A., and Cochrane, C. G., *J. Exp. Med.* **121**, 215 (1965).
34. Kniker, W. T., and Cochrane, C. G., *J. Exp. Med.* **122**, 83 (1965).
35. DeShazo, C. V., Henson, P. M., and Cochrane, C. G., *J. Clin. Invest.* **51**, 50 (1972).
36. Block, K. J., Kourilsky, F. M., Ovary, Z., and Benacerraf, B., *J. Exp. Med.* **117**, 965 (1963).
37. Boyden, S., *J. Exp. Med.* **115**, 463 (1962).
38. Ward, P. A., Cochrane, C. G., and Müller-Eberhard, H. J., *J. Exp. Med.* **122**, 327 (1965).
39. Ward, P. A., Cochrane, C. G., and Müller-Eberhard, H. J., *Immunology* **11**, 141 (1966).
40. Ward, P. A., *J. Exp. Med.* **126**, 189 (1967).
41. Bokisch, V. A., Müller-Eberhard, H. J., and Cochrane, C. G., *J. Exp. Med.* **129**, 1109 (1969).
42. Ward, P. A., and Newman, L. J., *J. Immunol.* **102**, 93 (1969).
43. Shin, H. S., Pickering, R. J., Mayer, M. M., and Cook, C. T., *J. Immunol.* **101**, 813 (1968).

44. DeShazo, V., McGrade, M., Henson, P. M., and Cochrane, C. G., *J. Immunol.* **108**, 1414 (1972).
45. Cochrane, C. G., and Aikin, B. S., *J. Exp. Med.* **124**, 733 (1966).
46. Hawkins, D., *Fed. Proc.* **26**, 744 (1967).
47. Janoff, A., and Zeligs, J., *Science* **161**, 702 (1968).
48. Lazarus, G. S., Brown, R. S., Daniels, J. R., and Fullmer, M. M., *Science* **159**, 1483 (1968).
49. Janoff, A., and Scherer, J., *J. Exp. Med.* **128**, 1137 (1968).
50. Barnhart, M. I., Quintana, C., Lenon, H. L., Bluhm, G. B., and Riddle, J. M., *Ann. N.Y. Acad. Sci.* **146**, 527 (1968).
51. Prokopowicz, J., *Thromb. Diath. Haemorrh.* **19**, 84 (1968).
52. Prokopowicz, J., *Biochem. Biophys. Acta* **154**, 91 (1968).
53. Ziff, M., Gribetz, H. S., and Lospalluto, J., *Clin. Invest.* **39**, 405 (1960).
54. Janoff, A., and Blondin, J., *Proc. Soc. Exp. Biol. Med.* **135**, 302 (1970).
55. Davies, D. T. P., Krakauer, K., and Weissmann, G., *Fed. Proc.* **29**, 784 (1970).
56. Davies, D. T. P., and Wiessmann, G., *J. Cell Biol.* **43**, 29a (1969).
57. Wintroub, B. V., Goetzl, E. J., and Austen, K. F., *J. Exp. Med.* **148**, 812 (1974).
58. Janoff, A., Schaeffer, S., Scherer, J., and Bran, M. A., *J. Exp. Med.* **122**, 841 (1965).
59. Ranadive, N. S., and Cochrane, C. G., *J. Exp. Med.* **128**, 605 (1968).
59a. Curnutte, J. T., Kipnes, R. S., and Babior, B. M., *N. Engl. J. Med.* **293**, 628 (1975).
60. Henson, P. M., and Cochrane, C. G., *J. Exp. Med.* **133**, 554 (1971).
61. Hawkins, D., and Cochrane, C. G., *Immunology* **14**, 665 (1968).
62. Cousor, W. G., Stilmant, M., and Lewis, E. J., *Lab. Invest.* **22**, 236 (1973).
63. Rassos, H. C., Siqueira, M., Martinez, O. C., and Bier, O. G., *Immunology* **26**, 407 (1974).
64. Hawkins, D., and Cochrane, C. G., *Immunology,* **14**, 665 (1968).
65. Cochrane, C. G., and Henson, P. M., *J. Immunol.* **107,** 321 (abstr.) (1971).
66. Gerber, M. A., and Paronetto, F., *Lancet,* **1**, 1097.
67. Roy, P. L., Westberg, N. G., and Michael, A. F., *J. Clin. Invest.* (1974).

Chapter Four

Lymphokine-Mediated Reactions

STANLEY COHEN AND TAKESHI YOSHIDA

Department of Pathology, University of Connecticut Health Center, Farmington, Connecticut

The previous chapters have concerned themselves with reactions involving antibodies. In many cases, such as those involving anaphylaxis or Arthus reactions, the immunopathologic responses are consequences of the action of nonantibody mediator substances, and the antibodies merely serve as triggering agents. These mediators, for the most part, are not products of lymphocytes. Immunologic responses based upon this kind of mechanism have been termed "immediate hypersensitivity." In contrast, "delayed hypersensitivity" involves reactions that are dependent upon the activity of sensitized lymphocytes themselves rather than conventional antibody. For this reason, this class of response is now known as cellular immunity or cell-mediated immunity. The phrase "delayed hypersensitivity" is often restricted to a description of the classic cutaneous manifestation of cellular immunity, the tuberculin-type reaction. This is a slowly evolving inflammatory reaction at the site of injection of antigen into a previously sensitized individual. The reaction reaches maximal size in 24 to 48 hours. The gross appearance is that of a raised, erythematous, indurated lump; the most familiar example is a positive tuberculin reaction in man. Microscopically, in man and in the guinea pig the reaction has a rather typical appearance, being composed predominantly of lymphocytes and macrophages. Since in routine histologic sections it is not always possible to distinguish between lymphocytes and macrophages, they are usually collectively referred to as "mononuclear" cells.

The delayed hypersensitivity reaction can be passively transferred to a normal, nonimmune recipient by sensitized lymphocytes, but not by antiserum.

The original studies described in this chapter were supported by N.I.H. Grants AI-12477, AI-12225, AI-13258, CA-19286, and HL-19711.

The above represents a textbook definition of delayed hypersensitivity. Although it is useful as a starting point for our discussion of the mechanism of lymphocyte-mediated reactions, it is true only in a general way. Thus, although the reaction is delayed, it is not any more delayed than reactions mediated by reaginic antibody that have latent periods of 48 to 72 hours. Moreover, the classic time course of 24 to 48 hours for delayed hypersensitivity is merely a function of its traditional site for elicitation, the skin. As we shall see, in other locations such as the peritoneal cavity, these reactions may reach maximal intensity in as little as four hours. There are a number of biologically important situations in which the major infiltrating cell population is granulocytic rather than mononuclear. Finally, this class of immunologic reaction is no more nor no less cell-mediated than antibody-dependent reactions that are ultimately due to the participation of a lymphocyte or plasma cell. With the exception of those reactions that involve direct cell killing, most reactions of cell-mediated immunity are dependent, not upon the lymphocyte as effector, but rather upon soluble lymphocyte products known as lymphokines.

In this chapter, we will focus on the role of lymphokines in so-called cell-mediated immunity. Lymphocyte-dependent cytotoxicity will be discussed in a subsequent chapter.

THE NATURE OF THE CELLULAR INFILTRATE

It was originally thought that the bulk of the mononuclear cells comprising the infiltrate of delayed reactions represented sensitized cells possessing some sort of immunologic specificity directed toward the antigen and that there was some mechanism that served to attract such cells to the reaction site. However, it is now known that only a small number of infiltrating cells are specifically sensitized cells. Moreover, the bulk of the available evidence suggests that there is little, if any, preferential accumulation of these sensitized cells at the specific test site. The evidence for these contentions is based mainly on transfer experiments or on experiments involving animals immunized with two unrelated antigens either at different times or at different sites and whose proliferating cells of one specificity are labeled by strategically timed or placed injections of tritiated thymidine. These studies have been extensively reviewed (1,2).

Another misconception about the nature of the inflammatory response is related to the indurated nature of the delayed hypersensitivity reaction site. This has been considered to be a microscopic reflection of the vast numbers of infiltrating inflammatory cells. Some time ago, however, it was shown (3,4) that one could suppress cutaneous delayed hypersensitivity reactions by treating the experimental animals with anticoagulants. In our studies (3), it was found that this suppression involved only the effector arm of the response and not the state of immunization. The suppression was noted mainly as a decrease in induration; histologic observation using routine hematoxylin- and eosin-stained sections demonstrated substantial though reduced mononuclear cell infiltration in the suppressed animals. Moreover, the cellular inflammatory response to nonspecific irritants was not affected in these animals. These early studies have been brought into focus by the recent studies by Dvorak and his associates (5).

Using modern morphologic investigative techniques, they have unequivocally demonstrated deposition of fibrin in delayed hypersensitivity sites. In comparative studies involving nonindurated, basophil-rich, cell-mediated lesions, they have shown that the induration of delayed hypersensitivity reactions is not due to the infiltrating cells, but rather is due to the deposition of fibrin, possibly in association with bound extravascular water.

Even the nature of the cellular inflammatory infiltrate itself is not as clear-cut as is generally believed. It is certainly true that the typical cutaneous manifestation of cell-mediated immunity in the guinea pig and man is a lesion that is composed predominantly of mononuclear cells, with macrophages representing the great majority of these cells and lymphocytes present in lesser numbers. However, in the guinea pig and man it is possible to induce cell-mediated immune lesions in which the predominant cell is the basophil. These reactions, known as Jones-Mote hypersensitivity or cutaneous basophil hypersensitivity (CBH), occur when the immunizing stimulus is weak, for example, when antigen is incorporated into incomplete Freund's adjuvant. Also, many contact allergies of man seem to be of the CBH variety.

In certain circumstances, the eosinophil may play an important role. If one skin tests a guinea pig, allows the reaction site to heal, and then reinjects antigen at that site, the second reaction is more intense, evolves more rapidly, and is largely composed of eosinophils. This is known as a "retest" reaction.

Even the classic delayed hypersensitivity reaction may have a different morphologic appearance in different species. For example, in the mouse (6), the lesion contains large numbers of neutrophils. Finally, in certain experimental autoimmune disorders in which cell-mediated immunity is thought to play a pathogenetic role (such as thyroiditis or encephalomyelitis), the predominant infiltrating cell appears to be the lymphocyte.

These histologic patterns will be discussed more fully in the next chapter. They serve as examples to demonstrate that the typical macrophage-rich reaction represents but one manifestation of delayed hypersensitivity reactions. The central feature common to all is that a small number of specifically sensitized lymphocytes interact with antigen locally. As a consequence of that interaction, a set of events occurs which leads to the generation of an inflammatory response at the reaction site. As will be discussed later, those events are known to involve the production and release of soluble mediator substances that are collectively referred to as lymphokines.

INDUCTION OF DELAYED HYPERSENSITIVITY

It was long believed that delayed hypersensitivity occurred only in response to antigens of microorganisms, but it is now known that this type of reactivity may develop toward purified proteins or simple chemicals (haptens) chemically conjugated to such proteins (carriers). Moreover, under certain circumstances, the direct cutaneous application of various low-molecular-weight substances with reactive chemical groups can produce a similar response. This latter phenomenon, which is known as "contact sensitivity," is essentially a delayed hypersensitivity response in which the chemical becomes conjugated in vivo to certain of the animal's own proteins. In addition, reactions involving cellular immunity are believed to play a role in certain autoimmune diseases, in allograft reactions, and in host defense against infection or neoplasms.

The cutaneous delayed hypersensitivity reaction remains the best-studied model of cell-mediated immunity. In general, intradermal injections of antigen are most effective in the induction of this form of immunologic reactivity, and intravenous injections are least effective (7). Moreover, under appropriate experimental conditions, intravenous administration of antigen can lead to the development of tolerance with respect to delayed hypersensitivity in the face of continued immunologic reactivity as indicated by antibody formation. This phenomenon has been called "partial tolerance" or "immune deviation" (8,9,10).

Delayed hypersensitivity is produced most readily when the antigen is incorporated into an adjuvant. The first observation bearing on this point was made by Dienes (11), who showed that when ovalbumin was injected into foci of tuberculous infection in the guinea pig, delayed hypersensitivity was more likely to develop than following injection into normal animals. Raffel and his associates found that mixtures of ovalbumin with the wax isolated from tubercle bacilli are effective in producing delayed hypersensitivity (12). Currently, the most effective method of producing delayed reactivity is by means of the emulsion of an aqueous solution of antigen with Freund's complete adjuvant, which consists of oil, a surfactant, and killed tubercle bacilli. If tubercle bacilli are not present, the mixture is known as "incomplete adjuvant." The reactivity resulting from immunization with incomplete adjuvant is more transient than when complete adjuvants are used. The skin reactions, though grossly similar to those elicitable after immunization with complete Freund's adjuvant, have a somewhat different histologic appearance; as was described in the previous section, they are characterized by the presence of basophils as well as mononuclear cells in the infiltrate.

Although adjuvants enhance the formation of a delayed response, they are not essential. Good sensitivity can be produced by the injection of small amounts of protein in saline (13) or by the injection of antigen-antibody complexes prepared in antibody excess (14).

These procedures for producing delayed hypersensitivity are effective only when the antigen is a protein. Polysaccharides, in contrast, though capable of inducing antibody formation, do not produce delayed hypersensitivity. This may be related to the phenomenon of "carrier specificity." As stated previously, delayed hypersensitivity may be produced by an antigen that consists of a simple hapten conjugated to a protein carrier. If, for example, guinea pigs are immunized with dinitrophenylated bovine gamma globulin (DNP-BGG) and are skin tested with that antigen one week later, they exhibit strong delayed reactions. If they are tested with the same hapten coupled with a non-cross-reacting protein such as ovalbumin, delayed reactions are usually not observed. Conversely, skin tests with an unrelated hapten such as *O*-chlorobenzoyl chloride (OCBC) conjugated to the original protein sometimes give positive reactions (15–17). This is the opposite of the situation for reactions mediated by antibody, namely the Arthus reaction or anaphylaxis. In these cases, the haptenic group is the important determinant for reactivity. In the case of polysaccharide antigens, it is thought that these substances function as complex haptens and are conjugated with host proteins in vivo. Since the carrier is therefore unknown and unavailable, and polysaccharides do not have groups as reactive as those of skin-sensitizing low-molecular weight substances that produce contact sensitivity, delayed reactivity cannot be demonstrated to polysaccharides.

Although haptens are capable of combining with preformed antibody, they are not in themselves immunogenic. It is only when they are conjugated to a protein carrier that they are capable of inducing an immune response. The carrier specificity involved in eliciting a delayed reaction indicates that the triggering antigen must also be immunogenic, even though the animal has already been immunized. This requirement was demonstrated directly with the aid of polypeptides (18). For this purpose, dinitrophenylated polylysine molecules of various sizes were studied. It was found that the smallest antigen capable of inducing either antibody formation or delayed hypersensitivity was a single DNP molecule conjugated to a polylysine molecule containing seven lysine residues. The antibody response was directed in large measure against the DNP determinant, and, as expected, even DNP conjugated to a single lysine was capable of combining with the antibody so formed. Similarly, molecules containing fewer than seven lysines were capable of eliciting Arthus or anaphylactic reactions in the experimental animals. On the other hand, a molecule containing a minimum of seven lysines was required to elicit a delayed reaction. In other words, only the immunogenic molecule would suffice for the elicitation of delayed hypersensitivity. This distinction between delayed hypersensitivity and antibody-mediated reaction supports the widely accepted interpretation that the former reaction is not due to the presence of conventional antibody. Moreover, the requirement for immunogenicity shows that the triggering event for the delayed reaction must involve recognition mechanisms similar to those involved in antibody induction. These concepts, taken together with the observation that only a small percentage of the infiltrating cells at the delayed hypersensitivity reaction are specifically sensitized, provided the first clues as to the underlying mechanisms of these reactions.

DESENSITIZATION AND ANERGY

As stated previously, systemic administration of antigen alone prior to footpad injection of antigen in complete Freund's adjuvant can lead to the development of tolerance with respect to delayed hypersensitivity without diminution of antibody formation. Under appropriate conditions, intravenous administration of antigen after immunization temporarily suppresses delayed reactivity as well. This is known as "desensitization."

It was first shown by Uhr and Pappenheimer (19) that a single intravenous injection of 1 to 2 mg of antigen will suffice to desensitize guinea pigs immunized to purified proteins by the previous injection of immune complexes. The state of desensitization typically lasts for several days and is somewhat more prolonged if very large doses of antigen are used.

It is also possible to desensitize in vitro in a transfer system by preincubating the sensitized lymphoid cells with antigen prior to transfer. The mechanism of this reaction is not clear but is probably related either to the blocking of antigen-combining sites on the cells prior to their arrival at the skin site, or to antigen-triggered release of mediator substances in vitro with subsequent "exhaustion" prior to transfer. In any case, it is clear that desensitization, both in vitro and in vivo, is a consequence of the interaction of sensitized cells and antigen.

The immune unresponsiveness found in experimental desensitization has been compared to clinical anergy seen in various granulomatous diseases, Hodgkin's disease, and disseminated cancer.

Anergy differs from classical immunologic tolerance in that it is, in most cases, nonspecific and usually transient, and occurs in the presence of serum antibodies against antigens to which the patient is anergic. Sensitization is a precondition for anergy (20), whereas tolerance is more readily induced in the nonsensitized animal. Tolerance is usually specific to the inducing antigen and is long-lasting, although dose-dependent (19,21). Although tolerance suggests a specific suppression of immune responsiveness at the cellular level, desensitization or anergy appears to work in part via an active environmental factor(s) in the anergic animal's cellular environment (22). Thus, it has been established that it is not possible to transfer delayed hypersensitivity responses with immunologically competent lymphocytes into desensitized guinea pigs; the presence of a circulating humoral factor capable of interfering with the response of these cells has been postulated to explain these findings. This hypothesis received support from experiments in which attempts were made to transfer delayed-type hypersensitivity responses with cells from desensitized animals. The results suggested that such cells, once removed from the desensitized environment, rapidly recover their responsiveness to antigen (22).

Recent studies directly implicate the lymphokines in some of these manifestations of desensitization and anergy. This will be discussed in a later section.

PASSIVE TRANSFER OF DELAYED HYPERSENSITIVITY

We have already alluded to the fact that it is possible to effect a passive transfer of the state of delayed hypersensitivity to a nonimmunized animal. This can be accomplished by means of the administration of lymphocytes from a sensitized donor.

The success of transfer depends on the source of the cells, the species, and the sensitivity of the donor, but in any case, large numbers of cells (several hundred million) are required. Furthermore, even with the use of large numbers of cells from highly sensitized donors, transfer is not always successful. When cells are injected intravenously, there is no latent period before the appearance of a reaction of delayed sensitivity in the recipient. In contrast, anaphylactic antibodies cannot be detected for at least two days following transfer of cells from animals with both delayed and anaphylactic sensitivity. Transferred delayed sensitivity usually lasts only several days in the recipient; its termination appears to depend on the destruction of the donor cells by the homograft reaction. When an inbred strain is used, transferred sensitivity persists indefinitely. Furthermore, in inbred animals, sensitivity can be transferred with a relatively small number of cells, in which case it becomes apparent only during the second or third week after transfer.

Transfer cannot be achieved between species and is not even always successful between two different strains of inbred guinea pigs.

The immediate appearance of delayed sensitivity in the recipient and its rapid disappearance (except in inbred strains) indicated that transfer is not due to active sensitization.

The best available evidence indicates that in experimental animals intact living cells are required for transfer of delayed sensitivity. Treatment of the cells with mitomycin C, or actinomycin, which arrests the synthesis of RNA, abolishes their capacity to effect transfer. Although sporadic reports of successful transfer of delayed sensitivity in animals with subcellular fractions, or "transfer factors," have appeared in the literature, these observations have not been confirmed. It is possible that such "transfers" can be the result of nonspecific inflammatory reactions. The one apparent exception involves production of delayed-type lesions by local administration of lymphokines. This procedure involves bypass of the need for sensitization, rather than a need for passive transfer of sensitization per se.

IN VITRO CORRELATES OF CELL-MEDIATED IMMUNITY

Initially, delayed hypersensitivity reactions such as those described in the previous section were the focus of most of the studies aiming at the elucidation of the mechanisms involved in this class of immunologic phenomena. The subsequent discovery of a variety of assay systems that represented in vitro correlates of delayed hypersensitivity markedly extended the range of experiments that could be performed and thus led to the development of much of our current information in this field.

In vitro studies on delayed hypersensitivity were initiated by Rich and Lewis (23), who demonstrated that tuberculin preparations inhibited the migration of cells from spleen fragments or peripheral blood taken from actively immunized animals. This assay was simplified by George and Vaughan (24), who developed the modern capillary tube method. Bloom and Bennett (25) and David (26) independently demonstrated that the inhibition of migration of peritoneal exudate macrophages from such tubes was due to the release of a soluble factor (MIF) from sensitized lymphocytes reacting with antigen in the exudate suspension. The migration inhibition reaction could be demonstrated using peritoneal exudate cells from nonimmunized animals, provided that a source of MIF was included in the incubating mediums. The best source proved to be supernatant fluids from cultures of sensitized lymphocytes incubated with specific antigen.

MIF is of great historical importance since it was the first of the nonantibody, lymphocyte-derived soluble factors to be described. It was the first lymphokine. Several important general properties of this class of mediator were first discovered in studies of MIF. These factors are of relatively small molecular weight as compared to conventional immunoglobulins, and they lack immunologic specificity. In other words, although the lymphokines are generated by specific immunologic reactions between antigen and sensitized lymphocytes, they themselves, once formed, do not require interaction with antigen for the expression of their biologic activity. Thus, they are not antibody-like. The few known situations (to be discussed later) in which mediators have apparent specificity are not exceptions to this rule; in those circumstances, the specificity is due to the association of antigenic fragments with the mediators.

Three important methodologic principles were explicitly formulated in the early studies of MIF. First, control supernatants, which were obtained from the sensitized cells incubated in the absence of antigen, were always reconstituted with antigen prior to use. Second, controls for viability were also included. Third, reversibility of effect was demonstrated. By this is meant that if the migration inhibition preparations are allowed to remain in culture, the cells escape from inhibition and ultimately begin to migrate. These last two principles are of great practical importance. As a simple *reductio ad absurdum,* anything that kills a macrophage will prevent it from migrating. Since it is only in the very recent past that lymphokines have begun to be characterized and identified in precise physicochemical ways, the distinction between toxicity and migration inhibition remains a very important one to make. A surprisingly large number of experiments in the literature are difficult to interpret because this distinction was not always appreciated.

KINDS OF LYMPHOKINE ACTIVITIES

For the most part, the lymphokines have been defined in terms of in vitro bioassays. They fall into three main categories: lymphokines that damage their target cells (lymphotoxins), lymphokines that cause cell proliferation (mitogenic factors), and lymphokines that modulate the inflammatory response. In the first category are included not only factors that kill or injure cells but also factors that suppress certain of their biologic activities. One such example is "proliferative inhibitory factor" (PIF). Certain "helper" substances involved in T cell-B cell cooperation may fall into the second category. MIF, already described, is a member of the third category.

At last count, over 50 lymphokine activities had been described, all falling into one or another of the above categories. It seems likely that at least some of these activities were found because different assay systems detected different properties of the same molecular species "artifactors." One alternate suggestion that has been made (Janicki, B., personal communication) is that there is a (small) set of basic building block factors, the "mother factors" from which all the observed lymphokines are derived. A third possibility is that the lymphokines possess a distinct subunit structure, and that the various possible permutations of a small number of discrete subunits give rise to the observed diversity.

Inflammatory Lymphokines

The best-studied of the lymphokines involved in inflammatory responses are those that affect macrophages. In general, these fall into well-defined categories. Lymphokines have been described that affect the general metabolic properties of these cells. In addition, there are lymphokines that affect cell surface properties, lymphokines that affect the migration properties of the cell, and lymphokines that activate the macrophages for phagocytosis and killing functions. These activities have been exhaustively reviewed in a number of recent publications (27,28) and will not be discussed in further detail here. It is obvious, however, that MIF falls into the category of a lymphokine affecting cell migration properties. Another important lymphokine in this category is the "macrophage chemotactic factor" (MCF), first described by Ward et al. (29). By definition, chemotaxis is directed movement. A chemotactic factor converts random cell movement to enhanced movement in the direction of an increasing concentration gradient of the factor.

The usual assay system involves the Boyden double chamber technique in which the test substance is placed in the lower compartment and the target cell suspension in the upper compartment. The two compartments are separated by a micropore filter with pore size large enough to allow cell migration through the filter. The number of cells migrating through the filter after a given period of incubation in the test preparation is compared to the number migrating in a control preparation not containing the test substance. Increased numbers of cells in the presence of the gradient are taken as evidence of a positive chemotactic response. An important additional control here is to include a chamber with test substance in *both* compartments so as to abolish the gradient and so exclude the possibility that one is detecting nonspecific enhancement of random motility in the presence of the test substance, rather than true chemotaxis.

Since the above-mentioned lymphokine activities are defined in terms of bioassay rather than chemical identification, whether or not they are ascribable to discrete and therefore theoretically separable molecular species remains an open question. Certain lymphokines, such as MIF and MCF, appear to be different, but the case for others, such as MIF vs "macrophage activating factor" (MAF), remains unclear.

The effects of lymphokines on other inflammatory cell types have been less well studied than their effects on macrophages. There is a migration inhibitory factor for neutrophils "LIF." This appears to be distinct from MIF, in part on the basis of inactivation studies using simple monosaccharides (30). Also, there is at least one chemotactic factor for each granulocyte type and for lymphocytes. These, mainly on the basis of indirect evidence, appear to be distinct from one another. One such lymphokine, the "eosinophil chemotactic factor" (ECF), has unusual properties that are worth describing in detail.

As background, it is worth recalling that eosinophils are conspicuous components of inflammatory infiltrates at sites of various kinds of immunologic reactions. They are found in the nasopharynx and bronchi of patients with allergic conditions such as hay fever or asthma, and in the intestinal tract as a consequence of parasitic infestations. In experimental situations, they are present in peritoneal exudates following multiple injections of foreign protein, in lymph nodes draining sites of antigen administration, in skin following injection of antigen-antibody complexes into normal animals, and in skin of delayed hypersensitive animals following multiple injections of antigen at the same site. In addition, eosinophils may be found in certain autoimmune lesions that involve cell-mediated responses, such as experimental autoimmune thyroiditis. All these observations (reviewed in ref. 28) show a relationship between the eosinophil and the immune system, and the last two findings cited suggest that this relationship, in part, involves cell-mediated immunologic reactions.

The various observations described above led us to the suspicion that a lymphokine with chemotactic activity for eosinophils exists. Preliminary studies of

MIF-rich supernatant fluids from antigen-stimulated lymphocyte cultures failed to detect such a factor. We soon discovered (31,32), however, that these supernatants contained an inactive precursor substance (ECFp) which could be activated by reaction with specific preformed immune complexes in vitro to generate a potent eosinophil chemotactic factor (ECF). Studies using antigen- and antibody-coupled immunoadsorbent columns have demonstrated that ECFp behaves as though it is associated with a "piece" of antigen and that its activation to ECF is associated with a loss of that piece. These findings have led to the model for activation in which ECFp combines with a free antibody site in the immune complex by coprecipitation. As a consequence of this interaction, a modified, active, antigen-free mediator molecule (ECF) is then released. It should be noted that ECF, on injection into guinea pig skin, produces an inflammatory reaction in which the predominant cell type is the eosinophil. We have presented indirect evidence that suggests that ECF may play a role in the cutaneous "retest" reaction (33) and in experimental autoimmune thyroiditis (34).

KINDS OF CELLS THAT MAKE LYMPHOKINES

Lymphocytes

On the basis of much indirect evidence, mostly based upon the fact that cell-mediated immune reactions appear to be manifestations of T lymphocyte function, it was assumed that T cells were the source of all lymphokines. Indeed, this was one of the major unquestioned answers of lymphokine biology. However, when we explored this problem using surface markers such as the complement receptor on lymphocyte membranes as a basis for cell separation, we obtained quite different results (35). With conventional soluble protein antigens, only T cells could make MIF. When PPD was used as antigen, however, B as well as T cells could make MIF. If nonimmunized animals were used, the T cells did not produce MIF, as expected; however, the B cells again produced MIF. A variety of controls demonstrated that the observed activity could not be due to the contaminant T cells in the B cell preparations.

In all cases, B cell-derived MIF and T cell-derived MIF were identical by all available physicochemical and biologic characterization procedures. These results were put into perspective for us by the report that commercial preparations of PPD are B cell mitogens. We repeated these experiments using endotoxin lipopolysaccharide (LPS), another known B cell mitogen, with identical results. These results have been confirmed in many laboratories. Thus, the respective capabilities of human B cells to make MIF (36), human (37) and guinea pig (38) B cells to make MCF as well as MIF (39), and human B cells to make (mitogen-induced) interferon (40), have all been recently described. In most of these studies, a requirement for B cell activation by mitogenic factors has been demonstrated, although in one report (36) specific antigen was found capable of serving as inducing agent as well.

In retrospect, studies demonstrating MIF-like activity in long-term lymphocyte cultures may have detected a similar effect, since some of those lines may have been B cell-derived. We explored this by specifically looking at a number of B cell- and T cell-derived lines and found that both were capable of spontaneous MIF production (41). They also had strong neutrophil chemotactic factor (NCF) activity.

The reports by ourselves and others that B cells are capable of producing MIF as well as other lymphokines raise an interesting paradox. The evidence for the association of cellular immunity and T cell function is overwhelming. There is also good evidence that many, if not all, of the manifestations of cell-mediated immunity are due to lymphokine-dependent mechanisms (28). Since B cells can make lymphokines in vitro, it is at first glance difficult to understand the apparent requirement for T cells in cell-mediated immunity. Part of the explanation for this paradox lies in the difference in the requirements for lymphokine induction by T and B cells. T cells can be activated by either specific antigen or mitogens. B cells, with the exception of one report to the contrary (36), appear to require mitogenic activation. In those instances where specific antigen appears to induce B cells to produce MIF, this activity requires the simultaneous presence of T cells (42), and it may well be that under those circumstances the T cells are providing an endogenous mitogenic factor.

This difference in the activation requirements for T and B cells cannot provide the whole explanation, since many substances such as PPD can function both as antigen and as B cell mitogen. One clue comes from the fact that the conditions under which B cell lymphokine production occurs in vitro involve the use of purified subpopulations of lymphocytes, from which T cells are purposely removed. We have recently reported that T cells are capable of suppressing the ability of B cells to engage in lymphokine production (43). This effect is mediated by a soluble T cell-derived factor which we have defined as (migration inhibition factor) inhibition factor, or MIFIF.

Although a number of prior studies have provided evidence for the regulation of various manifestations of cell-mediated immunity by suppressor cells, MIFIF appears to be the first example of suppressor activity with respect to the lymphokines themselves. It may well be that mechanisms similar to those described here will be found operative with respect to conventional T cell-derived MIF as well, and that these mechanisms play an important role in the regulation of cell-mediated immune reactions in vivo.

Nonlymphoid Cells

Work in our laboratory has demonstrated that the infection of a variety of cells by viruses such as mumps and Newcastle disease virus in vitro or in vivo, and simian virus 40 (SV40) in vitro, leads to the production of lymphokine-like substances that we have defined as cytokines (reviewed in ref. 44). Similar data have been obtained by others in the SV40 system (45). The mediators from these sources have physicochemical properties strikingly similar to those of lymphokines with corresponding biologic properties. As will be discussed later, it is possible to prepare antisera against culture supernatants obtained from antigen-activated cultures of sensitized lymphocytes (46,47). We found (48) that sepharose bead columns conjugated with an antibody prepared against lymphocyte-derived MIF were capable of adsorbing cytokine MIF (derived from SV40-infected African green monkey kidney cells). Columns conjugated with an antibody prepared against control supernatants had no such effect. Moreover, we found that cytokine MIF could substitute for lymphocyte-derived MIF in certain in vivo model systems involving desensitization. These results all suggest the identity of MIF from virus-infected nonlymphoid cells to conventional MIF. Furthermore, they raise the interesting possibility that lymphokine production per se may be a general biologic phenomenon and that what is unique to the immune system is the way in which lymphoid cells can be activated for such production either by mitogen or specific antigen.

IN VIVO ACTIVITY OF LYMPHOKINES

As has already been alluded to, very little is known about the fine details of lymphokine structure and chemistry. All the lymphokines have been defined in terms of complex, semiquantitative biologic assays. Thus, although it is widely held that the lymphokines are the mediators of many of the manifestations of cellular immunity in vivo, it is not surprising that direct evidence for this contention has been difficult to obtain. The initial demonstrations that MIF-rich supernatants could produce inflammatory infiltrates when injected into guinea pig skin provided evidence on this point, and the observed activity was ascribed to "skin reactive factor" (SRF). The significance of those observations was unclear because of the essentially nonspecific nature of the inflammatory response. Since that time, much attention has been devoted to the problem of demonstrating in vivo roles of the lymphokines. This is a rather complex issue, and we will illustrate the experimental approaches with examples taken mainly from our own studies.

Macrophage Disappearance Reaction

One can readily induce a nonspecific peritoneal inflammatory exudate in delayed hypersensitive guinea pigs by the intraperitoneal injection of glycogen. Three or four days after the injection of this irritant, these exudates consist mainly of mononuclear cells; and of these, macrophages predominate. The intraperitoneal injection of specific antigen at this time causes a prompt reduction in the macrophage content of such exudates; five hours following antigen administration, there is a drop of approximately 90% in the absolute number of these cells recoverable in the peritoneal fluid. There is a slow recovery of macrophage content over the next 24 to 48 hours. This reaction is known as the macrophage disappearance reaction (MDR) and has been shown to be a manifestation of cellular immunity (49,50).

The MDR is a consequence of increased macrophage adhesiveness induced by specific antigen. This leads to clumping and sticking of macrophages to peritoneal surfaces, with a subsequent drop in the number recoverable from the peritoneal fluid. The bulk of the experimental evidence favors the view that the macrophage disappearance reaction is an in vivo analogue of the migration inhibition reaction in vitro. It provides an especially suitable model system with which to explore lymphokine activity in vivo.

The results of experiments (51) using this model have provided evidence for such a role. It is possible to transfer passively an MDR in nonimmune animals by intraperitoneal injections of sensitized lymphocytes and specific antigen. This procedure is successful even when lymphocytes are enclosed in micropore chambers (which can be demonstrated to remain cell-impermeable during the five-hour time course of the experiment). Moreover, the MDR can be passively transferred using only cell-free MIF-rich supernatants from antigen-stimulated lymphocyte cultures. In these experiments, the supernatants were subjected to Sephadex chromatography to exclude the presence of immunoglobulins.

These results provide strong evidence that the MDR, which as stated above is a manifestation of cellular immunity, is mediated by a soluble, lymphocyte-derived factor.

Extracts of Skin Reaction Sites

Many investigators have attempted to detect MIF activity in extracts of delayed hypersensitivity skin reaction sites. These attempts have been uniformly unsuccessful. There are several possible explanations for this failure, the most obvious one being that MIF might not play a role in the evolution of the delayed hypersensitivity reaction in the skin. Another and less heretical possibility is that only small amounts of MIF are produced and released at these sites, and that this material is rapidly adsorbed onto cells or other tissue constituents. The adsorbed MIF might not be released into the medium by the relatively crude extraction procedures currently in use.

Our own efforts to find MIF activity in extracts of skin delayed reaction sites were also unsuccessful. However, armed with the knowledge that the lymphocyte culture supernatants could induce an MDR, we injected some of our skin extract fluids into nonimmunized guinea pigs bearing peritoneal exudates. To our surprise, we achieved a macrophage *appearance* reaction with a two- to threefold increase in macrophage content consistently observed. The MDR is thought to be an in vivo manifestation of MIF activity. Thus, it seemed likely that the anomalous macrophage accumulation caused by the skin extracts might be due to the chemotactic activity of MCF, acting under conditions where no MIF was available to induce cell stickiness and clumping. This expectation was confirmed (52) when the extracts of sites of delayed reactions to various protein antigens or of sites of contact reactions to *O*-chlorobenzoyl chloride, a potent sensitizing agent, were examined by means of the Boyden double chamber assay system for the presence of in vitro chemotactic activity. Chemotactic activity toward macrophages and lymphocytes, but not neutrophils, could be detected in these extract fluids. Extracts prepared from normal skin or from skin sites of nonspecific inflammatory reactions did not show such activity. Physicochemical properties of these chemotactic factors were similar to those of respective factors previously obtained from supernatant fluids from lymphocytes cultured with specific antigen. Thus, at least two lymphokines, or at least lymphokine-like activities, could be recovered from sites of cell-mediated reactions.

Serum Lymphokine Activity in Experimental Animals

Yoshida et al. (53) have shown that rats or guinea pigs immunized with various antigens in complete Freund's adjuvant showed increases in peripheral blood monocytes for at least two weeks following immunization, in agreement with previous studies. However, when specific antigen was injected intravenously into such immunized animals, there was a prompt reduction in the number of circulating monocytes.

The maximal disappearance from the circulation occurred at six hours following antigen administration, and there was a slow return to normal over the next 24 hours. It was shown in these studies that the effect of antigen on blood monocytes was a function of the state of delayed hypersensitivity of the animals, and that this reaction, like the MDR, was therefore a manifestation of cellular immunity.

Because of the analogies between this system and the MDR, we attempted to detect MIF in the serum of such animals (54). Guinea pigs were immunized by intramuscular injection of 0.5 mg of the BCG strain of tubercle bacilli and subsequently challenged intravenously with 0.5 mg of the BCG. This procedure induces an intense state of delayed hypersensitivity, and this state is associated with massive splenomegaly as well as peripheral lymphadenopathy. Sera were obtained from these animals at various times following intravenous challenge. MIF activity was detectable in the sera of these animals but never in unimmunized animals or those controls that were immunized but unchallenged. Activity was maximal at 6 to 12 hours, corresponding approximately to the times of greatest reduction in the numbers of circulating monocytes.

Injection of Exogenous Lymphokines

The detection of MIF in guinea pig serum following a systemic antigenic challenge in delayed hypersensitive animals and the temporal relationship between that serum MIF activity and the drop in circulating monocytes in such animals prompted a study of the consequences of administering preformed, exogenous lymphokines to experimental animals (54). It was found that the intravenous injection of MIF-containing, but not control, supernatants into normal animals resulted in a drop in circulating monocytes comparable in magnitude to that observed in immunized animals challenged with specific antigen. Of even greater interest was the observation that lymphokine-treated animals developed anergy; if immunized animals were treated with lymphokines systemically, they became transiently incapable of mounting a skin reaction to the test antigen. Appropriate controls excluded participation of antigen or antibody in the suppressive effect. These results again confirmed the finding that lymphokines could play in vivo roles. Moreover, they provided a hint as to one possible mechanism for desensitization. During desensitization by specific antigen, serum MIF becomes detectable, and this may be as effective as the exogenously administered lymphokines in the above experiment. In support of this contention is the observation that desensitization is often nonspecific (a multiply immunized animal desensitized with large doses of one antigen often shows anergy to the others). More direct evidence comes from recent studies (52) in which we have shown that it is possible to transfer passively the state of desensitization with (lymphokine-containing) serum of desensitized animals.

Serum Lymphokine Activity in Man

The detection of MIF in the serum of experimental animals raised the possibility that MIF could be found in human sera during the course of certain diseases. The ability of exogenous MIF-containing supernatants to suppress cutaneous reactivity suggested that diseases associated with anergy might be good candidates. Accordingly, we initiated studies of patients with various lymphoproliferative disorders, such as chronic lymphatic leukemia, multiple myeloma, Hodgkin's disease, non-Hodgkin's lymphoma, and the Sézary syndrome. We found that the large majority of such patients had detectable serum MIF (55,56). MIF was thus found in B cell as well as T cell disease in accordance with the observations already discussed on the ability of B cells to make lymphokines. Healthy individuals and patients with a variety of illnesses such as bronchopneumonia, adenocarcinoma of the colon, astrocytoma, diabetes, osteoarthritis, myelofibrosis, etc., have a combined incidence of detectable serum MIF of less than 2%. The other disease process in which we are now finding serum MIF with great frequency is sarcoidosis. It is tempting to speculate that in these conditions one explanation for the cutaneous anergy frequently observed involves the circulating lymphokine itself, in analogy with our studies in experimental animals.

One additional situation in which serum MIF is detectable is the post-transplantation hepatic dysfunction syndrome (57). These patients have derangements in liver function that are often reflected in episodic variations in chemical parameters such as serum glutamic-oxaloacetic transaminase (SGOT) levels. Such patients also have transient elevations in serum MIF activity, and the appearance of serum MIF invariably precedes elevations in SGOT. The significance of this temporal relationship is unclear but the data nonetheless document another situation in which a lymphokine activity may be detected in vivo.

The Use of Antilymphokine Antibodies

As has already been mentioned, very little data are available as to the precise chemical nature of any of the known lymphokines. They are usually the products of T cells, although in special circumstances B cells may also be induced to produce lymphokines (35–42). In all these situations, multiple lymphokine activities are generated simultaneously. Moreover, these substances are present in small amounts and contaminated by a variety of other products of cellular metabolism. For all these reasons, the isolation and characterization of lymphokines have been extremely difficult, and indeed, even MIF, the best-studied of these factors, has been characterized only in terms of general physicochemical properties and response to enzyme treatment.

The general availability of antibody to any of the known lymphokines would have obvious importance for the purification of these, and eventually for studies on the mechanisms of cell-mediated immunity. However, such antibody production has been difficult to accomplish because of the impurity of the fluids that are the source of such factors. We have found it possible to circumvent this problem by means of a two-stage immunization procedure (46,47). Although the details of the procedure are beyond the scope of this discussion, it may be stated that it is possible to produce an antiserum in rabbits which, when conjugated to sepharose bead columns, can selectively remove MIF, MCF, and SRF activity from activated culture supernatants. Anti-control antibody does not have this property. The antisera so prepared do not have lymphocyte or macrophage cytotoxicity.

The antilymphokine antiserum has proved to be a useful tool in exploring the in vivo activity of lymphokines. As previously indicated, lymphokine-containing supernatants can induce mononuclear inflammatory infiltrates when injected into guinea pig skin. This activity has been ascribed to a "skin reactive factor" (SRF) that probably is in reality a mixture of the lymphokines that affect mononuclear cells in vitro. The antilymphokine antibody can remove SRF activity from activated supernatants. Of even greater significance is the observation that injection of antilymphokine, but not anti-control supernatant, antibody can profoundly suppress the ability of a previously immunized animal to respond to local antigenic challenge with a cutaneous delayed hypersensitivity reaction. This observation strongly implicates lymphokine involvement in the expression of delayed hypersensitivity.

THE SIGNIFICANCE OF THE LYMPHOKINES

We have seen that lymphokines and lymphokine-like factors that are identical with or very similar to conventional lymphokines may be produced by a variety of cell types and in a variety of in vitro and in vivo situations. It is possible to document their participation in the underlying mechanisms of a number of experimental models. Their general significance in the overall biology of the organism, however, remains to be elucidated. In this section we will touch briefly on three aspects of cellular immunity that focus on this point: the cutaneous delayed hypersensitivity reaction itself, infectious immunity, and tumor immunity.

The evidence for the participation of lymphokines in cutaneous reactions has already been summarized. This includes the detection of chemotactic lymphokines in extracts of such reaction sites, the induction of inflammatory skin reactions by local injection of lymphokines, the suppression of skin reactions by systemic administration of lymphokines, and the suppression of skin reactions by local administration of antilymphokine antibody. Note, however, that these data provide no information as to which lymphokine or lymphokines is specifically involved in the skin. Although most textbooks stress the role of MIF in this regard, this is probably based on historical grounds, since for many years MIF was the only lymphokine known. We are aware of no evidence implicating MIF in cutaneous reactivity. Indeed, our work provides suggestive evidence to the contrary. As already indicated, extracts of skin reactions have chemotactic but not migration inhibitory activity (52). The failure to detect MIF is probably not due to adsorption to cell surfaces, since such adsorption is very difficult to document convincingly even in vitro. It could be due to selective inactivation or destruction of MIF as compared to MCF. However, other evidence points to a role for MCF rather than MIF. Anticoagulants interfere with the expression of cutaneous reactivity (3,4). In vitro, heparin has no effect on the migration inhibition reaction, but in unpublished studies we have found that it can inhibit MCF activity. Finally, by appropriate choice of antigen, it is possible to desensitize an animal with respect to either cutaneous reactivity or the macrophage disappearance reaction (MDR). Similarly, one can prevent the appearance of MCF or MIF in such animals. Also, one can achieve either antigen-specific or nonspecific desensitization with respect to these parameters, depending upon experimental conditions. Correlations of these patterns of inhibition provide evidence that whereas the MDR appears to be an in vivo manifestation of MIF activity, the skin reaction seems to be more dependent upon chemotactic activity (58).

A great deal of work has also been done on the role of lymphokines in infectious immunity. Much of this deals with the relationship of activated macrophages to resistance against infection by such organisms as *Listeria monocytogenes*. This response was shown to be dependent upon T lymphocytes that secrete lymphokine mediators capable of activating macrophages for this role. This topic, which is beyond the scope of the present discussion, has been extensively reviewed (59).

Lymphokines play a role in tumor immunity, as well as in infectious immunity (reviewed in ref. 60). Certainly, the role of lymphotoxin in this regard has been exhaustively studied. Like other lymphokines, lymphotoxins, though induced by specific immunologic or mitogenic stimuli, are themselves capable of acting in a nonspecific manner. Although lymphotoxins are thus usually cytotoxic to a variety of both normal and malignant cultured cells, a few reports show that tumor cells are more susceptible to lymphotoxins than normal cells.

Lymphokines may also interact with tumor cells in an indirect manner by activating inflammatory cells. Just as injection of animals with microorganisms may lead to increased nonspecific resistance to certain other organisms by this mechanism, tumor cells may be killed by activated macrophages. For example, Churchill et al. have shown that supernatants from cultures of lymphocytes stimulated by soluble protein antigen activate normal macrophages, either as monolayers or in suspension culture (61). The responsible lymphokine was called macrophage activating factor (MAF). These "activated" macrophages exhibit enhanced cytotoxic capacity against syngeneic strain 2 hepatoma and MCA-25 sarcoma cells.

Little is known of the mechanism underlying the interaction of the lymphocyte mediator with the surface of the macrophage which results in enhanced cytotoxicity by the activated cells. However, a number of morphologic, biochemical, and functional alterations have been described when macrophages are activated by MAF. These include increased adherence to glass plastic, increased ruffled membrane movement, increased phagocytotic activity, increased glucose oxidation, decrease in lysosomal enzyme, acid phosphatase, cathepsin D, and β-glucuronidase, increased membrane enzyme adenylate cyclase, increased incorporation of glucosamine, and enhanced bacteriostasis to *Listeria*. It is interesting that present physicochemical characterization studies cannot distinguish

MAF from MIF, although there still remains the possibility that several different factors affecting macrophages exist.

As another possible direct effect of lymphokines in addition to cytotoxic killing of tumor cells, one can consider the effects of lymphokines on the mobility of tumor cells. It has been thought for many years that the mobility of individual tumor cells may be important in local tumor spread and in the establishment of metasis. It has, however, proved difficult to examine the mobility of tumor cells in in vitro systems.

Recently, however, we have adapted the capillary tube migration assay system to a study of tumor cells. Using this procedure, we have shown the existence of a lymphokine that can inhibit tumor cell migration in vitro (62). The responsible factor, which is probably distinct from MIF, is not cytotoxic for the target cell. The in vivo significance of this lymphokine activity awaits further exploration.

CONCLUSIONS

In this brief review, we have discussed the various manifestations of cell-mediated immunity that are attributable to lymphokine-dependent mechanisms. With the notable exception of lymphocyte-dependent cytotoxicity, most aspects of cellular immunity appear to fall into this category. Although we have paid much attention to lymphokines that act on inflammatory cells, many other lymphokine activities are known. Sensitized lymphocytes can release substances that affect vascular permeability, and these cells may participate in collagen synthesis and degradation as well. Thus, nonantibody, lymphocyte-derived soluble mediators play a pivotal role in various aspects of inflammatory and reparative processes.

Although it is now relatively easy to present a good case for the role of lymphokine-dependent responses in in vivo manifestations of immunity, it remains a difficult task to unravel the complexities of the regulatory events involved in these responses. A major area of current investigation relates to the control processes by which the expression of cellular immunity is modulated in normal and pathologic states. Progress in this area will provide us with new tools for clinical intervention both in situations where cell-mediated immunity is defective and in situations where cell-mediated immunity, acting in an aberrant or excessive manner, is itself responsible for disease.

The surprising discovery that nonlymphoid cells can be induced to make lymphokine-like mediators suggests that the lymphokines may be one manifestation of a general biologic phenomenon that is important in host defense and possibly other aspects of homeostasis. In this view, what is unique to the lymphocyte is that it has acquired some specialized means for triggering mediator production not available to other cells. If this notion is correct, then in an evolutionary sense, cell-mediated immunity may be the most primitive expression of immunologic reactivity that has developed out of even more general and nonspecific basic inflammatory responses.

Regardless of the means by which this complex system has developed, it is clear that nature has provided us with a remarkable "fail safe" system. From what has been said, it should be clear that many of the properties of the lymphokine system can be duplicated by some fragment derived from the complement pathway. Also, as we have seen, B cells have the capacity to make lymphokines, although under normal circumstances the expression of this capacity appears to be suppressed. Parenthetically, this may explain the ability of certain patients with T cell immunodeficiencies to mount good antibody responses to T-dependent antigens. Cytokines represent yet another means to the same inflammatory or immunologic end.

With this "redundancy" of mediator function, it might appear at first glance that the T cell is not terribly important in host defense. However, it is likely that mediators in the local environment near a lesion, such as those produced by the infected cells themselves, are not of prime importance in terms of initiating a protective inflammatory response. After all, one must first mobilize cells from the marrow and arrange for their migration through vessels, as well as for their attraction, immobilization, and activation. The lymphocyte is a perfect cell for these activities since it travels with the inflammatory crowd. It is a member of a population capable of rapid expansion; and it is capable of delivering a "shot" of mediators when and where it is most needed, at some proximity to the target cells for those mediators.

Viewed in these terms, the reactions of so-called cell-mediated immunity provide an important link between the immune system and the inflammatory system.

REFERENCES

1. McCluskey, R. T., and Cohen, S., *Pathobiol. Annu.* **2**, 111 (1972).
2. McCluskey, R. T., and Leber, P. D., in *Mechanisms of Cell-Mediated Immunity* (R. T. McCluskey and S. Cohen, eds.), John Wiley, New York, 1974, p. 1.
3. Cohen, S., Benacerraf, B., McCluskey, R. T., and Ovary, Z., *J. Immunol.* **98**, 351 (1967).
4. Nelson, D. S., *Immunology* **9**, 219 (1965).
5. Dvorak, H. F., Mihm, M. C., Dvorak, A., Johnson, R. A., Manseau, E. J., Morgan, B. A., and Colvin, R. B., *Lab. Invest.* **31**, 111 (1974).
6. Cohen, S., *Hum. Pathol.* **7**, 249 (1976).
7. Leskowitz, S., and Waksman, B. H., *J. Immunol.* **84**, 58 (1960).
8. Borel, Y., Fauconnet, M., and Miescher, P. A., *J. Exp. Med.* **123**, 585 (1966).
9. Asherson, G. L., and Stone, S. H., *Immunology* **9**, 205 (1965).
10. Dvorak, H. F., Billote, J. B., McCarthy, J. S., and Fish, M. H., *J. Immunol.* **94**, 966 (1965).
11. Dienes, L., *J. Immunol.* **17**, 531 (1929).
12. Raffel, S., Arnaud, L. E., Dukes, C. D., and Huang, J. S., *J. Exp. Med.* **90**, 53 (1949).
13. Salvin, S. B., *J. Exp. Med.* **107**, 109 (1958).
14. Uhr, J. W., Salvin, S. B., and Pappenheimer, A. M., *J. Exp. Med.* **105**, 11 (1957).
15. Benacerraf, B., and Gell, P. G. H., *Immunology* **2**, 53 (1959).
16. Benacerraf, B., and Gell, P. G. H., *Immunology* **2**, 219 (1959).
17. Salvin, S. B., and Smith, R. F., *J. Exp. Med.* **111**, 465 (1960).
18. Schlossman, S. F., and Levin, H. A., in *Cellular Interactions in the Immune Response* (S. Cohen, G. Cudkowicz, and R. T. McCluskey, eds.), S. Karger, Basel, 1971, p. 153.
19. Uhr, J. W., and Pappenheimer, A. M., *J. Exp. Med.* **108**, 891 (1958).
20. Kantor, F. S., *N. Engl. J. Med.* **292**, 629 (1975).
21. Frey, J. R., de Weck, A. L., and Geleick, H., *Int. Arch. Allergy,* **30**, 521 (1966).
22. Dwyer, J. M., and Kantor, F. S., *J. Exp. Med.* **137**, 32 (1973).
23. Rich, A. R., and Lewis, M. R., *Bull. Johns Hopkins Hosp.* **50**, 115 (1932).
24. George, M., and Vaughan, J. H., *Proc. Soc. Exp. Biol. Med.* **111**, 514 (1962).

25. Bloom, B. R., and Bennett, B., *Science* **153**, 80 (1966).
26. David, J. R., *Proc. Natl. Acad. Sci.* (U.S.A.) **56**, 72 (1966).
27. Remold, H. G., and David, J. R., in *Mechanisms of Cell-Mediated Immunity* (R. T. McCluskey and S. Cohen, eds.), John Wiley, New York, 1974, p. 25.
28. Cohen, S., Ward, P. A., and Bigazzi, P. E., in *Mechanisms of Cell-Mediated Immunity* (R. T. McCluskey and S. Cohen, eds.), John Wiley, New York, 1974, p. 331.
29. Ward, P. A., Remold, H. G., and David, J. R., *Cell. Immunol,* **1**, 162 (1970).
30. Rocklin, R. E., *J. Immunol.* **116**, 816 (1976).
31. Cohen, S., and Ward, P. A., *J. Exp. Med.* **133**, 133 (1971).
32. Torisu, M., Yoshida, T., Ward, P. A., and Cohen, S., *J. Immunol.* **111**, 1450 (1973).
33. Leber, P. D., Milgram, M., and Cohen, S., *Immunol. Commun.* **2**, 615 (1973).
34. Cohen, S., Rose, N. R., and Brown, R. C., *Clin. Immunol. Immunopathol.* **2**, 256 (1974).
35. Yoshida, T., Sonozaki, H., and Cohen, S., *J. Exp. Med.* **138**, 784 (1973).
36. Rocklin, R. E., MacDermott, R. P., Chess, L., Schlossman, S. F., and David, J. R., *J. Exp. Med.* **140**, 1303 (1974).
37. Mackler, B. F., Altman, L. C., Rosenstreich, D. L., and Oppenheim, J. J., *Nature* **249**, 834 (1974).
38. Wahl, S. M., Iverson, G. M., and Oppenheim, J. J., *J. Exp. Med.* **140**, 1631 (1974).
39. Bloom, R. R., Stoner, G., Gaffney, J., Shevach, E., and Green, I., *Eur. J. Immunol.* **5**, 218 (1975).
40. Epstein, L. B., Kreth, H. W., and Herzenberg, L. A., *Cell. Immunol.* **12**, 407 (1974).
41. Yoshida, T., Kuratsuji, T., Takada, A., Takada, Y., Minowada, J., and Cohen, S., *J. Immunol.* **117**, 548 (1976).
42. Bloom, B. R., and Shevach, E., *J. Exp. Med.* **142**, 1306 (1975).
43. Cohen, S., and Yoshida, T., *J. Immunol.* **119**, 719 (1977).
44. Cohen, S., *Hum. Pathol.* **7**, 249 (1976).
45. Hammond, M. E., Roblin, M. O., Dvorak, A. M., Selvaggio, S. S., Black, P. H., and Dvorak, H. F., *Science* **185**, 955 (1974).
46. Yoshida, T., Bigazzi, P. E., and Cohen, S., *J. Immunol.* **114**, 688 (1975).
47. Kuratsuji, T., Yoshida, T., and Cohen, S., *J. Immunol.* **117**, 1985 (1976).
48. Yoshida, T., Bigazzi, P. E., and Cohen, S., *Proc. Natl. Acad. Sci.* (U.S.A.) **72**, 1641 (1975).
49. Nelson, D. S., and Boyden, S. V., *Immunology* **6**, 284 (1963).
50. Sonozaki, H., and Cohen, S., *J. Immunol.* **106**, 1401 (1971).
51. Sonozaki, H. and Cohen, S., *Cell. Immunol.* **2**, 341 (1971).
52. Cohen, S., Ward, P. A., Yoshida, T., and Burek, C. L., *Cell. Immunol.* **9**, 363 (1973).
53. Yoshida, T., Benacerraf, B., McCluskey, R. T., and Vassall, P., *J. Immunol.* **102**, 804 (1969).
54. Yoshida, T., and Cohen, S., *J. Immunol.* **112**, 1540 (1974).
55. Cohen, S., Fisher, B., Yoshida, T., and Bettigole, R. E., *New Engl. J. Med.* **290**, 882 (1974).
56. Yoshida, T., Edelson, R., Cohen, S., and Green, I., *J. Immunol.* **114**, 915 (1975).
57. Torisu, M., Yoshida, T., and Cohen, S., *Clin. Immunol. Immunopathol.* **3**, 369 (1975).
58. Sonozaki, H., Papermaster, V., Yoshida, T., and Cohen, S., *J. Immunol.* **115**, 1657 (1975).
59. North, R. J., in *Mechanisms of Cell-Mediated Immunity,* (R. T. McCluskey and S. Cohen, eds.), John Wiley, New York, 1974, p. 185.
60. Yoshida, T., and Cohen, S., in *Mechanisms of Tumor Immunity,* (R. T. McCluskey, I. Green, and S. Cohen, eds.), John Wiley, New York, 1977, p. 87.
61. Churchill, W. H., Piessens, W. F., Sulis, C. A., and David, J. R., *J. Immunol.* **115**, 781 (1975).
62. Cohen, M. C., Zeschke, R., Bigazzi, P. E., Yoshida, T., and Cohen, S., *J. Immunol.* **114**, 1641 (1975).

Chapter Five

Role of Granulocytes in Cell-Mediated Immunity

ROBERT B. COLVIN AND HAROLD F. DVORAK

Departments of Pathology, Massachusetts General Hospital and Harvard Medical School, Boston, Massachusetts

The granulocytes are polymorphonuclear leukocytes that circulate in the blood of all mammals and that originate in the bone marrow by differentiating from immature precursors. Three types of granulocytes are recognized: neutrophils, eosinophils, and basophils. This classification is based on the staining properties of the prominent cytoplasmic granules that characterize these cells, although it is recognized that in different species these granules vary considerably in their morphology and staining reactions with Romanowsky dyes. Neutrophils are the most numerous of the granulocytes and may account for half or more of circulating leukocytes. Eosinophils, and particularly basophils, are much less frequent in the blood of most species and usually represent 2% or less of leukocytes. However, the level of these cells in the circulation should not necessarily be taken as an index of their importance to homeostasis and immunologic defense mechanisms, because additional stores of these cells are present in the bone marrow and these can be quickly mobilized and expanded.

It has long been known that granulocytes have a prominent role in humoral antibody-mediated immune reactions. Basophils, like fixed tissue mast cells, specifically bind homocytotropic antibodies (e.g., IgE in man) and are triggered to sudden massive release of pharmacologic mediators on contact with specific antigen, leading to the clinical syndrome of anaphylaxis (1). One such mediator, eosinophil chemotactic factor of anaphylaxis (ECF-A), is thought to be responsible for attracting eosinophils, and eosinophils are, in fact, prominent in atopic states where they may inactivate certain basophil/mast cell products such as slow-reacting substance of anaphylaxis (2). Finally, neutrophils are prominent in

This work was supported by USPHS Awards AI-09529, AI-10,496, and CA-20822-01.

a variety of clinical states involving antibodies that fix complement and thereby generate factors chemotactic for these cells.

That a chapter on granulocytes is required in a monograph dealing with cellular immunity is attributable to the tremendous progress that has been made in the last ten years in our understanding of the biology, histology, and pathogenesis of these complex and heterogeneous reactions. It will be our purpose to acquaint the reader with newer studies dealing with the function of granulocytes in delayed reactions, to indicate the mechanisms by which granulocytes may be attracted to sites of immunologic reactivity, and, finally, to call attention to areas where new work and new insights are required for a clearer understanding of the expanding role that granulocytes may have in cell-mediated hypersensitivity.

BASOPHILS

Basophils are the least numerous of the granulocytes in most mammalian species, generally constituting $< 1\%$ of leukocytes (3). (The rabbit is an exception in that basophils may comprise up to 10% of circulating white blood cells.) Interest has focused on their prominent cytoplasmic granules, which are thought to contain proteoglycans (responsible for metachromatic staining), as well as low-molecular-weight mediators with potent pharmacologic activities. Two of these, histamine and eosinophil chemotactic factor of anaphylaxis (ECF-A), are stored preformed within the cell; two others, slow-reacting substance of anaphylaxis (SRS-A) and platelet activating factor, are generated after cell stimulation (4). Recently, both trypsin- and chymotrypsin-like esterase-protease enzymes have been found in the granules of guinea pig basophils (5,6), and a plasminogen activator has been localized to their plasma membrane (6, 133). The abundant literature describing the capacity of basophils to bind homocytotropic antibodies and to undergo anaphylactic degranulation and mediator release in response to specific antigen will not be summarized here. Rather, the interested reader is referred to review articles dealing with the function of basophils in immediate hypersensitivity reactions mediated by antibodies (1,3,7,8). We will focus here on the role that basophils play in cellular immunity.

CUTANEOUS BASOPHIL HYPERSENSITIVITY

Guinea pigs immunized by procedures that avoid the use of mycobacterial adjuvants develop a systemic form of lymphocyte-mediated, delayed-onset reactivity termed cutaneous basophil hypersensitivity (CBH) (9–12). In contrast to the reactions in classic, tuberculin-type delayed hypersensitivity (DH), CBH skin reactions are relatively nonindurated, are characterized by extensive infiltrations of basophilic leukocytes in addition to mononuclear cells, are effected by lymphocytes that are difficult to render tolerant (and that have lower average avidity for antigen), lack extensive fibrin deposits, and, with many antigens, can be elicited only at early intervals after immunization. Originally recognized as a response to soluble protein antigens (so-called "Jones-Mote" reactivity) (13), reactions having a similar histology are characteristic of the guinea pig's response to a variety of other biologically more important immunogens, including contact allergens, vaccinia virus, allogeneic tumor cells, insect bites, and skin allografts. As a result, CBH has come to be recognized as a distinct form of immunologic response, separate both from DH and from the well-known antibody-mediated reactions.

In fact, CBH may represent the primary form of cell-mediated immune response to many biologically important antigens, including contact allergens (14), vaccinia virus (15), tumor cells (16), schistosomes (17, Colvin, R. B., unpublished data), tick bites (18), and skin allografts (19).

The immunogenic requirements necessary to induce DH and CBH are generally similar and are under the genetic control of histocompatibility-linked immune response genes (20). Moreover, hapten- and carrier-specific forms of both types of hypersensitivity exist (9,21). With the hapten-carrier combinations studied thus far, the antigen skin test requirements for eliciting CBH and DH are similar and are those necessary for lymphocyte activation rather than for a passive combination with preformed antibody. Although a close correlation exists between the appearance of circulating antibody and the decline of Jones-Mote reactivity, it is not yet clear that antibody itself "turns off" the basophil-rich, delayed-onset type of response. Passive antibody does not interfere with the induction of CBH but is capable of interfering with its expression, apparently in a nonspecific manner (22). It is important to emphasize that CBH reactions need not be transient. The CBH response persists indefinitely following immunization with antigens (e.g., vaccinia virus, dinitrochlorobenzene (DNCB), tumor cells) which do not initiate a significant antibody response.

Basophil-rich, delayed-onset reactions may also be elicited at early intervals after immunization with soluble protein antigens in complete Freund's adjuvant, but later these evolve into indurated, mononuclear cell-rich DH reactions having few basophils (10). This transition, is not, however, invariant since the basophil-rich response to certain tumor cells persists for months following immunization with mycobacteria (16).

Histologic Manifestations of CBH

The reactions of CBH in the guinea pig are similar in their time course, evolution, and distribution in the skin to those of delayed hypersensitivity (DH), beginning several hours after skin testing as perivascular accumulations of lymphocytes. Venules are dilated and compacted, accounting for the "red spot" that is characteristic of CBH as well as DH. In contrast to the reaction in tuberculin-type DH, basophils are abundant in CBH, emigrating from blood vessels, and with time they undergo a dramatic increase both in absolute and in relative frequency to reach a maximum at 24 to 48 hours (10). In typical lesions, basophils are present in concentrations of 300 to 600 per linear millimeter of skin surface and comprise 20% to 60% of infiltrating cells. This concentration is remarkable in that basophils normally account for less than 1% of circulating leukocytes in the guinea pig, a fraction not significantly altered by usual techniques of immunization and skin testing. Basophils were not appreciated in earlier histologic descriptions of Jones-Mote reactions because improved morphologic techniques, involving fixation and embedding of the type used in electron microscopy, are required for visualizing these cells reliably. Guinea pig, but apparently not human, basophils may also be recognized in Giemsa-stained paraffin sections if mercuric fixatives are employed (23).

With all antigens studied, basophils are preferentially localized to the upper (papillary) dermis in the guinea pig, where they may account for as many as 90% of cells; by contrast, deeper areas of the dermis contain relatively more mononuclear cells and fewer basophils (10). Localization of basophils may thus correspond poorly to the distribution of antigen in the skin, a point emphasized by Stadecker and Leskowitz (24), who were able to follow residual particulate skin test antigen (formalinized sheep erythrocytes) in the deep dermis and subcutis, well away from the more superficial basophil response. However, basophils do infiltrate deeper portions of the dermis in response to testing with *syngeneic* tumor cells, and intimate associations between partially degranulated basophils and damaged tumor cells are common in the reticular dermis in these animals (16). To account for the predominance of basophils in the papillary dermis of the guinea pig, we have postulated that the microvasculature of this layer of the skin is specialized in some way to facilitate the diapedesis of basophils. Evidence supporting this view comes from studies of systemic CBH. Animals primed for CBH and challenged parenterally with a large dose of specific antigen develop a delayed-in-time, systemic rash, characterized histologically by a basophil-rich infiltrate confined to the papillary dermis (25).

Eosinophils may be present in variable numbers in CBH skin reactions but are generally not prominent. Neutrophils and monocytes/macrophages are extremely rare. Fibrin deposition, edema, and induration, characteristic features of DH (26,27), are conspicuously absent. After 48 hours, reactions are faded grossly, but the cellular infiltrate disappears more slowly over the course of a week. During this time, remaining basophils are observed to be phagocytosed by histiocytes.

Basophil Specificity in CBH

There is substantial evidence indicating that basophil function in many immunologic reactions is controlled by cell-bound, homocytotropic antibodies whose interaction with specific antigen leads to the release of basophil granules and their pharmacologic contents (1). In the guinea pig, homocytotropic IgG_1 and IgE-like antibodies have been described (28–30), and absorption of either or both of these to basophils could render these cells specific for antigen. Moreover, substantial levels of circulating antibodies have now been unexpectedly described in animals primed for contact sensitivity to DNCB, a form of CBH thought to be antibody independent (31). It had been thought that animals so primed developed few or no antibodies.

To date, there is little evidence that the basophils participating in CBH-type reactions need have specificity for sensitizing antigen. Typical CBH reactions may be elicited at four days after sensitization, before antibodies can be detected by systemic or passive or active cutaneous anaphylaxis or by serologic methods. In fact, animals primed for CBH with certain antigens develop little or no detectable antibody at any interval after immunization. Moreover, intravenous or local injections of sensitizing antigens in guinea pigs bearing mature (24-hour) basophil-rich CBH reactions to human serum albumin (4) or to ovalbumin (Dvorak, H. F., unpublished data) failed to induce vascular permeability alterations characteristic of histamine release; nor did they lead to overt basophil degranulation when skin testing was performed four to five days after sensitization. However, occasional basophils participating in CBH reactions do exhibit anaphylactic-type degranulation (10,16). It is certainly possible, therefore, that cell- and antibody-mediated forms of hypersensitivity may cooperate in synergistic fashion in at least certain types of CBH, the former bringing sensitized basophils to a site where they may interact with specific antigen (14). This might be especially true in more chronic expressions of CBH, such as tumor rejection, where antigen (tumor cells) persists at a reaction site for one to two days before it is totally killed.

In order to determine whether nonhistamine-releasing antibodies might be present on the surface of basophils participating in early CBH, direct interactions between basophils and antigen were studied by means of a sensitive rosetting technique (21). Basophils were isolated from the blood or teased from skin reactions of CBH-primed animals and exposed to appropriate specific cell-bound antigens. Under these conditions, the overwhelming majority of basophils circulating in the blood or accumulating in skin reactions of CBH failed to form rosettes (less than 2%, 8%, and 1% of basophils recovered in guinea pigs sensitized to sheep erythrocytes, human albumin, and allogeneic tumor cells, respectively). By contrast, more than 75% of circulating basophils from hyperimmunized animals and one-third of basophils teased from "late reactions" formed specific rosettes. Finally, a substantial proportion of basophils teased from CBH reactions was able to acquire rosetting capacity following exposure to immune serum in vitro.

Taken together, these studies provide strong evidence that neither the attraction of basophils nor their subsequent function in CBH reactions is *necessarily* mediated by homocytotropic antibodies. In fact, an animal's capacity to produce basophil-rich, delayed-onset skin reactions seems inversely related to the presence of basophils coated with specific antibody. It is likely, therefore, that control mechanisms other than homocytotropic antibodies must be sought to explain the accumulation and behavior of basophils in CBH reactions; lymphocytes and/or their products are likely candidates for such a role. However, it is also probable that homocytotropic antibodies may affect the function of basophils participating in CBH reactions. Indeed, the occasional basophils isolated from CBH reactions that form rosettes with specific antigen may correspond to the infrequent basophils that exhibit anaphylaxis-like discharge of their cytoplasmic granules as observed in the electron microscope (10,16).

Role of Lymphocytes in CBH Reactions

Although basophils are a prominent component of CBH reactions, lymphocytes are the cells essential to the induction and expression of this form of hypersensitivity, just as they are in classic DH. Animals primed for CBH exhibit an expansion of the thymus-dependent paracortical zones of draining lymph nodes

(32), reactivity may be inhibited by antilymphocyte serum (33), and reactions may be passively transferred to normal recipients by viable sensitized lymph node cells (14). Moreover, recent studies with a highly specific rabbit antibasophil serum suggest that lymphocytes, *not* basophils, are responsible for the erythema observed at local test sites (134). Thus, animals primed for CBH and treated with antibasophil antibodies at the time of skin testing developed normal appearing, delayed-onset skin reactions nearly devoid of basophils but containing normal numbers of lymphocytes. It is presumed that lymphocytes in CBH, as in DH, secrete a vasodilatory factor (skin reactive factor) responsible for inducing local erythema and hence the characteristic "red spot."

The exact nature of the lymphocytes responsible for mediating CBH and their relation to those that mediate classic DH have not as yet been established. The finding that an anti-T lymphocyte serum strikingly inhibits the expression of CBH in vivo (33) is in agreement with morphologic data implicating T cell expansion in the draining lymph nodes and indicates that the lymphocytes mediating CBH, like those affecting DH, are probably T cells. Further support for this conclusion comes from genetic studies indicating that "nonresponder" guinea pigs cannot develop CBH reactivity to certain defined polymers (20). The immunologic defect of "nonresponder" guinea pigs is thought to reside in their T and not in their B cells.

Evidence that lymphocytes may be responsible not only for the expression of CBH but also for its *termination* comes from studies of Neta and Salvin (34). They demonstrated that adoptive transfer of spleen and peritoneal exudate cells from guinea pigs whose Jones-Mote reactivity was on the wane suppressed the expression of CBH in sensitized recipients that would have been expected to respond maximally; moreover, this suppression was immunologically specific. Katz and co-workers (35,36) have likewise presented evidence that a balance between discrete "effector" and "suppressor" populations of lymphocytes may determine whether an animal will respond to skin test challenge with DH or CBH. Further experiments with defined populations of T and B lymphocytes, and/or their respective subsets, will be required to determine the respective roles and possible interactions of each cell type in both DH and CBH.

As in DH, the lymph node cells stimulated in CBH-primed animals incorporate increased amounts of ^{3}H-thymidine and undergo blast transformation in cultures containing specific antigen (37). This response parallels CBH skin test reactivity, occurring only at early intervals (i.e., one week) after sensitization in the case of a soluble protein antigen, human serum albumin (HSA). Lymphocyte activation in DH-primed animals, in turn, parallels DH skin test reactivity and consists of a persistent and evolving response elicitable at later intervals (i.e., six weeks) after immunization.

The lymphocytes of CBH-sensitized animals are also capable of secreting mediators or lymphokines on subsequent exposure to specific antigen in vitro. A basophil chemotactic factor (BCF) (38,39), migration inhibition factor (MIF) (40), and a factor stimulating macrophage glucosamine incorporation have all been detected in supernatants from such lymphocyte cultures (40). The possibility of a vasodilatory factor was discussed above but has not yet been looked for in culture supernatants.

The mechanisms of basophil chemotaxis are particularly relevant to this discussion. Basophil chemotactic factor (BCF) is a nondialyzable macromolecule liberated by draining lymph node cells from either CBH- or DH-primed animals that have been cultured in the presence of specific antigen (39). It is only moderately heat-sensitive and bands on sucrose density gradients in a biphasic pattern similar to that of monocyte chemotactic factor. Absorption of lymphokine fluids with monocytes results in a loss of detectable chemotactic activity for basophils but not for monocytes; however, absorption with basophils has no effect on either activity. This dissociation of effect suggests that the chemotactic factors for basophils and monocytes are distinct. BCF has been detected in fluids lacking MIF and neutrophil chemotactic activities.

A basophil chemotactic activity has also been described in culture fluids of stimulated human peripheral lymphocytes (41). Both B and T cell mitogens and specific antigens led to the appearance of activity. The amount of BCF released was independent of lymphocyte proliferation and occurred as early as 24 hours of culture, well before increased thymidine incorporation became detectable. As in the guinea pig, human BCF was physicochemically similar to monocyte chemotactic factor and was not separable from this activity by column chromatography. Lett-Brown et al. (41) suggest, in fact, that the same molecule may possess separate and chemically distinct active sites for attracting basophils and monocytes. Human BCF has a molecular weight of approximately 15,000 daltons and is stable at 56°C for 60 minutes.

Modification of the basophil chemotactic response has been achieved by incubation of basophils with appropriate agents prior to chemotactic assay. Boetcher and Leonard (38) showed that the chemotactic response of human basophils to C5a could be augmented five- to tenfold by preincubation with lymphokine-containing fluids. These human lymphocyte culture supernatants, therefore, contain a second activity, basophil chemotaxis augmentation factor (BCAF), which modulates basophil migration. Conversely, Ward and associates (39) have shown that chemotaxis of guinea pig basophils to both lymphocyte culture supernatants and to the C5 fragment is substantially reduced by prior exposure to an antigen to which these basophils had specificity. Under the experimental conditions employed, the exposure of basophils to antigen did not lead to overt basophil degranulation.

These chemotactic data suggest a mechanism by which sensitized lymphocytes, interacting with specific antigen, may attract basophils to skin test sites in CBH. Also, the recognition that interaction with specific antigen substantially reduces the chemotactic responsiveness of sensitized basophils affords yet another possible explanation for the decline of CBH reactivity that is associated with the appearance of antibody.

Passive Transfer of CBH

It is well established that CBH reactivity may be passively transferred by means of draining lymph node cells at appropriate intervals after immunization with protein antigens in incomplete Freund's adjuvant (IFA) (14,42). Of interest, passive transfer of peritoneal or lymph node exudate cells from CFA-sensitized donors may prime normal recipients for a mixed type of delayed reactivity that is rich in basophils but is also indurated and infiltrated by numerous mononuclear cells. Animals immunized with CFA are known to develop CBH-type reactions at early intervals after immunization but at later times exhibit only classic DH (10,14). These experiments, therefore, have uncovered lymphocytes with the latent capacity of attracting basophils in donor animals able themselves only to express DH.

Recently, Askenase and co-workers (23,43–45) have succeeded in the passive transfer of basophil-rich reactions by means of immune serum. An important difference between their techniques and those of earlier workers who could not effect such transfers was the use of serum obtained from donors at early intervals after immunization, at the height of CBH reactivity, rather than the use of hyperimmune sera with higher antibody titers obtained at later times. Purification studies on immunoabsorbent and other columns have revealed that the active serum factor migrated with specific $7S\gamma_1$ antibody. Askenase et al. have proposed that the CBH response is itself heterogenous, like that of cell-mediated immunity in general, and that both B and T lymphocytes may play separate and distinct roles in basophil accumulations in cutaneous hypersensitivity.

CBH in Other Organs and Species

The expression of CBH has been most carefully studied in the skin of guinea pigs, but cell-mediated reactions rich in basophils also occur in other organs and species. Examples include peritoneal rejection of ascites tumor cells (16) and ocular reactions to protein antigens in guinea pigs (46); allergic contact dermatitis (26,47) and skin (19) and renal (48) allograft rejection in guinea pigs and man; experimental allergic encephalomyelitis in rats (49); the response to the Rous sarcoma virus (50) and to phytohemagglutinin in the chicken (51).

Significant species differences exist in the frequency with which basophils participate in cell-mediated reactions, and in some instances the distinction between CBH and DH is blurred. Basophil infiltration, both absolute and relative, is substantially greater in guinea pigs than in most species thus far studied. In comparison, mature lesions of allergic contact dermatitis in man contain basophils (26), but these seldom exceed 200 per linear millimeter and comprise $< 15\%$ (often $< 5\%$) of the infiltrate. Nonetheless, as would be predicted from guinea pig experiments, basophils are more numerous in allergic contact dermatitis in man than they are in classic delayed hypersensitivity reactions to microbial antigens.

BASOPHIL "DEGRANULATION" IN CELL-MEDIATED REACTIONS

Although occasional basophils in guinea pig CBH reactions exhibit degranulation of the anaphylactic type, the vast majority do not and appear unaltered even at 48 hours (10). In the case of immunologic tumor rejection, however, the cytoplasmic granules of basophils closely associated with hepatoma cells show a striking loss of affinity for the Giemsa stain, suggesting that a portion of the granules' substance had been lost (16). This conclusion was supported by electron-microscope evidence indicating a substantial but variable loss in the electron density of individual granules without fusion of granules or other configurations characteristic of anaphylaxis (16).

A similar type of change has been observed in human basophils infiltrating sites of allergic contact dermatitis (52). In the light microscope these changes consisted of a loss of metachromatic granule staining, and many granules came to appear as lucent cytoplasmic vacuoles. In the electron microscope the initial change was a loss of particles from localized portions of the granule periphery; these zones contained finely granular material of reduced electron density or appeared nearly electron-lucent. In favorable sections, such zones were found in open communication with localized evaginations of the granule membrane. These outpouchings appeared as vesicular structures attached to the granules by a narrow neck and were filled with finely granular material or, less commonly, with material resembling granule particles. Many granules exhibited an apparent diffuse loss of granule substance, manifest as a loose packing of remaining particles within the granule. In extreme form, granules were nearly or completely devoid of particles, appearing as slightly enlarged, electron-lucent, membrane-bound vacuoles. The derivation of these empty vacuoles from basophil granules was based on the identification of intermediate forms, basophil granules with focal areas of lucency. Also, even "empty" granules frequently contained small numbers of residual granule particles.

These qualitative impressions were substantiated by quantitative analysis of human contact dermatitis reactions performed at both the light- and electron-microscopic levels. Using defined criteria, it was found that approximately 40% of basophils were fully granulated in 24-hour reactions and less than 10% were largely degranulated; by contrast, in 72-hour reactions these frequencies had more than reversed and were 7.3% and 60.2%, respectively. Degranulation was apparently not associated with cell death, as the vast majority of basophils, at all intervals studied, was viable by both light- and electron-microscopic criteria. However, the ultimate fate of basophils in these reactions was not established.

Another prominent feature of basophils participating in the reactions of contact dermatitis was the presence of abundant, membrane-bound cytoplasmic vesicles of the type we have called attention to in guinea pig basophils engaged in endocytosis (53). Many of these vesicles had the dimensions and appearance of 500 to 700 Å pinocytotic vesicles, but others were several times larger, though always substantially smaller than basophil granules. The majority of vesicles were free in the cytoplasm, but some were continuous with the cytoplasmic membrane; others were observed in association with the cells' cytoplasmic granules, forming tail-like appendages that were often constricted to form a neck at their junction with the granule membrane. At all levels some vesicles contained particles morphologically identical to those comprising the cytoplasmic granules, and others contained finely granular material similar to that found in the periphery of altered granules. The biochemical nature of the vesicle contents has not as yet been established.

Basophil degranulation of the type occurring in anaphylaxis is thought to involve a process of exocytosis in which adjacent granules fuse membranes with each other (to form multigranular aggregates), and with the plasma membrane, thereby creating direct communications between several granules and the extracellular space and permitting sudden explosive release of granule contents (3). That this anaphylactic mechanism can also explain the basophil degranulation occurring in allergic contact dermatitis is unlikely. Whereas extrusion of intact basophil granules has been noted occasionally in guinea pig CBH reactions (see above), it was never observed in the human reactions. Fusions between adjacent cytoplasmic granules were extremely rare, involving only about 2% of 685 granules in the 75 basophils we examined in the electron microscope. Moreover, continuities between individual granules and the plasma membrane were not observed, despite the fact that these basophils underwent a progressive loss of granule content over a period of several days. Therefore, if continuities between basophil granules and the plasma membrane do form in contact dermatitis, they must either be infrequent and/or of brief duration.

Taken together, our morphologic findings have led us to propose a "piecemeal" model of basophil degranulation that can account for the gradual loss of granule substance occurring in contact dermatitis. We propose that degranulation ordinarily occurs by means of the 500 Å or larger membrane-bound vesicles abundantly present in basophil cytoplasm. We suggest that exocytotic vesicles bud from the granule membrane, carrying with them small quanta of intact or dissolved granule material, and flow to the cell surface where they fuse with the plasma membrane and discharge their contents into the extracellular space. Thus, no fusion of granules with the plasma membrane is required. It is well established that such vesicles may transport tracers such as horseradish peroxidase in the opposite direction, from the cell exterior to the cytoplasmic granules (53). The details of this model, as well as alternative possible explanations of our data, have been presented elsewhere (3) and are currently the subject of experimental testing.

EOSINOPHILS

Eosinophils are conspicuous elements in the inflammatory infiltrates accompanying many types of immunologic reactions. They are found in the nasopharynx and bronchi of patients with allergic conditions such as hay fever or asthma, and in the intestinal tract as a consequence of parasitic infestations. In experimental situations, they are present in peritoneal exudates following multiple injections of foreign protein (54), in lymph nodes draining sites of antigen administration (54–56), in skin following injection of antigen-antibody complexes into normal animals (57), and in the skin of animals following a second injection of antigen into a subsiding delayed hypersensitivity reaction (58). In addition, eosinophils may be found in certain autoimmune lesions that involve cell-mediated immune responses, such as experimental autoimmune thyroiditis (59). All these observations point to a relationship between the eosinophil and the immune system.

Eosinophils are several times more numerous in circulating blood than basophils and have been available in highly purified form for some time. As a result, much has been learned about the chemical composition of eosinophils and of their characteristic cytoplasmic granules. Thus, eosinophils are known to contain a potent peroxidase (60), an aryl sulfatase capable of inactivating SRS-A

(61,62), an inhibitor of histamine release from basophils (EDI) (63), and possibly plasminogen (64). EDI is apparently a mixture of prostaglandins (65). Moreover, a small basic protein has been identified as a major component of guinea pig and human eosinophils, but no function has yet been found for this molecule (66,67). Experiments in vitro have demonstrated that eosinophils possess surface receptors for 7S immunoglobulins and perhaps for IgE, but not for complement, and are capable of phagocytosing antigen-antibody complexes, particularly those involving homocytotropic antibodies (63,68–70).

Despite this profusion of biologic and biochemical information, much less is known about the function of eosinophils in allergic reactions. Their content of EDI and aryl sulfatase suggests a role in modulating basophil/mast cell function, and it has been known for some years that eosinophils accumulate in skin test sites of atopic subjects (71–74). However, eosinophil accumulation in such reactions is delayed until many hours after testing, at a time when the wheal and flare reaction has subsided and mast cell degranulation has long been completed. Similarly, eosinophils may be a minor component in Arthus reactions but again are not prominent until 24 to 48 hours, long after the reaction has passed its peak (75).

Eosinophils in Delayed Hypersensitivity

The role of eosinophils in cell-mediated immunity remains, for the most part, at a descriptive stage, but recent developments from several laboratories suggest that this rather unsatisfactory state of affairs will not persist much longer.

Eosinophils have been described as incidental components in several types of cell-mediated hypersensitivity reactions. Thus, small numbers of these cells occur in allergic contact dermatitis reactions in man (26) and, irregularly, in CBH or DH reactions to several antigens in guinea pigs (10,23,46,76). Characteristically, eosinophils appear in such reactions after the arrival of basophils, suggesting that release of chemotactic factors such as ECF-A by basophils may be at least partly responsible for their accumulation. Similarly, the delayed (24-hour) appearance of eosinophils at sites of allergy skin tests in some individuals has been thought to involve cellular hypersensitivity, but recent evidence suggests that, in fact, IgE alone may mediate these "late" reactions (77). By the same token, eosinophils are numerous in a variety of disease states in man thought to involve a cell-mediated immune component, particularly certain of the collagen diseases, but perhaps including such common entities as "subacute" appendicitis.

Ponzio and Speirs (78) have shown that specific challenge of tetanus toxoid-primed mice elicits a cell-mediated response characterized by an accumulation of eosinophils at the injection site. This response, as well as a secondary rise in antitoxin production, could be passively transferred with spleen cells. Studies with anti-theta antibodies revealed that the eosinophil accumulation response was mediated by T lymphocytes, whereas both T and B cells were required for secondary antibody production.

Data of a similar nature have been presented by Schriber and Zucker-Franklin

(79). These authors immunized and challenged rats with intravenous injections of antigen-coated latex particles too large to pass through the pulmonary capillary bed. In sensitized animals, these particles induced a local inflammatory response in the lungs that was typical of delayed hypersensitivity, consisting largely of lymphocytes and monocytes. Eosinophils were also present, particularly at 48 hours, and the reaction was accompanied by a striking eosinophilia. Neutrophils were absent, and basophils and mast cells were extremely rare. Lymphocytes isolated from the blood of animals immunized in this manner were stimulated to incorporate thymidine in vitro by specific antigens that are thought to be T cell-dependent. No correlation was found in these studies between eosinophil levels and antibody.

Basten and associates (80,81) have shown that the capacity of rats to respond to parasitic infestation with peripheral eosinophilia is dependent on the presence of lymphocytes. They found further that this capacity could be transferred adoptively with lymphoid cells enclosed in diffusion chambers, suggesting that a diffusable factor released by lymphocytes was involved.

Eosinophils in Cutaneous Basophil Hypersensitivity

Recent data suggest that eosinophils may have a role in certain expressions of cutaneous basophil hypersensitivity. Studies of ocular reactions to protein antigens in guinea pigs primed for CBH reveal the development of basophil-rich, delayed-onset infiltrations in the eye as well as in the skin (46). However, basophils accounted for a substantially small fraction of cells infiltrating the eye, whereas eosinophils, generally uncommon in CBH reactions in flank skin, were relatively much more frequent, constituting about 20% of cells infiltrating the limbus. Eosinophils were even more numerous in the iris.

A prominent role for eosinophils has also been found in the recently described state of systemic cutaneous basophil hypersensitivity (SCBH) (25). In this entity, guinea pigs primed for CBH develop a systemic, delayed-onset, maculopapular rash when challenged parenterally with large doses of specific antigen five to seven days after immunization. Although the rash itself contained numerous basophils and only a few eosinophils, it was accompanied by a striking circulating eosinophilia, and infiltrates of eosinophils were observed in other organs, including the lungs, spleen, and thymus. Taken together, these findings suggest that eosinophils have a role in CBH and indicate that the same antigen may induce a distinctly different inflammatory infiltrate in different regions of the body. It is likely that local factors account at least in part for these differences. The nature and mode of action of these postulated local factors are presently unknown, but Waksman (82) and we (11,12,25,46) have suggested that the distribution and character of the microvasculature may contribute significantly to differences in local inflammatory reactions. This could occur, for example, if the endothelium of the microvasculature in different portions of the body were specialized to permit the attachment of certain types of inflammatory cells, but not of others, and thereby favored diapedesis of the former and retention within the circulation of the latter.

The "Retest" Reaction

Arnason and Waksman (58) observed accelerated reactivity on reinjection of antigen at skin sites of prior (healed) delayed hypersensitivity. These "retest" reactions reached maximal intensity at about eight hours and were characterized by the presence of large numbers of eosinophils. Recent studies have clarified the mechanism of this reaction. First, Leber et al. (76) demonstrated that retest reactions could be elicited in animals primed for CBH as well as for DH; in fact, eosinophils were three to four times as numerous in the former (animals primed with egg albumin in IFA) than in the latter (animals immunized with the same antigen in CFA). Of equal interest, the same authors demonstrated that the two characteristic features of the "retest" reaction, accelerated time course and eosinophil infiltration, were dissociable. Animals were immunized with an azobenzene arsonate conjugate of acetyl-tyrosine (ABA-tyr), which induces delayed hypersensitivity without detectable antibody formation. A retest reaction induced with ABA-tyr showed typical accelerated evolution but few eosinophils. It is likely that the failure to induce local eosinophilia in these animals may be related to the inability of ABA-tyr to induce antibody production (see below).

Eosinophil Chemotaxis in Cellular Immunity

Many chemotactic factors for eosinophils have been described, including those released by anaphylactic degranulation of basophils/mast cells or activation of the complement system. Of greater relevance to the present discussion is a lymphocyte-derived eosinophil chemotactic factor described by Cohen and Ward (83). In supernatants of sensitized lymphocytes cultured with specific antigen, these investigators found a precursor substance (ECFp) that could be activated by reaction with preformed immune complexes in vitro to generate a factor (ECF) strongly chemotactic for eosinophils both in Boyden chambers and in vivo following intradermal injection. Furthermore, ECF was generated only when the antigen used to form the immune complexes was the same as that used to stimulate the lymphocyte cultures (83,84). Generation of ECF would thus seem to require a unique synergism between cellular and humoral immune responses.

That ECF may have a role in vivo is suggested by studies of experimental autoimmune disease (59). Guinea pigs sensitized with thyroid extracts in CFA develop an autoimmune thyroiditis composed largely of mononuclear cell infiltrates; several pieces of experimental evidence suggest that cell-mediated immunity is largely responsible for this disease state. Of interest, many, but not all, affected animals had circulating antithyroid antibodies, and in these (and only these) animals, eosinophils were present in the thyroid lesions. The injection of immune sera from these animals did not lead to the appearance of eosinophils in the thyroids of normal guinea pigs, but it increased the incidence of eosinophil infiltration in the glands of animals with minimal thyroid mononuclear infiltrates and no detectable circulating antibody of their own. The requirement for both mononuclear infiltration and circulating antibody, and the distribution of eosinophils in what appeared to be interface regions between sites of access of antibody formed systemically and sites where lymphokine production could occur locally, suggested that ECF might be involved in the mechanisms of eosinophil accumulation in this model of thyroiditis.

Colley (85) and Greene and Colley (86) have described another eosinophil-active lymphokine, eosinophil stimulation promoter (ESP), that induces increased migration of eosinophils out of agarose microdroplets. ESP is apparently produced by an antithymocyte serum-sensitive, peripheral T lymphocyte population. ESP does not require immune complexes for its generation, and it appears to act by increasing eosinophil motility rather than by a specific chemotactic effect. Physicochemically, it is also distinct from ECF. That ESP may have a role in vivo is suggested by the finding that isolated, intact schistosome egg granulomas from the livers of infected mice release this mediator spontaneously in short-term tissue culture (87).

NEUTROPHILS

A wide variety of stimuli provoke neutrophil infiltration, including antigen-antibody complexes that fix complement (88), and endotoxin (89) and tissue necrosis. It is thus not surprising that neutrophils have been noted in delayed-type hypersensitivity reactions by many investigators (90–100). Although it is apparent that neutrophils can occur in cell-mediated reactions, it is not clear whether their presence is due to the interaction of lymphocytes with antigen or to other factors. In many instances, necrosis, endotoxin, trauma, nonspecific "irritation," or a concomitant antibody-mediated reaction may account for the neutrophil infiltration. Only after these and perhaps other possibilities have been excluded may one safely conclude that neutrophils are indeed related to cell-mediated hypersensitivity.

Participation of Neutrophils in Delayed Reactions

The frequency of neutrophil participation in delayed reactions varies markedly depending on the particular antigen studied, the interval after skin testing at which measurements are made, the species tested, and, finally, the anatomic site of antigen challenge. In man there are few or no extravascular neutrophils at any interval after skin testing with tuberculin, Candida, streptokinase-streptodornase, mumps virus, or a variety of contact allergens in the absence of necrosis (26); as noted above, however, other granulocytes may be present. In DNCB reactions only four to eight hours old, very few or no infiltrating neutrophils were present, although they were observed within small vessel lumens (Dvorak, H. F., unpublished data, 1974). Thus, neutrophils would not appear to play a necessary role in DH reactions in man, even accepting the caveat that the importance of a particular cell type may not be proportional to its overall frequency.

Careful studies by Turk et al. (95) have indicated that neutrophils are a regular but minor component in DH reactions in guinea pigs, even when antibody production has been minimized by sensitizing animals with antigen-antibody complexes. Even stronger evidence comes from passive transfer experiments, in which it has been found that guinea pig recipients of sensitized lymphocytes develop an infiltrate that includes neutrophils three hours after challenge with tuberculin or ovalbumin (101). Finally, neutrophil participation in delayed reactions in guinea pigs depends to a considerable extent on the site of antigenic challenge. Thus, guinea pigs sensitized with egg albumin in complete Freund's adjuvant and tested six weeks later in both the eye and flank skin develop reactions differing strikingly in their neutrophil content. Indeed, at 24 hours nearly 80% of cells infiltrating the eye were neutrophils, whereas the corresponding figure in the skin was less than 20% (46).

The mouse has presented a special problem in that delayed hypersensitivity reactions in this species commonly have abundant neutrophils even at 24 hours. This had led to debate as to whether true delayed skin reactions can be elicited in this species (reviewed in ref. 102). However, neutrophils are equally numerous in the DH reactions of mice that have received adoptive immunity by passive transfer of sensitized lymphocytes (101). Others have made similar observations in the rat (103). Furthermore, the infiltration of neutrophils in some mouse reactions (e.g., contact hypersensitivity reactions to oxazolone) can be abolished by thymectomy (104). These last studies are particularly instructive in that a "nonspecific" (nonimmunologic) cause of neutrophils was excluded; that is, the accumulation of neutrophils was apparently dependent on the presence of sensitized lymphocytes. However, even here it is possible that the actual stimulus to neutrophil immigration is the tissue "injury" that resulted from the cell-mediated reaction.

Finally, it should be noted that DH reactions to certain antigens, generally those associated with the development of cellular immunity (as opposed to hypersensitivity alone), are particularly likely to have a prominent neutrophil infiltrate (96,100–102). One such example is that of DH reactions to *Candida* antigens in mice where neutrophils may predominate even as late as 18 hours (101). Participation of antibody was unlikely because neutrophils were predominant not only in actively sensitized animals but also in passive recipients of sensitized lymphoid cells. In guinea pigs, however, the situation is somewhat different. Although neutrophils are present at sites of cutaneous infection, they were found to an equal extent in both immune and nonimmune animals. Moreover, immune animals were distinguished from their nonimmune counterparts by a largely mononuclear cell infiltrate of the dermis and an increased epidermal scaling (not associated with inflammatory cells) that apparently was instrumental in ridding the host of *Candida* organisms (105).

Dextran has also been noted to elicit neutrophil-rich DH reactions in actively sensitized mice and in recipients of sensitized cells (102). The variation in the frequency of neutrophils in DH reactions to different antigens has not been satisfactorily explained but might be related to differences in the subpopulations of lymphocytes that respond to different antigens. Also, the possibility exists that neutrophils have functions in certain species (e.g., the mouse) that are performed by another granulocyte, the basophil, in species such as man or the guinea pig. According to this view, lymphocyte-mediated, neutrophil-rich, delayed-onset reactions in the mouse or rat might be analogous to CBH in the guinea pig.

We are unaware of any studies that consider the question of whether neutrophils are *necessary* for DH reactions in species such as the mouse, rat, or guinea pig. It is known from the work of McCluskey and associates (106) and Lubaroff and Waksman (107) that bone marrow-derived cells are essential for the expression of DH in guinea pigs and rats. Apparently these "nonspecific" cells are primarily monocytes; whether neutrophils are also essential is not known.

Influence of Lymphocytes and Other Mononuclear Cells on Neutrophils

The possibility that neutrophils might have an integral role in DH reactions has been strengthened by recent findings that products of lymphocytes ("lymphokines"), and, possibly, products of monocytes/macrophages, may significantly modulate neutrophil function. These products include a neutrophil chemotactic factor (108), leukocyte inhibitory factor (LIF) (109,110), skin reactive factor (SRF) (111–113), and migration enhancement factor (MEF) (114).

Ward et al. (108) have described a lymphokine that is chemotactic for neutrophils. This factor was separable from both MIF and a factor chemotactic for monocytes by polyacrylamide-gel electrophoresis. It was considerably less potent than the monocyte chemotactic factor in the Boyden double chamber assay. Both neutrophil and monocyte chemotactic factors were obtained from antigen-stimulated guinea pig lymphocyte cultures (108).

LIF is produced by incubation of human blood mononuclear cells with specific antigen (109) or with concanavalin A (110). Rocklin has characterized LIF produced by Con A as a chymotrypsin-sensitive, DFP-inhibitable esterase of approximately 68,000 daltons and with an electrophoretic motility similar to that of albumin (110). The material inhibits the migration of neutrophils from capillary tubes or agarose drops but has little or no effect on monocytes or macrophages. Its larger molecular size, sensitivity to DFP, and insensitivity to neuraminidase distinguish LIF from MIF, a factor produced by human and animal lymphocytes that inhibits macrophage migration. LIF is also the only known lymphokine with enzymatic activity. Its sensitivity to DFP is characteristic of serine esterases and is similar to that of a plasminogen activator secreted by virus-transformed cells which is involved in macrophage migration inhibition (115). It will be of considerable interest to determine whether LIF is also a plasminogen activator.

Increased migration of human neutrophils was found by Weisbart et al. (114) to be effected by factor(s) released from sensitized human mononuclear cells challenged with PPD in the first two days of culture. The factor responsible was termed migration enhancement factor or MEF and is an alpha or beta globulin that has not been completely characterized. By contrast, later (five- to seven-day) supernatants inhibited migration. Thus, lymphocytes stimulated with antigen may produce MEF and LIF, both of which affect neutrophil locomotion and/or cell interaction.

SRF, skin reactive factor, first described by Bennett and Bloom (111), is found in the supernatants of human or guinea pig lymphocyte cultures stimulated with specific antigen or mitogens. Injection of concentrates of partially purified fractions of serum-free culture supernatants into the skin of guinea pigs produces an indurated, erythematous reaction, maximal at three to nine hours, which is rich in neutrophils and mononuclear cells. Pick and co-workers have further characterized SRF from guinea pigs as sharing many properties with MIF (112), although their relationship is still uncertain. Mice may react with primarily a neutrophil infiltrate (113). Recent work suggests that LIF and SRF derived from PPD-stimulated human mononuclear cells may be separate molecules (116). In contrast to SRF fractions, supernatants with LIF activity produced a marked neutrophil infiltration. Several groups have confirmed the activity of SRF(s), but controversy has centered on the abundance and significance of neutrophils that SRF regularly elicits. Attraction of neutrophils might be due to nonspecific toxic effects of stimulated lymphocyte cultures or might indeed be a biologically important consequence of lymphocyte-antigen interaction. Resolution of the controversy will require further characterization of SRF.

A neutrophil immobilizing factor (NIF), derived from monocytes/macrophages, has been described by Goetzl and Austen (117) and Goetzl et al. (118). Endotoxin, phagocytosis, or low pH caused the release of a 4,000 to 5,000-dalton peptide from human monocytes in culture. This substance irreversibly decreased both the random motility of neutrophils and their response to a variety of chemotactic stimuli but did not alter phagocytosis or adherence. Motility of eosinophils, but not monocytes, was also reduced. The authors postulate that NIF may serve to retain neutrophils early in inflammatory reactions and that at later stages, if the concentration of NIF increases further, migration of neutrophils may be inhibited, allowing mononuclear cells to predominate (118).

One plausible mechanism of neutrophil attraction to cell-mediated reaction sites is by means of the clotting system. Fibrin is extensively deposited in the extravascular space during cell-mediated reactions in animals and man (11,12,26,27,46,47). Since fibrin split products are chemotactic for neutrophils (119–121), factors such as plasminogen activators from macrophages (122) or basophils (133) might initiate enough digestion of the fibrin deposits to cause neutrophils to accumulate. Several other components of the clotting system known to attract neutrophils might similarly participate, such as kallikrein (123) or plasma plasminogen activator (124), but there has been no direct demonstration of their role in cell-mediated reactions.

Neutrophil Products That Affect Lymphocytes

It is well known that neutrophils contain an abundance of proteolytic, oxidative, and other degradative enzymes (e.g., see ref. 125), and it is probable that whatever role the neutrophil may have in cell-mediated reactions is related to this digestive function. Proteolytic enzymes can induce mitogenesis in a variety of cells (126), including lymphocytes. Vischer et al. (127) incubated human and mouse lymphocytes with purified neutral proteases derived from human neutrophil granules. The enzymes that had esterase and a chymotrypsin-like activity stimulated DNA synthesis by human blood lymphocytes and mouse spleen cells, but not mouse thymocytes. The enzymes also stimulated an increase in the percentage of blast cells having surface Ig, as well as cells having cytoplasmic Ig. Thus, these enzymes would appear to act as B cell stimulants. Similarly, trypsin stimulates DNA synthesis in mouse B lymphocytes (128) and has been reported to be able to substitute for helper T cells by stimulating antibody-producing cells in Mishell-Dutton chambers (129). Yoshinaga et al. found that after one hour of culture the supernatants of casein-induced, neutrophil-rich (94%) mouse peritoneal exudates had the ability to augment ^{3}H-thymidine uptake by phytohemagglutinin (PHA)-stimulated thymocytes (130). Supernatants from macrophages contained a similar activity that has not been further characterized. Even less clear is the role of the SH-dependent protease derived from rabbit neutrophils that cleaves a 14,000-dalton fragment from rabbit IgM that is chemotactic for rat thoracic duct lymphocytes (113). Ward also noted that neutrophil lysates were chemotactic for lymphocytes (132). Whether the early migration of neutrophils may thus enhance later mononuclear infiltration and/or proliferation is an old hypothesis still awaiting proof. The significance of the neutrophil mitogenic factor and the neutrophil proteolytic enzymes in lymphocyte function is not yet clear, but it will no doubt receive increased attention as one aspect of the more general phenomenon of cell surface interactions with proteases.

In summary, it appears that although neutrophils are often present in DH reactions as a result of nonspecific stimuli, in some instances their presence has been related to the activity of sensitized lymphocytes. Several lymphocyte- or monocyte-derived factors can influence neutrophil function, and, possibly, neutrophils may influence migration and proliferation of mononuclear cells. What is now needed is a better characterization of lymphocyte/monocyte interactions with granulocytes, coupled with convincing evidence of the biologic significance of the phenomena observed in vitro.

REFERENCES

1. Ishizaka, T., and Ishizaka, K., in *The Biological Role of the Immunoglobulin E System,* (K. Ishazaka and D. H. Dayton, eds.) U. S. Government Printing Office, Washington, D.C., 1973, p. 33.
2. Soter, N. A., and Austen, K. F., *J. Invest. Dermatol.,* **67**, 313 (1976).
3. Dvorak, H. F., and Dvorak, A. M., *Clin. Haematol.* **4**, 651 (1975).
4. Lewis, R. A., Goetzl, E. J., Wasserman, S. I., Valone, F. H., Rubin, R. H., and Austin, K. F., *J. Immunol.* **114**, 87 (1975).
5. Orenstein, N. S., Hammond, M. E., Dvorak, H. F., and Feder, J., *Biochem. Biophys. Res. Commun.* **72**, 230 (1976).
6. Dvorak, H. F., Orenstein, N. S., Dvorak, A. M., Hammond, M. E., Roblin, R. O., Feder, J., Schott, C. F., Goodwin, J., and Morgan, E., *J. Immunol.* (in press).
7. Lichtenstein, L. M., in *Biochemistry of the Acute Allergic Reactions,* (K. F. Austen and E. L. Becker, eds.), F. A. Davis, Philadelphia, 1968, p. 153.
8. Lichtenstein, L. M., Gillespie, E., and Bourne, H., in *The Biological Role of the Immunoglobulin E System* (K. Ishizaka and D. H. Dayton, eds.), U.S. Government Printing Office, Washington, D.C., 1973, p. 165.
9. Richerson, H. B., Dvorak, H. F., and Leskowitz, S., *J. Exp. Med.* **132**, 546 (1970).
10. Dvorak, H. F., Dvorak, A. M., Simpson, B. A., Richerson, H. B., Leskowitz, S., and Karnovsky, M. J., *J. Exp. Med.* **132**, 558 (1976).

11. Dvorak, H. F., and Dvorak, A. M., in *Progress in Immunology,* II (L. Brent and E. J. Holborow, eds.), North Holland, Amsterdam, 1974, vol. 3, p. 171.
12. Dvorak, H. F., *J. Allergy Clin. Immunol.* **58**, 229 (1976).
13. Jones, T. D., and Mote, J. R., *N. Engl. J. Med.* **210**, 120 (1934).
14. Dvorak, H. F., Simpson, B. A., Bast, R. C., Jr., and Leskowitz, S., *J. Immunol.* **107**, 138 (1971).
15. Dvorak, H. F., and Hirsch, M. S., *J. Immunol.* **107**, 1576 (1971).
16. Dvorak, H. F., Dvorak, A. M., and Churchill, W. H., *J. Exp. Med.* **137**, 751 (1973).
17. Askenase, P., Hayden, B., and Higashi, G., *J. Allergy Clin. Immunol.* **55**, 111 (1975) (abstr.).
18. Allen, J. R., *Int. J. Parasitol.* **3**, 195 (1973).
19. Dvorak, H. F., *J. Immunol.* **106**, 279 (1971).
20. Stadecker, M., and Leskowitz, S., *J. Exp. Med.* **143**, 206 (1976).
21. Dvorak, H. F., Colvin, R. B., and Churchill, W. H., *J. Immunol.* **114**, 507 (1975).
22. Colvin, R. B., Pinn, V. W., Simpson, R. B., and Dvorak, H. F., *J. Immunol.* **110**, 1279 (1973).
23. Askenase, P. W., *J. Exp. Med.* **138**, 1144 (1973).
24. Stadecker, M. J., and Leskowitz, S., *Proc. Soc. Exp. Biol. Med.* **142**, 150 (1973).
25. Dvorak, H. F., Hammond, M. E., Colvin, R. B., Manseau, E. J., and Goodwin, J., *J. Immunol.* **118**, 1549 (1977).
26. Dvorak, H. F., Mihm, M. C., Jr., Dvorak, A. M., Johnson, R. A., Manseau, E. J., Morgan, E., and Colvin, R. B., *Lab. Invest.* **31**, 111 (1974).
27. Colvin, R. B., and Dvorak, H. F., *J. Immunol.* **114**, 377 (1975).
28. Benacerraf, B., Ovary, Z., Bloch, K., and Franklin, E., *J. Exp. Med.* **117**, 937 (1963).
29. Levine, B. D., Chang, H., and Vaz, N. M., *J. Immunol.* **106**, 29 (1971).
30. Margni, R. A., and Hajos, S. E., *Immunology* **25**, 323 (1973).
31. DeHurtado, I., and Osler, A. G., *Proc. Soc. Exp. Biol. Med.* **149**, 628 (1975).
32. Dvorak, A. M., Bast, R. C., Jr., and Dvorak, H. F., *J. Immunol.* **107**, 422 (1974).
33. Stadecker, M. J., and Leskowitz, S., *Fed. Proc.* **34**, 1040 (1975) (abstr.).
34. Neta, R., and Salvin, S. B., *Cell. Immunol.* **9**, 242 (1973).
35. Katz, S. I., Heather, C. J., Parker, D., and Turk, J. L., *J. Immunol.* **113**, 1073 (1974).
36. Katz, S. I., Parker, D., Sommer, G., and Turk, J. L., *Nature* **248**, 612 (1974).
37. Bast, R. C., Jr., Simpson, B. A., and Dvorak, H. F., *J. Exp. Med.* **133**, 202 (1971).
38. Boetcher, D. A., and Leonard, E. J., *Immunol. Commun.* **2**, 421 (1973).
39. Ward, P. A., Dvorak, H. F., Cohen, S., Yoshida, T., Data, R., and Selvaggio, S. S., *J. Immunol.* **114**, 1523 (1975).
40. Hammond, M. E., Selvaggio, S. S., and Dvorak, H. F., *J. Immunol.* **115**, 914 (1975).
41. Lett-Brown, M. A., Boetscher, D. A., and Leonard, E. J., *J. Immunol.* **117**, 246 (1976).
42. Salvin, S. B., *J. Exp. Med.* **107**, 109 (1958).
43. Askenase, P. W., and Hayden, B. J., *Fed. Proc.* **34**, 1039 (1975) (abstr).
44. Haynes, J. D., Kantor, F. S., and Askenase, P. W., *Fed. Proc.* **34**, 1039 (1975) (abstr.).
45. Askenase, P. W., Haynes, J. D., and Hayden, B. J., *J. Immunol.* **117**, 1722 (1976).
46. Friedlaender, M. H., and Dvorak, H. F., *J. Immunol.* (in press).
47. Dvorak, H. F., and Mihm, M. C., Jr., *J. Exp. Med.* **135**, 235 (1972).
48. Colvin, R. B., and Dvorak, H. F., *Lancet* **1**, 212 (1974).
49. Hoenig, E. M., and Levine, S., *J. Neuropathol. Exp. Neurol.* **33**, 251 (1974).
50. Burton, A. L., and Higginbotham, R. D., *J. Reticuloendothel. Soc.* **3**, 314 (1966).
51. Stadecker, M., Lukic, M., Dvorak, A. M., and Leskowitz, S., *J. Immunol.* **118**, 1564 (1977).
52. Dvorak, A. M., Mihm, M. C., Jr., and Dvorak, H. F., *J. Immunol.* **116**, 687 (1976).
53. Dvorak, A. M., Dvorak, H. F., and Karnovsky, M. J., *Lab. Invest.* **26**, 27 (1972).
54. Litt, M., *Ann. N.Y. Acad. Sci.* **116**, 964 (1964).
55. Cohen, S. G., Sapp, T. M., and Gallia, A. R., *Proc. Soc. Exp. Biol. Med.* **113**, 29 (1963).
56. Cohen, S., Vassali, P., Benacerraf, B., and McCluskey, R. T., *Lab. Invest.* **15**, 1143 (1966).
57. Cohen, S. G., and Sapp, T. M., *J. Allergy* **36**, 415 (1965).
58. Arnason, B. G., and Waksman, B. H., *Lab. Invest.* **12**, 737 (1963).
59. Cohen, S., *Clin. Immunol. Immunopathol.* **30**, 454 (1971).
60. Cotran, R. S., and Litt, M., *J. Exp. Med.* **129**, 1291 (1969).
61. Parmley, R. T., and Spicer, S. S., *Lab. Invest.* **30**, 557 (1974).
62. Wasserman, S. I., Goetzl, E. J., and Austen, K. F., *J. Immunol.* **114**, 645 (1975).

63. Hubscher, T. *J. Immunol.* **114**, 1379 (1975).
64. Barnhart, M. I., and Riddle, J. M., *Blood* **21**, 306 (1963).
65. Hubscher, T., *J. Immunol.* **114**, 1389 (1975).
66. Gleich, G. J., Loegering, D. A., Kueppers, F., Bajaj, S. P., and Mann, K. G., *J. Exp. Med.* **140**, 313 (1974).
67. Gleich, G. J., Loegering, D. A., Mann, K. G., and Maldonado, J. E., *J. Clin. Invest.* **57**, 633 (1976).
68. Rabellino, E. M., and Metcalf, D., *J. Immunol.* **115**, 688 (1975).
69. Litt, M., *J. Cell Biol.* **23**, 355 (1964).
70. Ishikawa, T., Wicher, K., and Arbesman, C. E., *Int. Arch. Allergy* **46**, 230 (1974).
71. Kline, B. S., Cohen, M. D., and Rudolph, J. D., *J. Allergy* **3**, 531 (1932).
72. Green, G. R., Zweiman, B., Beerman, H., and Hildreth, E. A., *J. Allergy* **40**, 224 (1967).
73. Fowler, J. W., and Lowell, F. C., *J. Allergy* **37**, 19 (1966).
74. Feinberg, A. R., Feinberg, S. M., and Lee, F., *J. Allergy* **40**, 73 (1967).
75. Gell, P. G. H., and Hinde, I. T., *Int. Arch. Allergy* **5**, 23 (1954).
76. Leber, P. D., Milgrom, M., and Cohen, S., *Immunol. Commun.* **2**, 615 (1973).
77. Solley, G. O., Gleich, G. J., Jordon, R. E., and Schroeter, A. L., *J. Clin. Invest.* **58**, 408 (1976).
78. Ponzio, N. M., and Speirs, R. S., *Immunology* **28**, 243 (1975).
79. Schriber, R. A., and Zucker-Franklin, D., *J. Immunol.* **114**, 1348 (1975).
80. Basten, A., Boyer, M. H., and Beeson, P. B., *J. Exp. Med.* **131**, 1271 (1970).
81. Basten, A., and Beeson, P. B., *J. Exp. Med.* **131**, 1288 (1970).
82. Waksman, B. H., *Am. J. Pathol.* **37**, 673 (1960).
83. Cohen, S., and Ward, P. A., *J. Exp. Med.* **133**, 133 (1971).
84. Torisu, M., Yoshida, T., Ward, P. A., and Cohen, S., *J. Immunol.* **111**, 1450 (1973).
85. Colley, D. G., *J. Immunol.* **115**, 150 (1975).
86. Greene, B. M., and Colley, D. G., *J. Immunol.* **116**, 1078 (1976).
87. James, S. L., and Colley, D. G., *J. Reticuloendothel. Soc.* **18**, 283 (1975).
88. Cochrane, C. G., *Adv. Immunol.* **9**, 97 (1968).
89. Stadecker, M. J., and Leskowitz, S., *J. Immunol.* **113**, 496 (1974).
90. Dienes, L., and Mallory, T. B., *Am. J. Pathol.* **8**, 689 (1932).
91. Gell, P. G. H., and Hinde, I. T., *Br. J. Exp. Pathol.* **32**, 516 (1951).
92. Broughton, B., and Spector, W. G., *J. Pathol. Bacteriol.* **85**, 371 (1963).
93. Wiener, J., Spiro, D., and Zinku, H. O., *Am. J. Pathol.* **47**, 723 (1965).
94. Kolin, A., Johanorsky, J., and Pekarel, J., *Int. Arch. Allergy* **26**, 167 (1964).
95. Turk, J. L., Heather, C. J., and Diengdoh, J. V., *Int. Arch. Allergy* **29** , 278 (1966).
96. Collins, F. M., and Mackaness, G. B., *J. Immunol.* **101**, 830 (1968).
97. Wiener, J., Lattes, R. G., and Spiro, D., *Am. J. Pathol.* **50**, 485 (1967).
98. Lenzini, L., and Barnabe, R., *Int. Arch. Allergy* **35**, 402 (1969).
99. Dietrich, F. M., and Hess, R., *Int. Arch. Allergy* **38**, 246 (1970).
100. Claflin, J. L., and Larson, C. L., *Infect. Immun.* **5**, 311 (1972).
101. Rowlands, D. T., Crowle, A. J., and Russe, H. P., *Int. Arch. Allergy* **28**, 328 (1965).
102. Crowle, A. J., *Adv. Immunol.* **20**, 197 (1975).
103. Basman, C., and Feldman, J. D., *Am. J. Pathol.* **58**, 201 (1970).
104. deSousa, M. A. B., and Parrot, D. M. V., *J. Exp. Med.* **130**, 671 (1969).
105. Sohnle, P. G., Frank, M. M., and Kirkpatrick, C. H., *J. Immunol.* **117**, 523 (1976).
106. McCluskey, R. T., Benacerraf, B., and McCluskey, J. W., *J. Immunol.* **90**, 466 (1963).
107. Lubaroff, D. M., and Waksman, B., *J. Exp. Med.* **128**, 1425 (1968).
108. Ward, P. A., Reinold, H. G., and Dand, J. R., *Cell. Immunol.* **1**, 162 (1970).
109. Rocklin, R. E., *J. Immunol.* **112**, 1461 (1974).
110. Rocklin, R. E., *J. Immunol.* **114**, 1161 (1975).
111. Bennett, B., and Bloom, B. R., *Proc. Natl. Acad. Sci.* **54**, 756 (1968).
112. Pick, E., Krejci, J., and Turk, J. L., *Int. Arch. Allergy Appl. Immunol.* **41**, 18 (1971).
113. Yoshida, T., Nagai, R., and Hashimoto, T., *Lab. Invest.* **29**, 329 (1973).
114. Weisbart, R. H., Bluestone, R., Goldberg, L. S., et al., *Proc. Natl. Acad. Sci.* **71**, 875 (1975).
115. Hammond, M. E., Roblin, R. O., Dvorak, A. M., et al., *Science* **185**, 955 (1974).
116. Warrington, R. J., Buehler, S. K., and Roberts, K. B., *Int. Arch. Allergy Appl. Immunol.* **51**, 186 (1976).
117. Goetzl, E. J., and Austen, K. F., *J. Exp. Med.* **136**, 1564 (1972).

118. Goetzl, E. J., Gigli, I., Wasserman, S., et al., *J. Immunol.* **111**, 938 (1973).
119. Barnhard, M. I., in *Chemical Biology of Inflammation* (J. C. Houck and B. Forescher, eds.) Pergamon Press, New York, 1968, p. 205.
120. Stecher, V. J., *Fed. Proc.* **33**, 336 (1974) (abstr.).
121. Kay, A. B., Pepper, D. S., and Ewart, M. R., *Nature New Biol.* **243**, 56 (1973).
122. Unkeless, J. C., Gordon, S., and Reich, E., *J. Exp. Med.* **139**, 834 (1974).
123. Kaplan, A. P., Kay, A. B., and Austen, K. F., *J. Exp. Med.* **135**, 81 (1972).
124. Kaplan, A. P., Goetzl, E. J., and Austen, K. F., *J. Clin. Invest.* **52**, 2591 (1973).
125. Bagglioni, M., *Enzyme* **13**, 132 (1972).
126. Zetter, B. R., Chen, L. B., and Buchanan, J. M., *Cell* **7**, 407 (1976).
127. Vischer, T. L., Bretz, U., and Baggiioni, M., *J. Exp. Med.* **144**, 863 (1976).
128. Vischer, T. L., *J. Immunol.* **113**, 58 (1974).
129. Gisler, R. H., Vischer, T. L., and Dukor, P., *J. Immunol.* **116**, 1354 (1976).
130. Yoshinaga, M., Nakamura, S., and Hayashi, H., *J. Immunol.* **115**, 533 (1975).
131. Higuchi, Y., Horda, M., and Hayashi, H., *Cell. Immunol.* **15**, 100 (1975).
132. Ward, P. A., *J. Exp. Med.* **128**, 1201 (1968).
133. Dvorak, H. F., Orenstein, N. S., Rypysc, J., Colvin, R. B., and Dvorak, A. M., *J. Immunol,* **120,** 766 (1978).
134. Galli, S. J., Colvin, R. B., Verderber, E., Galli, A. S., Monahan, R., Dvorak, A. M., and Dvorak, H. F., *J. Immunol.,* in press (1978).

Chapter Six

Aging and Immunity

EDMOND J. YUNIS, BARRY S. HANDWERGER,
HELEN M. HALLGREN, ROBERT A. GOOD,
AND GABRIEL FERNANDES

Sidney Farber Cancer Institute, Harvard Medical School, Boston, Massachusetts; Departments of Laboratory Medicine and Pathology and Medicine, University of Minnesota, Minneapolis, Minnesota; and Sloan-Kettering Cancer Institute, New York, New York

Studies in mice, and to a limited extent in man, have provided evidence that the development of age-associated diseases and the causative factors of aging may be controlled by immunologic factors that are influenced by inherited characteristics. Three distinct immunologic mechanisms may be important in the etiology and pathogenesis of aging: (1) thymic involution and cell-mediated immune dysfunctions; (2) viral infection and resistance to viral infection and replication; and (3) a genetically programmed system for immunologic control that probably involves genes that control immune recognition.

In mice, evidence indicates that longevity is influenced by factors that are to some degree susceptible to manipulation. In man, circumstantial evidence links deficits in body defense processes to age-related diseases such as cancer. This view derives in part from the observed age-associated decrease in cell-mediated immune function and increase of the incidence of cancer and in part from the occurrence of lymphoreticular malignancies in high frequency in patients with congenital or acquired immunologic deficiencies (1).

The documentation that deficiency in immunologic function is central to the pathogenesis of many of the diseases associated with aging, e.g., autoimmunity, vascular degeneration and insufficiency, renal deficiency, amyloidosis, and even central nervous system insufficiency, may establish an approach to manipulation and control of these diseases (2).

Of course, the ideal way of studying the aging process would be to follow a given population from birth to death. Since this is not possible during the lifetime of one investigator, the only alternative is to examine families with persons of all ages to correlate physiologic, endocrinologic, pathologic, and immunologic parameters with aging and disease. These studies should provide information concerning inherited bases of long life, and a sequential study will help determine whether screening of immunologic defects in late adult life has predictive value for longevity. If such is the case, then health care programs directed at the prevention of age-associated diseases, and perhaps, to a certain extent, the aging process itself, might be developed in an immunologic perspective.

GENERAL ASPECTS OF AGING

In the most general sense, life span is defined for any one person as the length of his survival, and for a population either as the median survival or the length of life of the longest survivors among the cohorts. Aging is understood as the collective changes that occur during these life spans that set limits upon them. As with many biologic phenomena, ample evidence supports the view that both genetic and environmental influences are important in determining both life span and aging (3).

The interaction between genotype and environment must exist at different levels and occur at different times during the life of a person. Therefore, the understanding of aging involves an analysis of an extremely complex interaction between hereditary and external environment. Any understanding of aging must involve knowledge of the control mechanisms of morphogenesis, differentiation, and metabolism. These control mechanisms, which regulate the internal and external environment in which cellular interactions occur, are influenced by the coordinated activity of the neurologic and endocrine systems. These controls change during life from fertilization to senescence (4). Since all processes of life are regulated at various levels through a sequence of interactions, some operating during embryogenesis, differentiation, and growth and others during senescence, it is not surprising that no single theory of aging is adequate in itself to define the aging process in its entirety.

Generally, there is no difficulty in including as a part of the aging process conditions such as graying of the hair and wrinkling of the skin while excluding embryogenesis and processes involved in maturation. However, aging and death of individual cells occur at all stages of development, and organs develop and involute according to a specific timetable within a particular genetic framework.

The timetable of organ development and involution in a species, as well as the limits reflected by a preordained proliferative capacity of cells after birth (5), strongly suggests that the life span of a species is under genetic control mediated through the existence of cellular and organ clocks. However, since life span is also the result of adaptation of all regulatory mechanisms of the animal (including embryogenesis and maturation) to the environment, it is not possible to exclude stochastic theories of aging (6,7).

In humans, it appears that many environmental factors can be manipulated by medicine, sanitation, and nutrition and that the survival curves are progressively approaching a rectangular shape. Consequently, at approximately 80 to 85 years of age, the remaining population (approximately 5 to 8% of original cohort) are the few individuals of maximum genetically determined life span. This group is therefore composed of the only examples of man wherein the entire process of life leading to senescence could be described (primary aging) (3).

It is also known that approximately 20% of the general population have genetic defects that shorten life span (8) and contribute significantly to the death of persons below age 60 to 70 years. These observations argue in favor of the importance of different, individually determined physiologic clocks which, because they run down at different rates in different persons, determine individual life span. It is important to determine which of these physiologic clocks plays a crucial role in determining or defining maximal life span. Understanding these controls individually or collectively may establish which one or which combination is the most important in defining the supergenotype with the extremely long life.

It is extremely important to consider as diseases of aging those disturbances that result in decline and death of individuals or strains of animals not so perfectly endowed as the supergenotypes, and to understand the waning of physiologic controls that predisposes to the diseases in question. It seems possible that one might alter and control the diseases of aging by manipulation of relatively few physiologic functions, including perhaps those involved in involution of thymus and the T cell lymphoid system. If such were the case, much disease and suffering associated with old age in man might be effectively addressed.

In this discussion, we will examine evidence, both old and new, that supports the view that the life span and aging of a species are under genetic regulation, depending in a major way on an intact immune system for maintenance of internal integrity and protection against the external environment.

THE IMMUNE SYSTEM AND AGING

The Immunologic Theory of Aging

The immunologic theory of aging, first clearly stated by Walford (3), has been extensively promulgated by Burnet (2). This theory states that the immune system is essential to maintenance of health and that, to a major extent, the aging process per se may reflect a genetically programmed decline in immune function.

In our studies, the decline of effective immunologic function during the aging process in man and mouse has been associated with the same diseases and immunologic perturbations that plague man and other animals that lack a normal T cell immunity system (1). Observations consistent with the clonal selection theory of immunity have provoked Burnet (5) to maintain that clones of cells, ordinarily forbidden expression by an intact immunity system, appear by somatic mutation and can persist when immunity functions are defective. This, he feels, accounts for the frequent autoimmunity observed in aging and immunodeficient man and animals (2).

On the other hand, Good and Yunis (1) have interpreted the association of autoimmunity with immune deficiency states, as seen in aging and following neonatal thymectomy, to be consistent with a forbidden antigen theory of autoimmunity (see Chapters 7 and 8). We have argued that as a consequence of immunodeficiency, antigens that otherwise would be prohibited from entering the body, or else would be promptly eliminated from it, are not eliminated. These antigens then induce the production of cross-reacting autoantibodies and autoimmunity. From either perspective, because of the decrease in cellular immunity that occurs with aging, autoimmunity phenomena might be expected to occur (as they do) with greater frequency in aging.

Gatti and Good (9) and Greenberg and Yunis (10) have reviewed the relationship between the various components of the aging process and the functional state of the immune system. They have classified aging according to its primary and secondary events and proposed that the primary component be considered separately from the secondary ones. They have argued that the primary components of immunologic aging are embodied in a chronologic process that is genetically programmed to result in a decline in effective function and control of immunity. According to this view, the genetically programmed clock operates at a rate consistent with the median life span of the species and perhaps reflects limits imposed by the Hayflick (11) formulation. To conform to this limitation, it is probable that the thymic process of spawning T lymphocytes ceases through loss of central nervous system or endocrine support because of its intrinsic temporal limitations. An involuted thymus would thus impose an essential limit on the immunologic vigor of the T cell system because of the limited programmed potentiality for replication of T lymphoid elements found in the peripheral systems (12).

All other immunologic aspects of the aging process can be viewed as events secondary to the genetically programmed failure of the thymic clock (10). These secondary immunologic components of aging encompass certain disease processes and pathology commonly associated with aging, but not directly a function of the aging process per se. These include cancer, autoimmune phenomena, arthritis, amyloidosis, hyalinization of blood vessels and other tissues, hyalinization and sclerosis of the renal glomeruli, increased frequency of serious infections due to pathogens of low-grade virulence, and the varying degrees of immunodeficiency (13,14).

Burnet (15) has recently presented an interpretation of aging that combines genetic programming with the stochastic random error theory proposed by Orgel (6,7). Under this concept, random accumulation of error in cells results from genetically determined degrees of error-proneness in DNA polymerases and from enzymes that are responsible for the fidelity with which DNA is replicated or reconstituted after damage and repair. The accumulation of errors on thymus-derived lymphocytes could result in age-dependent loss of T cell function. Since T lymphocytes play a major role in tumor immunity, in the host defense against infection, and in the preservation of self-tolerance, the genetically programmed failure of thymic function could well play a major role in the pathogenesis of aging and age-related diseases, such as autoimmunity and cancer (16).

Immunity and Aging

Specific thymic alterations related to aging have been described and extensively discussed by Hammar (17) and reviewed by many others (18). It has been known for many years that, beginning at the time of sexual maturation, there begins in the central lymphoid organs a process of apparently programmed involution, which is succeeded by a period of gradual involution of the peripheral lymphoid apparatus and declining vigor of immunologic function (19–22). In both mice and man, the rate of this immunologic involution is highly variable, but nevertheless proceeds according to a schedule that in a broad framework is characteristic of the species.

Among inbred strains of mice, the rates of aging in general, and immunologic aging in particular, have clearly defined time constraints. CBA mice tend to be very long-lived and to maintain immunologic function longer than other strains when measured by several standards. Like CBA mice, C57B1 mice are long-lived and sustain their immunologic processes well into the third year. By contrast, NZB and (NZB × NZW)F_1 mice are short-lived and develop immunodeficiencies and immunologic abnormalities early in life (21–24). It is important to note that we are primarily discussing age-related changes within the species, without attempting to explain the possible evolutionary processes determining the life span of each species (25). For instance, both survival and maintenance of immunologic function seem very short when CBA mice are compared to man, yet survival time and the duration of immunologic function of NZB mice may seem long by standards that could be applied to the Snell-Bagg or Ames dwarf mice (26).

Thus, aging, diseases of aging, and thymic and immunologic involution may occur early in certain inbred strains of mice and much later in others; but in all strains studied, even the very long-lived strains, evidence of immunologic involution may be found as the animals age.

T Cell Immune Function

A number of studies have demonstrated that a decline in cell-mediated immune function occurs with aging. In 1944, Tuft and co-workers showed a very sharp decrease in cell-mediated allergy to food or plant allergens in persons over 50 (27). Gross showed that old persons bearing neoplasms have very markedly reduced delayed responses to 2,4 dinitrochlorobenzene (DNCB); old persons free of neoplasms also showed significantly less frequent sensitization to 2,4 DNCB than did 14- to 15-year-old children (28).

Giannini and Sloan (29) studied active immunization to 2,4 DNCB and skin reaction to tuberculin and showed that they were markedly defective in aged populations as compared to reactions in younger persons of the same geographic areas. Responses of peripheral lymphocytes to phytohemagglutinin (PHA), which are primarily a reflection of response of the thymus-dependent cell population, are also deficient in aged persons (30,31) (see Table 1 and Fig. 1).

Table 1. Alteration of Immune Parameters in Aging Man

	Age Group	
	Young (20–39 years)	Aged (80–99 years)
Cellular Immunity:		
Response to phytohemagglutinin	Normal	Decreased
Response to Concanavalin A	Normal	Decreased
Response to allogeneic cells	Normal	Decreased
Suppressive action of Concanavalin A-stimulated lymphocytes	Normal	Decreased
Percentage of peripheral T cells	Normal	Normal
Humoral Immunity:		
Antibody response to heterologous antigens	Normal	Decreased
Autoantibody production	Normal	Increased
Serum levels of IgG and IgA	Normal	Increased
Percentage of peripheral B cells	Normal	Normal

Diminished T cell-mediated immunity has also occurred in aging mice, as evidenced by (1) defective rejection of allografts and heterografts of tumor and skin (32,33); (2) diminished ability to respond to allogeneic cells in mixed lymphocyte reactions; (3) diminished graft-versus-host (GVH) activity; and (4) depressed PHA reactivity (34–37). These deficiencies occur subsequent to a decline in serum thymic hormone levels (38,39). Yet, despite the profound functional T cell deficiency, the percentage of lymphocytes bearing T cell markers does not appear to decline or declines only minimally with age in both mouse (40) and man (41). This implies that either each cell is less efficient in its function, possibly because of changes in its microenvironment, or that a shift in subsets of lymphoid populations occurs with aging which results in the profound defect in

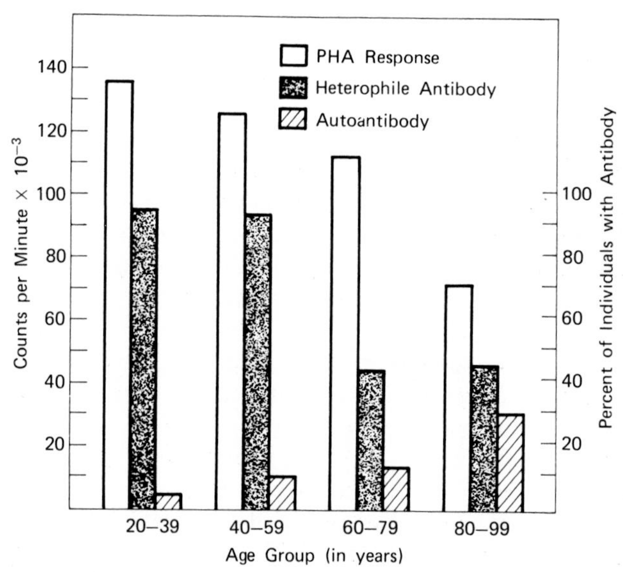

Figure 1. Relationship of lymphocyte response to phytohemagglutinin (PHA), frequency of heterophile antibodies, and appearance of autoantibodies during human aging.

function of the T cell system as a whole.

Mice of autoimmune susceptible strains show a very early decline in several parameters of cell-mediated immunity, such as ability to induce GVH reaction, PHA blast transformation, development of killer lymphocytes, and spread of tumors in hosts challenged by tumors (Table 2). These findings can be accelerated by neonatal thymectomy, emphasizing the importance of the thymus in the pathogenesis of autoimmunity and cancer development (42).

Humoral Immune Function

It is now well documented that humoral immune responses also decline with age (43,44). Approximately 10% of this decline can be accounted for by extrinsic factors, i.e., by changes in the environment or "milieu" in which lymphoid cells are found (45). Thus, the antibody-forming capacity of cells grafted to young recipients is greater than that of cells grafted to old recipients, regardless of the age of the donor; this suggests a role for extrinsic factors in determining the level of humoral immune activity. About 90% of the reduction in antibody-forming capacity observed in old mice, however, is a consequence of changes in cells of the immune system (46). The ability to mount a humoral immune response is dependent on the interaction or collaboration of T lymphocytes (both helper T cells and suppressor T cells), macrophages, and B lymphocytes (the precursors of the antibody-forming cells).

Although the decline in antibody-forming capacity that occurs with aging could be due to an alteration in the number or function of any of these cell populations, the predominant factor appears to be a decrease in T helper cell function, and not a decrease in B cell or macrophage function (47). Thus, the ability of mice to respond (by antibody production) to T-dependent antigens appears to decline to a greater degree and at an earlier age than the ability to respond to T-independent antigens. Moreover, the relative preservation of B cell function with aging is supported by studies evaluating mitogenic response of murine spleen cells (48). As in the case of antibody production, B cell activity appears to decline to a lesser extent and at a later age than does T cell activity.

In mice, the ability of macrophages to collaborate with T and B cells in antibody production is not impaired with age (49). Investigations of other macrophage characteristics and functions, however, have not been performed.

Humoral immune function is also altered in aging man. Antibody response to heterophile antigens decreases markedly with age, whereas the production of autoantibodies increases. The percentage of peripheral B cells, however, remains fairly constant throughout adult life (Table 1 and Fig. 1).

The age-related alterations in humoral immunity in both mouse and man can be explained on the basis of a primary deficit in the function of the T cell system, characterized by decreased T helper cell function, resulting in a diminished antibody response to heterologous antigens, and by decreased T suppressor cell activity, allowing the production of antibodies reactive with self-antigens. Diminished suppressor cell activity has been documented in an aged human population (50) and NZB mice (51).

Recently, increased suppressor cell activity has been related to impaired im-

Table 2. Alteration of Immune Functions in Autoimmune Susceptible and Resistant Strains of Mice

Mouse Strain	Age (mos.)	Response to Mitogens		Antibody-Forming Cells (SRBC)	Cellular Immune Function (GVH)	Suppressor T cells or Thymic Hormone	Resistance to Allogeneic Tumor Cells
		PHA (T cell)	LPS (B cell)				
NZB	2	Normal	Normal	High	High	Low	High
(autoimmune susceptible)	12	Low	Low	Low	Low	Low	Low
(NZB × NZW) F_1	2	Normal	Normal	High	Normal	Low	High
(autoimmune susceptible)	10	Low	Normal	Low	Low	Low	Low
CBA/H	2	High	High	Normal	Normal	High	High
(autoimmune resistant)	12	High	High	Normal	High	Low	High
	24	Low	Normal	Low	Normal	Low	Normal

munoglobulin synthesis in common variable hypogammaglobulinemia (52) and in multiple myeloma (53). Whether this mechanism plays a role in the immunodeficiency that occurs in aging remains to be established.

The preceding observations suggest that the primary age-related effect on the immune system is a decrease in T cell functional capacity. That this deficiency may be important in humans in the pathogenesis of diseases of the aged gains support by the findings that old people with defective cell-mediated immunity have a decreased life expectancy, as compared to those with normal T cell function (19).

VIRAL INFECTION, RESISTANCE, AND AGING

Several reports suggest a possible relationship between immunologic deficits and viral infection (54–56). During the past several years, a great deal of attention has been focused on the possible role of viruses (endogenous and exogenous) in the pathogenesis of aging (57), and of age-related diseases such as autoimmunity (58–61) and malignancy (62).

On the basis of these studies, Levy has postulated a possible role of virus infection in the regulation of the thymic clock (58). The following discussion will emphasize the difficulties in separating which is the primary event: genetics of thymic involution and/or environmental or intrinsic vertically transmitted factor, such as viral infection.

A relationship between persistent viral (slow virus) infection and a multitude of autoimmune phenomena is now well documented (58–61). Hotchin (57,59) and Oldstone (60) have demonstrated that mice neonatally or congenitally infected with lymphocytic choriomeningitis (LCM) virus have a shortened life span and develop evidence of autoimmune pathology, including glomerulonephritis, chronic hepatitis, and arteritis. In addition, infected mice demonstrate neurologic changes, degenerative skin changes, ruffled fur, blepharitis, hunched posture, and marked hair loss, giving them an "aged, dilapidated appearance" (57). Adult mice inoculated with large doses of LCM virus develop antiviral antibodies and antibodies directed against both LCM-infected and normal liver, kidney, spleen, and brain tissues (i.e., true autoantibodies) (57,60). Tissue injury in LCM-infected mice occurs as a result of the interaction of the anti-LCM immune response with virus and virus-infected cells (57,60), rather than as a consequence of direct virus-induced injury per se.

The major animal models for the study of autoimmunity are the NZB and (NZB × NZW)F_1 mouse strains. These mice have a high incidence of Coomb's positive hemolytic anemia, immune complex glomerulonephritis, (LE) cell phenomena, and antibodies to nucleic acids (58,60,61). In addition, they have an increased incidence of neoplasms, especially of the lymphoreticular system (58,61). NZB mice are infected with at least three different RNA viruses: a Gross-type murine leukemia virus (GLV) (58); a Maloney murine leukemia virus (58,63); and a xenotrophic C-type RNA virus (58). A role for the xenotrophic virus in the etiology of NZB autoimmunity has been postulated (58) but not yet documented. NZB and (NZB × NZW)F_1 mice mount a strong immune response to the Gross murine leukemia (64). A significant proportion (5 to 18%) of the IgG eluted from NZ nephritic kidneys has specificity for GLV (64,65). Thus, deposition of GLV-anti-GLV immune complexes in the kidneys of NZ mice may play a role in the pathogenesis of the lupus-like glomerulonephritis seen in these animals.

The major cause of nephritis in these animals, however, appears to be the glomerular deposition of DNA-anti-DNA complexes (65). Although the exact etiology of the anti-DNA antibody response in NZ mice is not clear, it appears likely that the immune imbalance that occurs in NZB and (NZB × NZW)F_1 mice and results in immunologic hyperreactivity to nucleic acid antigens (66,67) is an important contributory factor. An effect of the presence of RNA tumor viruses in NZ mice on antinuclear antibody (ANA) production has been suggested (68). Persistent viral infection from birth with either lymphocytic chromomeningitis virus or polyoma virus enhances ANA formation, immune complex glomerulonephritis, and increases mortality in NZ mice (66,69). Inoculation of Rauscher or Graffi leukemogenic virus into (BALB/c × C57B1/6)F_1 or (C3H × C57B1/6)F_1 mice induces the production of ANA antibodies (70). Purified virus obtained from an NZB tumor line induces ANA, glomerulonephritis, and lymphoma when injected into newborn (BALB/c × NZB)F_1 mice (71). These data strongly suggest a role for RNA viruses in induction of murine lupus-like autoimmunity.

Genetic control of susceptibility to virus-induced autoimmunity in mice has been suggested (70,71) but has not been well studied. The level at which genetic control is exerted, moreover, remains unknown, but is likely to be related either to the nature of the immune response to the inducing agent (virus) or to susceptibility of the host and possibly of the host's immune system to infection with the etiologic virus.

One of the first animal models used for the study of systemic lupus erythematosus (SLE) was Aleutian mink disease, a commonly occurring disease of ranch-bred mink, characterized by immune complex glomerulonephritis, vasculitis, Coomb's positive hemolytic anemia, thrombocytopenia, hypergammaglobulinemia, and widespread lymphoreticular hyperplasia (72,73). A small (approximately 25-nm), ether-resistant, heat- and formalin-sensitive virus has been isolated from these animals and appears to be important in the pathogenesis of the disease (73,74).

Equine infectious anemia (EIA) is a disease of horses characterized by lymphoid hyperplasia, glomerulonephritis, vasculitis, hemolytic anemia, chronic hepatitis, hypergammaglobulinemia, and hypocomplemententemia. A filtrable virus (the equine infectious anemia virus) has been isolated and has been shown to be capable of initiating the disease (75). As in LCM infection, in both Aleutian mink disease and EIA, pathology is thought to result from the effects of the antiviral immune response and interaction with virus and virus-infected tissue (73,75), rather than from direct viral injury, per se.

Lewis and his co-workers have described the existence of a systemic lupus erythematosus-like illness in dogs characterized by autoimmune hemolytic anemia, thrombocytopenia, arthritis, glomerulonephritis, positive LE cell tests, hypergammaglobulinemia, and the presence of ANA antibodies (76). Breeding studies have suggested that the transmission of this disease is by an extragenetic mechanism, i.e., by vertical or horizontal transmission of an infectious agent (77). Lewis and co-workers have recently reported that canine SLE can be transmitted to normal puppies or mice by cell-free filtrates prepared from spleens or lymph nodes of seropositive dogs. The disease, in fact, could then be transferred serially in murine recipients by cell-free extracts (78). Some of the mice injected with canine filtrates developed malignant lymphomas that contained numerous C-type RNA viral particles. When the C-type virus was partially purified and injected into newborn mice, ANA antibodies were produced (78), strongly implicating C-type virus in the etiology of murine autoimmunity.

Several recent reports have suggested an association between slow virus infection and autoimmunity in man. Antibodies have been produced in rabbits purified against C-type RNA virus obtained from a murine neoplasma induced by a cell-free filtrate prepared from the spleen of a dog with SLE. After appropriate absorption, this antiserum reacted with peripheral blood lymphocytes of human patients with SLE, suggesting the presence of C-type RNA viral antigens on the membrane of human SLE lymphoid cells. Lymphocytes from normal human subjects did not react with the anti-C-type virus and serum (78). Several laboratories have reported the presence of "myxovirus-like particles" in tissues of patients with SLE and polymyositis (80–82). Strand and August, furthermore, have recently described the presence of C-type RNA viral antigens in the spleens of human SLE patients (83), and Panem et al. have demonstrated the presence of C-type RNA virus antigens and antiviral antibodies in the immune complexes deposited in human SLE kidneys (84). The deposition of Australia (Au) antigen-antibody complexes in the arteries of some patients with polyarteritis has recently been demonstrated (85), suggesting a role for human hepatitis virus in the pathogenesis of this autoimmune disease.

The data presented above have documented a pathogenic role for virus in murine, canine, equine, and mink autoimmunity, and have suggested that this pathogenic mechanism may be involved in human autoimmunity. Persistent or slow virus infection has been implicated as an etiologic factor in a multitude of other animal and human diseases (86–90). The ability of both DNA and RNA viruses to induce a variety of malignancies in animal model systems is now well documented and has been recently reviewed (62). Of particular interest is the increased incidence of malignancies in animals with virus-associated autoimmunity (58,61,91,92).

Thus, immune function, genetics, and viral infection all may be of major importance in the pathogenesis of aging, autoimmunity, and malignancy. The exact interrelationship of these factors is complex and not well understood. Immune function has been shown to affect the course of viral oncogenesis (54,55) and viral-induced autoimmune disease (59,60,63,65,68,73). Immune reactions to nonviral antigens may enhance viral-associated neoplasia by activating oncogenic viruses (54). Oncogenic and nononcogenic viruses, in turn, may have profound inhibitory effects on immune function (56,58,93–95), the exact mechanism of which is unknown. Virus infection of lymphoid cells may in and of itself produce alterations in the functional capacity of those cells. Expression of viral antigens or virus-directed neoantigens on the surface of lymphoid cells may induce an antilymphocyte immune reaction, which, in turn, could secondarily lead to immunodeficiency. The nature of the alteration in immune function may be a consequence of lymphocyte subpopulations (helper T cells, suppressor T cells, cytotoxic T cells, antibody-forming cells, etc.) which are actually infected with virus. The elucidation of the exact interrelationship of immune function, viral infection, and genetics is of paramount importance to the understanding of the pathogenesis of autoimmunity, malignancy, and aging.

IMMUNOGENETICS OF AGING

It remains to be determined whether or not the decline of immunologic vigor, which seems to be centrally and genetically determined, is directly or indirectly controlled by the major histocompatibility complex (MHC) linkage group of chromosome 6 of man and chromosome 17 of mouse. This linkage group can be considered as a "supergene," since it may well control individuality, cell surface antigenicity, complement function, and the capacity to initiate and vigorously produce an immune response to foreign antigens. The MHC is also a major determinant of susceptibility or resistance to diseases that are commonly linked to aging, e.g., arthritis, diabetes, demyelinating disease of the central nervous system, and malignancies (96). In addition, it is provocative to think that MHC must also be associated with the aging process, per se. McDevitt and Bodmer (97) have suggested that anomalies in MHC-linked immune response genes may explain the associations between HLA and diseases. The reliability of HLA antigens as markers of disease states, therefore, depends on the continuous cosegregation of the genes involved. Consequently, in some cases, HLA antigens will serve as reliable markers of disease states (or disease susceptibility), whereas in other instances, they may reflect resistance to disease and may provide a potential marker of longevity. A relationship between histocompatibility markers and longevity has already been observed in mice: in three different strains derived from three different stocks, $H\text{-}2^b$ appears to be associated with the longest-lived strains of mice (98). Moreover, in humans, Matthews (99) has postulated an association of HLA-B8 with mortality in several populations. We have demonstrated a decreased frequency of HLA-B8 in older women (100).

Recent evidence suggests that abnormal insulin-insulin-receptor interaction on plasma membranes of target tissues plays an important role in the pathogenesis of several diabetic syndromes. Because insulin is the anabolic hormone *par excellence,* and the cellular uptake of many nutrients including amino acids depends on it, it is tempting to speculate that its inefficiency could result in widespread malnutrition "from within," which could play a role in age-related disorders. The recent description of a diabetic syndrome—acanthosis nigricans with insulin resistance—in which the abnormal receptor function seems to be caused by antireceptor antibodies (101), suggests the fascinating possibility of antigenic receptors, perhaps resulting from impaired immune surveillance and/or environmental insults, such as viral infection. Whether or not mechanisms of this kind play a role in age-associated diseases remains to be seen.

CONCLUDING REMARKS

The study of the relationships between aging and immunity has great practical importance. Some goals based upon this approach include:

1. Attempts to achieve maximum life span by correction of major causes of death of the aged, namely, atherosclerosis-related diseases and neoplasia. The result of this could be a 20-year gain in life expectancy of newborns (102). The expected increase in the population, based on these considerations, could be checked by more efficient contraception and family planning. The mean age of the population will, however, increase as a consequence.
2. The finding that old people with defective cell-mediated immunity have decreased life expectancy, as compared to those with normal T cell function, will justify attempts to identify immune deficiencies in the aged and to institute control measures to correct these deficiencies and/or prevent the consequences of these deficiencies, e.g., infections, neoplasia, autoimmunity, etc. (103).
3. Mechanisms of aging at the cellular and molecular level will also be studied. Emphasis of the research will be on the characterization of abnormalities of cellular interaction in the immune system occurring during aging. Immunoregulation depends on the interaction of different subsets of lymphocytes (T suppressor, T helper, and B cells), macrophages, antibody feedback, and soluble factors. Cellular interactions in the immune system appear to be under genetic control that is related to the major histocompatibility system (104,105). In addition, the exact interrelationship of immune function and viral infection needs to be evaluated. Specific immunotherapy with cells or soluble factors to correct age-associated deficiencies can only be attempted after these interactions are understood.
4. In animals the roles of hypocaloric nutrition in prolonging life seem, from data already at hand, to be one of the most promising approaches to aging and diseases of aging (106). Not only will it be important to explain in both metabolic and immune contexts why low caloric intake prolongs life in rodents (4), interferes with tumor development (107), and alters progression of autoimmune diseases (108), but the use of dietary manipulation will help to dissect the different immune and metabolic functions that become perturbed in the aging individual (109).

REFERENCES

1. Good, R. A., and Yunis, E. J., *Fed. Proc.* **33**, 2040 (1974).
2. Burnet, F. M., *Lancet* **1**, 35 (1970).
3. Walford, R. L., *The Immunologic Theory of Aging,* Munksgaard, Copenhagen, 1969.
4. Comfort, A., *Mech. Ageing Dev.* **3**, 1 (1974).
5. Burnet, F. M., *The Clonal Selection Theory of Acquired Immunity,* Vanderbilt University Press, Nashville, Tenn.
6. Orgel, L. E., *Proc. Natl. Acad. Sci.* **49**, 517 (1963).
7. Orgel, L. E., *Nature* **243**, 441 (1973).
8. Greenberg, L. J., and Yunis, E. J., *Immunology and Aging* (T. Makinodan and E. J. Yunis, eds.), Plenum, New York.

9. Gatti, R. A., and Good, R. A., *Med. Clin. North Am.* **54**, 281 (1970).
10. Greenberg, L. J., and Yunis, E. J., *Gerontologia* **18**, 247 (1972).
11. Hayflick, L., in *Schock Perspective in Experimental Gerontology,* Charles C Thomas, Springfield, Ill., 1966, p. 195.
12. Good, R. A., and Finstad, J., *Natl. Cancer Inst. Monogr.* **31**, 1969, p. 41.
13. Good, R. A., in *Textbook of Medicine,* 14th ed. (P. B. Beeson and W. McDermott, eds.), W. B. Saunders, Philadelphia, 1975a, p. 104.
14. Hansen, J. A., and Good, R. A., *Hum. Pathol.* **5**, 567 (1974).
15. Burnet, F. M., *Intrinsic Mutagenesis.* MTP, Lancaster, England, and John Wiley, New York, 1974.
16. Yunis, E. J., Fernandes, G., and Greenberg, L. J., in *Immunodeficiency in Man and Animals* (D. Bergsma, R. A. Good, and J. Finstad, eds.), Sinauer, Sunderland, Mass., 1975.
17. Hammar, J. A., *Z. Mikrosk. Anat. Forsch.* **6**, 1.
18. Good, R. A., and Gabrielson, A. E., *The Thymus in Immunobiology,* Hoeber Div., Harper and Row, New York, 1964.
19. Roberts-Thomson, I., Whittingham, S., Youngchaiyud, U., and Mackay, I. R., *Lancet* **2**, 368 (1974).
20. Yunis, E. J., and Greenberg, L. J., *Fed. Proc.* **33**, 2017 (1974).
21. Stutman, O., Yunis, E. J., and Good, R. A., *Proc. Soc. Exp. Biol. Med.* **127**, 1204 (1968).
22. Yunis, E. J., Fernandes, G., and Stutman, O., *Am. J. Clin. Pathol.* **56**, 280 (1971).
23. Yunis, E. J., Teague, P. O., Stutman, O., and Good, R. A., *Lab. Invest.* **20**, 46 (1969).
24. Teague, P. O., Yunis, E. J., Rodey, G., Fish, A. J., Stutman, O., and Good, R. A., *Lab. Invest.* **22**, 121 (1970).
25. Krohn, P. L., *Proc. R. Soc. Lond. B.* **157**, 128 (1962).
26. Duquesnoy, R. J., in *Immunodeficiency in Man and Animals* (D. Bergsma, R. A. Good, and J. Finstad, eds.) (*Birth Defects* **11**, 1), Sinauer, Sunderland, Mass. 1975, p. 536.
27. Tuft, L., Hock, V. M., and Gregory, D. C., *J. Allergy* **26**, 359 (1955).
28. Gross, L., *Cancer* **18**, 201 (1965).
29. Giannini, D., and Sloan, R. S., *Lancet* **1**, 525 (1957).
30. Pisciotta, A. V., Westring, D. W., DePrey, C., and Walsh, G., *Nature* **215**, 193 (1967).
31. Hallgren, H. M., Buckley, C. E., III, Gilbertsen, V. A., and Yunis, E. J., *J. Immunol.* **111**, 1101 (1973).
32. Krohn, P. L., *Gerontologia* (Basel) **5**, 182 (1961).
33. Mariani, T., Martinez, C., Smith, J. M., and Good, R. A., *Ann. N. Y. Acad. Sci.* **87**, 93 (1960).
34. Gerbase-DeLima, M., Meredith, P., and Walford, R. L., *Fed. Proc.* **34**, 159 (1975).
35. Adler, W., Takiguchi, T., and Smith, R. T., *J. Immunol.* **107**, 1357 (1971).
36. Konen, T. G., Smith, G. S., and Walford, R. L., *J. Immunol.* **110**, 1216 (1973).
37. Hung, C.-Y., Perkins, E. H., and Yank, W.-K., *Mech. Ageing Dev.* **4**, 29 (1975).
38. Bach, J. F., Dardenne, M., and Salomen, J. C., *Clin. Exp. Immunol.* **14**, 274 (1973).
39. Dauphinee, M. J., Talal, N., Goldstein, A. L., and White, A., *Proc. Natl. Acad. Sci.* **71**, 2637.
40. Fernandes, G., Yunis, E. J., and Good, R. A., *Clin. Immunol. Immunopathol.* **6** (1976).
41. Hallgren, H., *et al.,* unpublished observations.
42. Yunis, E. J., Hong, R., Grewe, M. A., Martinez, C., Cornelius, E., and Good, R. A., *J. Exp. Med.* **125**, 947 (1967).
43. Price, G. B., and Makinodan, T., *J. Immunol.* **108**, 413 (1972).
44. Price, G. B., and Makinodan, T., *J. Immunol.* **108**, 403 (1972).
45. Makinodan, T., and Adler, W., *Fed. Proc.* **34**, 153 (1975).
46. Perkins, E. H., and Makinodan, T., in *Proc. First Rocky Mt. Symp. on Aging,* Colorado State University, Fort Collins, 1971, p. 80.
47. Hendrick, M. L., and Makinodan, T., *J. Immunol.* **111**, 1502 (1973).
48. Makinodan, T., and Adler, W., *Fed. Proc.* **34**, 153 (1975).
49. Hendrick, M. L., *Gerontologia* **12**, 28 (1972).
50. Hallgren, H., and Yunis, E. J., Submitted for publication.
51. Barthhold, D. F., Kysela, S., and Steinberg, A. D., *J. Immunol.* **112**, 9 (1974).
52. Waldmann, T. A., Durm, M., Broder, S., Blackman, M., Blaese, R. M., and Strober, W., *Lancet* **2**, 609 (1974).
53. Broder, S., Humphrey, R., Durm, M., Blackman, M., Meade, B., Goldman, C., Strober, W., and Waldmann, T., *N. Engl. J. Med.* **293**, 887 (1975).

54. Hirsh, M. S., in *The Role of Immunological Factors in Viral and Oncogenic Processes* (R. F. Beers, Jr., R. C. Tilghsman, and E. G. Busset, eds.), Johns Hopkins University Press, Baltimore, 1974, p. 177.
55. Allison, A. C., and Law, L. W., *Proc. Soc. Exp. Biol. Med.* **127**, 207 (1968).
56. Dent, P. B., Peterson, R. D. A., and Good, R. A., *Proc. Soc. Exp. Biol. Med.* **119**, 86 (1965).
57. Hotchin, J. E., in *Tolerance, Autoimmunity and Aging* (M. M. Siegel and R. A. Good, eds.), Charles C. Thomas, Springfield, Ill., 1972, p. 132.
58. Levy, J. A., *Am. J. Clin. Pathol.* **62**, 258 (1974).
59. Hotchin, J., *Am. J. Clin. Pathol.* **56**, 333 (1971).
60. Oldstone, M. B. A., *Am. J. Clin. Pathol.* **56**, 299 (1971).
61. Howie, J. B., and Heyler, B. J., *Adv. Immunol.* **9**, 215 (1968).
62. Gross, L.: *Oncogenic Viruses,* 2d ed., Perejamon Press, London, 1970.
63. Mellors, R. C., *Am. J. Clin. Pathol.* **56**, 270 (1971).
64. Mellors, R. C., Shirai, T., Aoki, T., Juebner, R. J., and Krauczynski, P., *J. Exp. Med.* **133**, 113 (1971).
65. Dixon, F. J., Oldstone, M. B. A., and Tonietti, G., *J. Exp. Med.* **134**, 65s (1971).
66. Lambert, P. H., and Dixon, F. J., *Clin. Exp. Immunol.* **6**, 829 (1970).
67. Chused, T. M., Steinberg, A. D., and Parker, L. M., *J. Immunol.* **111**, 52 (1973).
68. Talal, N., Steinberg, A. D., Jacobs, M. C., Chused, T. M., and Gazdar, A. F., *J. Exp. Med.* **134**, 52s (1971).
69. Tonietti, Oldstone, M. B. A., and Depon, F. J., *J. Exp. Med.* **132**, 89 (1970).
70. Cannat, A., and Varet, B., *Immunol. Commun.* **2**, 527 (1973).
71. Croken, B. P., Jr., Del Villano, B. C., Jensen, F. C., Lerner, R. A., and Dixon, F. J., *J. Exp. Med.* **140**, 1028 (1975).
72. Barnett, E. V., Williams, R. C., Kenyon, A. J., and Hanson, J. E., *Immunology* **16**, 241 (1969).
73. Porter, D. D., Larsen, A. E., Porter, H. G., *J. Exp. Med.* **130**, 575 (1969).
74. Chesebro, B., Bloom, M., Hadlow, W., and Race, R., *Nature* **254**, 456 (1975).
75. Hensen, J. B., and McGuire, T. C., *Am. J. Clin. Pathol.* **56**, 306 (1971).
76. Lewis, R. M., Schwartz, R., and Henry, W. B., Jr., *Blood* **25**, 143 (1965).
77. Lewis, R. M., and Schwartz, R. S., *J. Exp. Med.* **134**, 417 (1971).
78. Lewis, R. M., Andre-Schwartz, J., Harris, G. S., Hirsh, M. S., Black, P. H., and Schwartz, R. S., *J. Clin. Invest.* **52**, 1893 (1973).
79. Lewis, R. M., Tannenberg, W., Smith, Ce., and Schwartz, R. S., *Nature* **252**, 78 (1974).
80. Fresco, R., *N. Engl. J. Med.* **26**, 1231 (1970).
81. Goodman, J. R., Sylvester, R. A., Talal, N., and Tuffanelli, D. L., *Ann. Intern. Med.* **79**, 396 (1973).
82. Grimley, M., Decker, L., Michelitch, J., and Frantz, M. M., *Arthritis Rheum.* **16**, 313 (1973).
83. Strand, M., and August, J. T., *J. Virol.* **14**, 1584 (1974).
84. Panem, S., Ordonez, N. G., Kirstein, W. H., Katz, A. I., and Spargo, B. H., *N. Engl. J. Med.* **295**, 470 (1976).
85. Gocke, D. J., Hsu, K., Morgan, C., et al., *Lancet* **2**, 1149 (1970).
86. Hunter, G. D., *J. Infect. Dis.* **125**, 427 (1972).
87. Stone, L. B., Takenoto, K. K., and Marten, M. A., *J. Virol.* **8**, 573 (1971).
88. Marsh, R. F., and Hanson, R. P., *J. Virol.* **3**, 176 (1969).
89. Appel, M. J. G., *Am. J. Vet. Res.* **30**, 1167 (1969).
90. Gibbs, C. J., and Gajdusek, D. C., in *Membranes and Viruses in Immunopathology* (S. B. Day and R. A. Good, eds.), Academic Press, New York 1972, p. 411.
91. East, J., and Branca, M., *Clin. Exp. Immunol.* **4**, 621 (1969).
92. Mellors, R. C., *Blood* **27**, 435 (1966).
93. Cure, S. F., and Cremer, N. E., *J. Immunol.* **102**, 1349 (1969).
94. Dent, P. B., *Prog. Med. Virol.* **14**, 1 (1972).
95. Friedman, H., and Ceglowski, W. S., in *The Role of Immunological Factors in Viral and Oncogenic Processes,* Johns Hopkins University Press, Baltimore, 1974, p. 187.
96. Dausset, J., *Proc. First Int. Symp. on HLA and Disease,* Paris, 1976.
97. McDevitt, H. O., and Bodmer, W. F., *Lancet* **1**, 1269 (1974).
98. Walford, R. L., *Fed. Proc.* **33**, 2020 (1974).
99. Matthews, J., *Lancet* **2**, 681 (1975).
100. Greenberg, L. G., and Yunis, E. J., manuscript in preparation.

101. Kahn, C. R., Flier, J. S., Bar, R. S., et al., *N. Engl. J. Med.* **294**, 739 (1976).
102. Siegel, J. S., and O'Leary, W. E., Some demographic aspects of aging in the United States. In *Current Population Reports,* U.S. Bureau of the Census, Series 023, No. 43, pp. 1-30, U.S. Government Printing Office, Washington, D.C., 1973.
103. Walford, R., in *Immunology and Aging* (T. Makinodan and E. J. Yunis, eds.), Plenum, New York.
104. Dupont, B., Hanson, J. A., and Yunis, E. J., *Advances in Immunology,* Academic Press, New York (in press).
105. Benacerraf, B., Bluestein, H. G., Green, I., and Ellman, L., in *Progress in Immunology* (D. B. Amos, ed.), Academic Press, New York, 1971, p. 487.
106. Fernandes, G., Good, R. A., and Yunis, E. J., in *Immunology and Aging* (T. Makinodan and E. J. Yunis, eds.), Plenum Press, New York.
107. Fernandes, G., Yunis, E. J., and Good, R. A., *Nature* (in press).
108. Fernandes, G., Yunis, E. J., and Good, R. A., *Proc. Natl. Acad. Sci.* **73**, 1279 (1976).
109. Good, R. A., Fernandes, G., Yunis, E. J., Cooper, W. C., Jose, D. G., Kramer, T. C., and Hansen, M. A., *Am. J. Pathol.* **86**, 599 (1976).

Chapter Seven

Immunoregulation in Tolerance and Autoimmunity

MICHAEL V. DOYLE, D. ELLIOT PARKS, CAROLE G. ROMBALL, WILLIAM O. WEIGLE

Scripps Clinic and Research Foundation, Department of Immunopathology, La Jolla, California

The immune system may respond to the presence of antigen in several different ways. The host may (1) produce circulating antibody of various classes and avidities, (2) develop a delayed hypersensitivity response, (3) generate immunologic memory for the antigen, or (4) become unresponsive. The generation of immunologic unresponsiveness upon contact with antigen represents a major, critical aspect of the mechanisms controlling immune responses because of the duration of its effects on the immunocompetency of the host. A thorough investigation of the phenomenon of tolerance is basic to any attempt to increase our theoretical and experimental knowledge of both fundamental immunobiologic systems and pathologic states. Equally important is the fact that analysis of the tolerant state can lead to the development of clinically useful tools and techniques for therapeutic and prophylactic application to the treatment of human disease states.

To analyze and describe the phenomenon of immunologic tolerance, two basic approaches have been developed. Antigen-directed unresponsiveness to foreign substances is one of these major areas of research. This approach to the study of

This is Publication No. 1198 from the Department of Immunopathology, Scripps Clinic and Research Foundation. The experimental work was supported by United States Public Health Service Grant AI-07007, Atomic Energy Administration Contract E (04–3)–410, American Cancer Society Grant IM-42F, and National Institutes of Health Grant AI-12449. Michael V. Doyle was the recipient of a National Institutes of Health Fellowship Award AI-01023. D. Elliot Parks was the recipient of National Institutes of Health Fellowship Award AI-05012. William O. Weigle was the recipient of United States Public Health Service Research Career Award 5-K6-GM-6936.

tolerance is based in part upon the hypothesis of Burnet and Fenner (1) suggesting that animals can develop antigen-specific unresponsiveness as a consequence of contact with foreign and self-antigens during neonatal life. A variety of foreign antigens and animal species have subsequently been used to prove that under selective conditions, tolerance can be induced in adults as well as in neonates. Such investigations, in which tolerance to a foreign antigen is studied, present the researcher with the opportunity for manipulating and defining the details of the system, such as the type and dosage of the antigen, the animals to be used, and the nature of the immune response to be studied. The experimenter can obtain direct answers to precise questions as to the kinetics of the induction, maintenance, and termination of tolerance, and the cell types involved and their interactions. One inherent disadvantage of such controlled approaches is that, because of their structured nature, they may offer a less relevant application to analysis of clinical disease states than many systems that study tolerance to self-antigens. The second method for studying the tolerant state involves investigation into unresponsiveness to self-antigens and the acquisition of anti-self-immune reactivity. The state of immune responsiveness to self-antigens occurs naturally in certain disease or clinical situations and can also be induced experimentally. Such systems of self-tolerance are difficult to study and analyze experimentally because of the limitations in experimental manipulation. They do, however, offer the advantage that they may have more direct clinical significance.

The purpose of this chapter is to present experimental results from research employing both of these approaches to the study of tolerance and to discuss their interpretation with reference to our understanding of the mechanisms responsible for the induction, maintenance, and termination of the state of immunologic unresponsiveness. In addition, an experimental system is described in which alternating phases of enhancement and suppression occur during an immune response. The possible involvement of such fluctuations in some forms of autoimmunity and persistent infection is discussed.

TOLERANCE TO FOREIGN ANTIGENS

There exists an extremely broad diversity of systems and models for studying antigen-induced unresponsiveness in animals. Many of these have been recently reviewed in detail and will not be presented here (2,3). Rather, an attempt will be made to present a few of the mechanisms that have been postulated as being responsible for the control of tolerance and to describe some of the specific systems providing evidence for those models. Special attention will be directed to defining the roles of thymus-derived (T) cells and bone marrow-derived (B) cells in these systems.

Effector Cell Blockade

One cellular mechanism proposed to account for the phenomenon of tolerance is the blockade of receptors at the surface of antigen-reactive cells, particularly antibody-forming cells (AFC). Baker et al. (4) reported that supraoptimal, immunizing doses of the T-independent antigen type III pneumococcal polysaccharide (SIII) results in dose-dependent reduction in the magnitude of the antibody response in vivo, as well as the rate of antibody synthesis and release by AFC in vitro. The authors suggested, on the basis of this observation, that tolerance may represent a reduction in the rate of antibody synthesis by specific B cells. This proposal that tolerance to SIII is due to inactivation of AFC by surface-associated antigen is supported by the work of Howard (5). He showed that the number of cells able to bind SIII is greater in the spleens of unresponsive mice than in the spleens of normal mice. Also, transfer of tolerant spleen cells to irradiated recipients results in the immediate loss of unresponsiveness. This phenomenon of blockade of AFC with antigen has been examined by Schrader and Nossal (6) and by Klaus (7) using hapten-substituted, T cell-independent antigens such as 2,4-dinitrophenyl polymerized flagellin (DNP-POL). The experiments involved injecting animals with antigenic forms of hapten-substituted proteins or polysaccharides to generate AFC to the hapten, exposing the lymphocytes to the tolerance-inducing molecules in vivo or in vitro, and measuring the level of antihapten response. The results indicate that multivalent antigens can suppress the immune response to hapten by inhibiting the ability of AFC to secrete antibody.

The possibility that a similar mechanism of cell blockade may operate at the level of the B cell precursor for AFC has been investigated by Aldo-Benson and Borel (8). Mice were made tolerant to DNP by injection of DNP-mouse gamma globulin. The hypothesis that tolerance to the hapten is due to blockade of hapten-reactive cells by the tolerance-inducing substance was examined using ^{125}I-labeled anti-DNP antibody to detect cells with surface-bound hapten. The cells from animals made unresponsive to DNP bind significantly more anti-DNP antibody than normal, control animals, indicating the presence of DNP on those cells. One additional aspect of this model of tolerance is its reversibility. Spleen cells from tolerant animals remain unresponsive to antigenic challenge upon transfer to lethally irradiated, syngeneic mice. However, incubation of the cells in vitro for 24 hours prior to transfer results in the loss of unresponsiveness (9). The authors suggest that this is due to shedding or capping of the surface-bound hapten, resulting in liberation of the lymphocyte receptors for interaction with antigen and accessory cells. More recently, Scott (10) showed that rats injected with fluorescein-labeled tolerogen possess detectable antigen-binding cells only during the first ten days after injection. Furthermore, one week after the initial injection, reinjection of the fluoresceinated tolerogen does not result in the appearance of any labeled cells. These results suggest that antigen blockade may be a transient phenomenon and that the tolerant state is the result of a central unresponsive state independent of cell-associated tolerogen.

A system involving blockade of reactive cells by free hapten has been developed by Gronowicz et al. (11). They induced unresponsiveness in mice by injection of 3,5 dinitro-4-hydroxy-phenacetyl (NNP) azide. Treated animals do not respond to injection of NNP-horse red blood cells. Evidence that the tolerance is due to hapten blockade of the antigen-reactive cells was reported in a recent paper by these workers (12). They showed that the spleen cells of tolerant mice can be activated to produce normal levels of antihapten AFC by incubation in vitro with the B cell mitogen, lipopolysaccharide (LPS). The authors suggest that tolerance is maintained by hapten blockade of the antigen-reactive cells, but that these cells can be induced to differentiate under appropriate conditions. Möller et al. (13) reported a similar effect of LPS on the immune response of cells made tolerant to fluoroiso-thiocyanate-human gamma globulin (FITC-HGG). When cultured in vitro with high concentrations of LPS, the tolerant spleen cells produce as many anti-FITC AFC as do normal cells.

An important aspect of the model of tolerance by antigen blockade, when applying it to systems of self-tolerance, is its reversibility and its dosage requirements. This hypothesis would only appear to be valid for the maintenance of tolerance to self-antigens under conditions in which the lymphocytes are constantly exposed to large doses of the antigens. Such would be the case for many of the serum proteins. However, self-tolerance to antigens that are present in low amounts, that are sequestered, or to which the lymphocytes are not routinely exposed, as in the case of neuronal antigens, thyroglobulin, and hormones, may require additional hypotheses or explanations (see below).

Suppressor T Cells

Recently, a large body of information has accumulated from investigation of a model of tolerance in which T cells actively suppress the immune response. Since the early work of Claman and co-workers (reviewed in ref. 14) and Miller and Mitchell (reviewed in ref. 15), it has become clear that cooperation between thymus-derived cells and bone marrow-derived cells is necessary to produce AFC to many antigens. Those T cells that cooperate with AFC precursor cells and antigen to induce the differentiation to plasma cells or to memory cells are referred to as helper T cells. The regulatory role for T cells in the immune response to antigen has more recently been shown also to include an inhibitory capacity. Those T cells that cause an inhibition of the immune response can be thought of as acting in an opposing manner to the helper T cells and are referred to as suppressor T cells.

One of the first reports indicating the suppressive capacity of thymus-derived lymphocytes was that of Horiuchi and Waksman (16), who showed that intrathymic injection of bovine gamma globulin in rats induces a state of hyporesponsiveness to subsequent antigenic challenge as assayed by the AFC response in the spleen. Since then, the pioneering work of Gershon and Kondo (17) has clearly established the existence of suppressor T cells. They showed that the addition of thymocytes to thymectomized, lethally irradiated, bone marrow-reconstituted mice during treatment with large numbers of sheep red blood cells (SRBC) results in unresponsiveness to challenge with SRBC. The IgM and IgG AFC responses of these animals are suppressed when the recipients are injected with normal thymocytes and challenged with SRBC. In addition, the spleen cells of these specifically unresponsive animals can suppress the ability of normal thymocytes to cooperate with normal bone marrow cells when challenged with SRBC after transfer to naïve, irradiated recipients. More recent work indicates that the suppressive activity can be specifically abrogated by treatment of the tolerant spleen cells with anti-theta serum and complement (18).

The system employed by Droege (19) to study tolerance mediated by T suppressor cells has enabled him physically to separate subpopulations of T cells. The data demonstrate that if normal thymocytes are transferred to a normal chicken and if repeated injections of the antigen, *Brucella abortus,* are administered, the birds become specifically unresponsive. The normal thymocyte population is suggested to have developed a population of T suppressor cells. However, if the thymocytes are taken from previously bursectomized chickens, then the recipient animals are not tolerized by the administration of large doses of *B. abortus*. These thymocyte populations from bursectomized birds are proposed to be lacking in the subpopulation of T suppressor cells or their precursors. Using electrophoretic mobility and cell size as criteria for the separation of T cell subpopulations, Droege has demonstrated that the pattern produced by normal thymocytes from control birds differs from the pattern developed by the thymocytes from bursectomized animals. The former cell population contains an additional subpopulation of small, low-charge, dense cells. Since that subpopulation is present in the thymocyte population that develops suppressive activity, and is absent from the population that does not develop such activity, this cell type is suggested to be the T suppressor cell.

Suppressor T cells have also been generated and their activity demonstrated in vitro. Dutton and co-workers (reviewed in ref. 20) and Rich and Pierce (21) have shown that when spleen cells from mice are incubated in vitro in the presence of the T cell mitogen, concanavalin A (Con A), there is a marked inhibition of the AFC response to SRBC. Mixing Con A-treated spleen cells with normal spleen cells causes inhibition of the normal spleen cell response. This suppressive activity is sensitive to anti-theta serum and complement treatment, indicating the requirement for T cells. In addition, under certain conditions of Con A stimulation, a population of helper T cells is generated. Evidently, there is a balance or competition between the ability of Con A to induce T suppressor or T helper cells. In fact, depending on the conditions of cell treatment and the assay used, both T cell helper and T cell suppressor activities can be generated by Con A (22). Tse and Dutton (23) have reported the physical separation and biologic characterization of these stimulator and suppressor T cells using Ficoll velocity sedimentation gradients. In this situation, the helper activity is associated with a population of small cells, while the population of larger cells exhibits the suppressive activity. One important difference between this system of T cell suppression and most others is that the suppressive activity is not antigen-specific. This may reflect the fact that a nonspecific activator, in this case, Con A, is used to induce the T suppressor cells.

In all these systems of T suppressor activity, the AFC immune response that is inhibited is of the IgM or of the IgG antibody class or both. However, the production of IgE or reaginic antibody can also be inhibited by T cells. Takatsu and Ishizaka (24) demonstrated the presence of T suppressor cells in the spleens of mice that were primed with ovalbumin and then injected with urea-denatured ovalbumin. These T cells will inhibit the ability of normal spleen cells to produce either IgG or IgE anti-DNP antibodies upon challenge with DNP-ovalbumin. Tada et al. (25) have demonstrated the presence of T suppressor cells in antigen-primed animals. Using a number of different systems of antigens and injections, they showed that IgM, IgG, or IgE antibody production can each be inhibited by T cells.

The association of T suppressor cells with immunologically unresponsive cell populations has been investigated in several systems. The demonstration of such an association has important implications for any model of the mechanism for the maintenance of the tolerant state. A short review of some of these reports will serve to emphasize the variety of models of tolerance that have suppressive activity associated with them and the spectrum of approaches to research in this area.

Nachtigal et al. (26) have induced unresponsiveness to human serum albumin (HSA) by serial injections of high doses of the antigen. The ability of the mice to respond to HSA reaches a maximum after the fourth or fifth injection, and the responses to subsequent injections are markedly reduced. The spleen cells from these tolerant animals inhibit the AFC response of normal spleen cells when both are transferred to lethally irradiated recipients and challenged with HSA. This suppressive activity is abrogated if the tolerant spleen cells are treated with anti-theta serum and complement to remove T cells. Also present in the unresponsive spleen cell populations is a set of T helper cells. These two populations are distinguishable by their sensitivity to irradiation. The suppressive activity is sensitive to doses of irradiation between 400 R and 700 R, whereas the helper activity is inhibited between 700 R and 900 R.

An association between the phenomenon of genetically determined unresponsiveness in mice to the synthetic terpolymer L-glutamic acid^{60} -L-alanine^{30} -L-tyrosine^{10} (GAT) and T suppressor cells has been demonstrated by Kapp et al. (27). Treatment of a nonresponder strain of mice with free GAT produces a state of unresponsiveness to challenge with the normally immunogenic molecule GAT-MBSA (GAT covalently linked to methylated bovine serum albumin). The unresponsive spleen cell population can actively suppress the ability of an untreated spleen cell population to respond to GAT-MBSA.

The cells from animals made tolerant to contact sensitization by haptens also express suppressive activity in certain systems. Phanuphak and co-workers (28) can specifically prevent the generation of contact sensitivity in mice to DNP by pretreatment of the mice with DNB-sulfonate. This unresponsiveness to DNP is transferred to normal recipients with unresponsive lymph node or spleen cells and is sensitive to treatment with anti-theta serum and complement.

A similar system has been developed by Asherson and Zembala (reviewed in ref. 29). They have shown the presence of T suppressor cells in lymph node and spleen cells from mice made tolerant to sensitization by picryl chloride. An interesting aspect of their work is that they can demonstrate production of a suppressive factor by tolerant cells (see below). This factor is taken up by adherent cells that consequently become suppressive themselves. In addition, whereas the original, tolerant cell population is specifically inhibitory for the response of normal spleen cells to picryl chloride, the suppressive, adherent cells are nonspecifically inhibitory.

Finally, Basten and co-workers (30,31), Benjamin (32), and Weigle et al. (33–35) have reported the presence of suppressive activity and suppressor T cells in association with the spleen cells of mice made tolerant to human gamma globulin. The interpretation of these data and their relevance to the maintenance of immunologic tolerance are examined in detail below.

The mechanism responsible for the suppressive activity associated with T cells from tolerant (36,37) and from antigen-primed (38) cell populations has been investigated at the molecular level. These experiments are designed to isolate and to characterize the substance(s) responsible for the suppressive activity generated by T cells. The factors described in these reports all have similar characteristics. They have molecular weights ranging from 35,000 to 50,000 daltons, have affinity for the antigen used to generate the suppression, and carry determinants of the H-2 mouse histocompatibility locus. It is interesting that these characteristics also describe a helper factor that has been demonstrated by Munro et al. (39) to be able to replace helper T cells in the immune response to a synthetic polypeptide antigen. Investigations such as these give promise to the goal of describing in molecular and cellular terms the interactions between T cells, B cells, and accessory cells that lead to either an enhanced immune response or a suppression of that response. In addition, these data may have important clinical implications with regard to controlling responses such as the IgE-mediated, allergic response to allergens.

Clonal Deletion

A conceptually simple and appealing model of unresponsiveness is based on the clonal deletion theory proposed by Burnet and Fenner (1). To explain tolerance to self-antigens, they postulated that unresponsiveness was due to the elimination of lymphocytes that possess specific receptors for that antigen. Essentially, their theory proposes a negative clonal selection of antigen-reactive cells in which the specific lymphocytes are deleted rather than activated by contact with antigen (see ref. 40 for a discussion of the clonal selection theory). Evidence consistent with this proposal has been reported by Nossal and Pike (41). They suggest that there is an early stage in the differentiation of lymphocytes from stem cells in which the cells possess receptors for antigen and during which stage they are obligately eliminated by contact with antigen under the appropriate conditions. The authors refer to this proposal as the clonal abortion theory, since the cells are aborted prior to developing into fully competent lymphocytes. The results indicate that in vitro culture of mouse bone marrow cells in the presence of antigen results in the subsequent unresponsiveness of these cells to that antigen when they are transferred to lethally irradiated, syngeneic recipients. Extremely low concentrations of monomeric antigen are sufficient to induce a specific tolerance in the B cells of the bone marrow, though not in the B cells of spleen cell cultures. The kinetics of the induction of tolerance are similar to the kinetics of the generation of Ig-positive, small lymphocytes in the marrow cultures. Finally, the effect of the continuous presence of antigen is to prevent the emergence of new, competent, antigen-reactive cells, rather than to eliminate preexisting cells. The data are consistent with the clonal abortion hypothesis, although the results are subject to alternative interpretations, such as receptor blockade by antigen.

A similar study has recently been reported by Metcalf and Klinman (42), who can induce tolerance to DNP in neonatal, but not adult, spleen cells by incubation with the antigen in vitro.

Another approach to testing the clonal deletion hypothesis has been to determine whether immunologically unresponsive animals possess specific antigen-binding cells (ABC). Antigen-binding lymphocytes are detected using radiolabeled antigen and autoradiography. Unfortunately, experiments with several different systems have provided conflicting results. The work of Ada et al. (43), Cooper et al. (44), and Humphrey and Keller (45) shows a normal number of ABC to flagellin, to hemocyanin, and to a synthetic polypeptide antigen in specifically unresponsive animals. By contrast, Naor and Sulitzeanu (46), Katz et al. (47), and Louis et al. (48) have reported a reduced level of specific ABC in mice tolerant to bovine serum albumin (BSA), to DNP, or to human gamma globulin, respectively. A problem with the interpretation of these latter results is the possibility that the reduced number of ABC may be due to blockade of the specific cells with the tolerizing antigen which prevents binding by the radiolabeled molecules, rather than due to elimination of the specific cells.

In conclusion, although the theory of clonal deletion is intellectually attractive because of its simplicity, there is no compelling evidence to support it. This is due in part to an inherent problem in the study of this theory of tolerance, because it is difficult to design an experiment to distinguish between the physical deletion of antigen-reactive lymphocytes and their functional inactivation, either permanently or temporarily.

CELLULAR EVENTS IN UNRESPONSIVENESS TO SERUM PROTEINS

Heterologous serum proteins are extremely useful probes for the investigation of immunologic unresponsiveness. They can be purified in large quantities and equilibrate rapidly in vivo between the intra- and extravascular fluid spaces, thereby, theoretically, reaching all immunocompetent cells. The immune response to these antigens can be readily quantitated at the cellular level in terms of the number of plaque-forming cells (PFC) by a modification (49) of the Jerne plaque assay (50). This method circumvents the danger of serologic testing where free antigen can mask circulating antibody. Finally, changing the physical states of the gamma globulins renders them either immunogenic or tolerogenic (51). In heat-aggregated form, gamma globulins are immunogenic, whereas the removal of aggregated material by ultracentrifugation yields a tolerogenic, aggregate-free preparation (52).

A single injection of deaggregated human gamma globulin (DHGG) into adult A/J mice results in a state of complete, long-lived, and specific unresponsiveness. Tolerized mice are totally refractive to subsequent challenges with HGG in the heat-aggregated, immunogenic form (AHGG). These mice are specifically tolerant to HGG and are able to mount a normal immune response to unrelated antigens such as fowl gamma globulin (53,54).

Induction

The antibody response to AHGG is T-dependent, requiring helper T cell function (55). Thus, the investigation of the cellular site(s) of the induction, maintenance, and termination of immunologic unresponsiveness requires an analysis of the immune status of both the T and B cells. Isakovic et al. (56) and Taylor (57) were among the first to demonstrate that immunologic unresponsiveness can be induced at the T cell level using heterologous serum proteins. Subsequently, several workers have shown the induction of tolerance in the bone marrow cells (58,59). Chiller et al. (60) demonstrated that mice treated with tolerogen (DHGG) possess both specifically unresponsive thymus cells and bone marrow cells and that tolerance in the intact animal can be maintained by unresponsiveness in either population alone. In these experiments, tolerant thymus cells and normal bone marrow cells, or tolerant bone marrow cells and normal thymus cells, were transferred into lethally irradiated, syngeneic recipients. Such recipients are tolerant if either the thymus cells or bone marrow cells are obtained from an unresponsive donor because cooperation between antigen-reactive T and B cells is not possible. An animal can also be rendered unresponsive by removing either specifically responsive T or B cells using an antigen suicide technique (61).

The kinetics of the induction of tolerance, which are shown in Table 1, are not the same for all cell populations (62). Unresponsiveness is complete in the thymus cells by 24 hours following the injection of tolerogen. In contrast, responsiveness in bone marrow cells does not begin to wane until eight days after tolerization and is not completely absent until 21 days. Whereas the timing of tolerance induction in splenic T cells parallels that in thymus cells, unresponsiveness occurs much more rapidly in the splenic B cells (by three days) than in bone marrow cells (63). Thus, tolerance is established in the intact animal very soon after the injection of tolerogen, i.e., as T cells become unresponsive. This is possible because unresponsiveness to a T-dependent antigen can be maintained in an animal whose T cells are tolerant, but whose B cells are immunocompetent. A similar state of unresponsiveness also exists during the termination of the unresponsive state, as discussed below.

The dose of tolerogen employed to establish an immunologic unresponsive state can dictate both the cell types tolerized and the duration of the unresponsive state. Generally, the degree of unresponsiveness is directly proportional to the amount of material injected (64–66). Thymus cells and bone marrow cells differ markedly in their susceptibility to the induction of unresponsiveness by moderate doses of DHGG (67) and BSA (68). A dose of 10^{-2} mg of DHGG induces unresponsiveness in thymus cells, whereas 2.5 mg is necessary to induce complete tolerance in bone marrow cells. The susceptibility of splenic B cells to tolerance induction is intermediate to that of thymus cells and bone marrow cells, requiring at least 0.5 mg of DHGG (see Fig. 1). Furthermore, the unresponsive state of the splenic B cell population is of longer duration with increasing tolerogenic doses. Rajewsky and Brenig (69) have demonstrated similar differences in the dose dependency of peripheral T and B cells to the induction of unresponsiveness to serum albumins. Thus, a considerably higher dose of tolerogen and longer period of induction are required to tolerize bone marrow cells than to render thymus or peripheral T cells unresponsive.

The dose of tolerogen required to establish complete unresponsiveness also varies from one strain of mouse to another (66). For example, Das and Leskowitz have shown that while DBA/2 mice are tolerized by an injection of 0.2 mg of deaggregated bovine gamma globulin (BGG), BALB/c mice remain responsive after a 100-fold greater dose of tolerogen (70). It has been suggested that mac-

Table 1. Temporal Pattern of Immunologic Tolerance to Human Gamma Globulin (HGG) in Various Lymphoid Tissues of A/J Mice[a]

Tissue	Days of Induction	Days of Maintenance
Whole animal	<1	130–150
Thymus	<1	120–135
Bone marrow	8–15	40–50
Spleen: T cells	<1	120–150
B cells	2–4	40–50

[a]Based on accumulated data using A/J male mice given 2.5 mg deaggregated HGG.

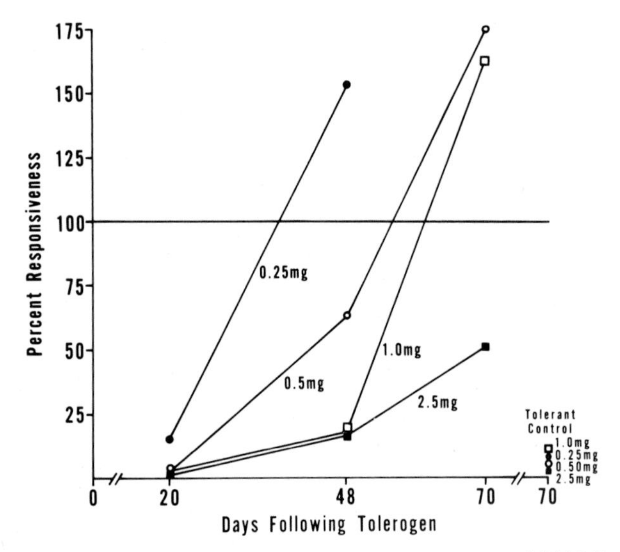

Figure 1. Adult A/J mice were tolerized with 0.25, 0.5, 1.0, or 2.5 mg of DHGG and challenged at various times following tolerogen with 400g of AHGG and 50g of LPS. Indirect plaque-forming cells were enumerated six days after challenge. Mice not given DHGG represent 100% responsiveness.

rophages play a major role in the establishment of unresponsiveness and may be the cells responsible for this resistance to tolerance induction in the BALB/c mouse. The active participation of macrophages favors the induction of immunity rather than tolerance (71,72). In addition, the role of macrophages, although nonspecific, is under genetic control (73). As antigen bound to macrophages can be more immunogenic than antigen in its soluble form (74), the macrophages of the BALB/c mice may process trace amounts of aggregates present in the tolerogen, thereby initiating an immune response before the unresponsive state can be established (75).

Interference with the Induction of Unresponsiveness

Nonspecific factors may modify the tolerogenic signal at the surface of either B or T cells, voiding that signal or rendering the signal immunogenic. Claman (76) demonstrated that the injection of bacterial lipopolysaccharide (LPS) with deaggregated BGG interferes with the induction of unresponsiveness to BGG. Similar experiments by Golub and Weigle (77) employing LPS and DHGG demonstrated that the temporal relationship between the injection of the tolerogen and LPS is critical. More recently, Louis et al. (78) have extended these observations. When LPS is injected with tolerogen (DHGG), it is found that (1) the induction of unresponsiveness in B cells is inhibited; (2) a primary antibody response is engendered; and (3) the secondary response of splenic B cells to subsequent AHGG challenge is T-independent in the face of an unresponsive state in the peripheral T cells (54,79).

The polynucleotide, poly A:U, also acts as a strong adjuvant for several antigens (80) and has been shown to interfere with the induction of unresponsiveness to BGG (81,82) and to HGG (83). Similar to the findings with LPS, tolerance induction is inhibited only when poly A:U is injected within 12 hours after the tolerogen (81). However, in contrast to the findings with LPS, both the adjuvanticity (84) and the interference with the induction of tolerance (83) by poly A:U are mediated by T cells rather than B cells, which are the target of the LPS effects. Thus, both T and B cells appear to remain responsive after treatment with poly A:U and tolerogen, contrary to the state of unresponsiveness induced by tolerogen and LPS where only the B cells remain immunocompetent.

Preparations of cobra venom factor (CoF) have also been implicated in the inhibition of the induction of tolerance. This anticomplementary protein enzymatically converts the complement component C3 to its active form when complexed with the C3 proactivator molecule (85). It has been reported that the injection of CoF into A/J mice three hours after the injection of DHGG will inhibit the induction of an unresponsive state to HGG and that this interference is attributable to the anticomplementary properties of CoF (86). However, it has also been reported that (1) CoF preparations that have lost their ability to activate C3 are still effective in interfering with the induction of tolerance (87); (2) certain preparations of highly purified anticomplementary CoF do not possess the ability to interfere with tolerance induction (88); and (3) the anticomplementary and interference activities of CoF can readily be dissociated by column chromatography on Sephadex G-200 (87). Therefore, it appears that the factor responsible for the inhibition of the unresponsive state is a contaminant in the CoF preparations.

Interference with the tolerogenic signal can also be accomplished by allogeneic cells when they are injected with DHGG (89). Inhibition of the induction of unresponsiveness with allogeneic cells apparently involves the activation of T lymphocytes during the graft-versus-host (GVH) reaction. This "allogeneic effect" can also interfere with the state of unresponsiveness induced in mice by the obligate tolerogen, DNP-D-GL (90). Under appropriate conditions, allogeneic cells can also terminate the unresponsive state, as will be discussed below.

Maintenance

The duration of the unresponsive state to HGG in mice varies among the T and B cells of various lymphoid compartments, as shown in Table 1. Thymus cells remain completely unresponsive for at least 120 days, which is reflected by tolerance in the intact animal (62). In contrast, while bone marrow cells require a longer period for tolerance induction than thymus cells, the unresponsive state in bone marrow cells is of relatively short duration and lasts no more than 50 days. The duration of the unresponsive state in peripheral T and B cells has been assessed by adoptive transfer (63) and by challenge with AHGG and LPS which renders the antigen T-independent (91). The kinetic pattern for the induction and duration of unresponsiveness in peripheral T cells is similar to the pattern observed in the thymus cells and the intact mouse. Splenic B cells, however, remain completely unresponsive for only 45 to 50 days, paralleling the bone marrow cells (92). They then gradually regain immunocompetency, as assessed by challenge with antigen and LPS, equaling the response of normal spleen cells approximately 90 days after tolerization (Fig. 2). Thus a period of time exists during the maintenance of unresponsiveness to HGG when the T cells are tolerant and the B cells are competent. It is at this time that the termination of the unresponsive state can be readily accomplished by bypassing the specificity of, or the need for, T cell help.

Additional insight into the induction and maintenance of the unresponsive state can be derived from the fate of antigen-binding cells. The patterns of ABC vary widely during the induction of unresponsiveness, depending on the experimental model employed (reviewed in ref. 93). The failure to demonstrate a reduction in the number of ABC with T-independent antigens (43,35) may reflect the presence of B cells that are capable of binding the radiolabeled antigen in vitro, but that are functionally masked by the persisting antigen in the unresponsive host. However, failure to show a decrease in ABC during unresponsiveness to T-dependent antigens may be due to the technical difficulty in detecting antigen-binding T cells. In tolerance to T-dependent antigens, which may be maintained solely by unresponsiveness at the T cell level, the ABC observed are most probably only in the B cell population that remains immunocompetent. The enumeration of ABC in the mouse to HGG helps resolve these conflicts under conditions where the unresponsive state in both the T and B cells can be monitored (48). There are no significant ABC detected in the spleens when both the T and B cells are unresponsive to HGG. The kinetics of the loss of ABC after injection of the tolerogen (DHGG) parallel the loss of function in B cells. Whether ABC have been eliminated or are still present, but their receptors have been either covered by antigen or stripped from the surface, cannot presently be answered.

Suppression

An alternative to clonal deletion as the mechanism for the maintenance of tolerance to HGG is the active suppression of antigen-reactive cells by other lymphocytes, especially T cells. Such a hypothesis could explain the inability of normal spleen cells to reconstitute the responsiveness of intact, tolerant hosts (see below).

Basten and co-workers (30,31) have reported results that show the presence of suppressive activity to be transiently associated with populations of HGG-tolerant spleen cells. Their system involved adoptive transfer to lethally irradiated recipients of a standard number of HGG-primed and DNP-primed

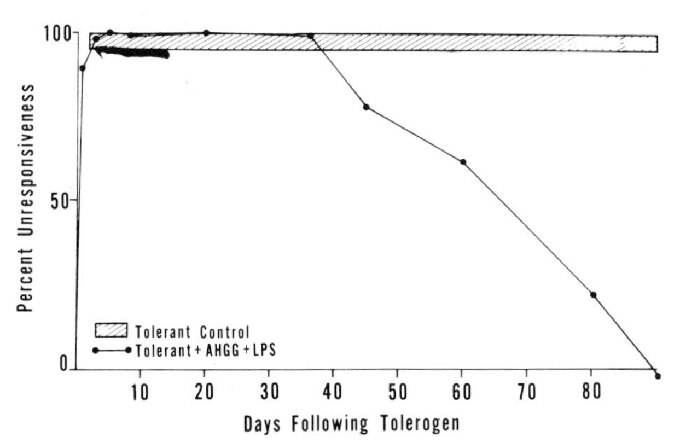

Figure 2. Adult A/J mice tolerized with 2.5 mg of DHGG were challenged and assayed as described in Fig. 1.

spleen cells with or without a variable number of HGG-tolerant cells. The animals were then challenged with DNP-HGG, and the PFC response to DNP was measured. The presence of the HGG-tolerant cells greatly reduces the anti-DNP response. The activity measured by this protocol is only present in the cells from animals made tolerant less than 15 days prior to adoptive cell transfer and is absent from cells of mice that have been tolerant for longer periods of time.

The work of Benjamin (32) also demonstrates suppressive activity associated with HGG-tolerant spleen cells. In this system the response of normal spleen cells to HGG can be inhibited by the presence of tolerant spleen cells when both types of cells are used to reconstitute irradiated recipients.

In an attempt to analyze and possibly resolve the differences between the results of Basten and Benjamin and the results of Chiller et al. (54), which showed the absence of suppressive activity under similar experimental conditions, a reexamination of the system of HGG tolerance was made. The results published by Weigle and co-workers (33–35) demonstrate that suppressive activity against the immune response of normal spleen cells to HGG can be found in tolerant spleen cells. In agreement with the work of Basten, this activity is only transiently present in the cells of tolerant animals and is lost by 40 days after DHGG treatment of the tolerant animals. The tolerant cells themselves remain unresponsive for at least 120 days after treatment. Benjamin (personal communication) has recently shown that in the cases of both low-dose tolerance to HGG and neonatally-induced tolerance, there is no detectable suppression. Such a dissociation of suppressor cell activity and unresponsiveness to HGG is an important consideration when analyzing possible mechanisms for the maintenance of the tolerant state and the relevance of suppression to those mechanisms. The protocol of Weigle and co-workers for demonstrating suppression involves the transfer of HGG-tolerant spleen cells or normal spleen cells or both to lethally irradiated, syngeneic mice. Recipient animals are challenged twice with AHGG, and their PFC response is measured by a modified Jerne plaque assay. The results show that 70×10^6 spleen cells from mice made tolerant ten days previously will suppress the immune response of 70×10^6 normal spleen cells by 75%. The suppression is antigen-specific, dependent on the presence of T cells and also adherent cells, and is active against the responsiveness of both B and T cells. Of particular interest from the standpoint of its relevance as a mechanism for controlling the tolerant state to HGG is the fact that the suppressive activity is only transiently present in the spleen cells of tolerant animals. Spleen cells from animals injected with DHGG ten days before cell transfer reduce the immune response of an equal number of normal spleen cells by 81%, whereas the cells from animals made tolerant 40 days earlier generate an insignificant level of suppression.

The results presented above indicate that active suppression of antigen-reactive lymphocytes is probably not responsible for controlling the unresponsive state to HGG. The mechanism responsible for suppression is, however, of interest in itself as a phenomenon associated with the tolerant state and as a means of controlling the immune response in general. Possibly the suppressive activity represents the induction of tolerance in the immunocompetent spleen cell population by tolerogen associated with the cells from tolerant animals. Such a possibility would be relevant to an understanding of the status of HGG-tolerant cells and is presently being investigated.

Termination

The experimental termination of unresponsiveness to HGG can be accomplished at a time when T cells are tolerant and B cells are competent. A variety of methods have been employed to circumvent the specifically unresponsive T cells. Using adoptive cell transfer, spleen cells taken from tolerant mice when B cells are no longer unresponsive respond upon transfer into lethally irradiated mice together with normal thymocytes (63). Immune responsiveness is not reconstituted by the transfer of normal thymus cells and spleen cells obtained from tolerant donors when both the T and B cells are unresponsive.

The maintenance of the unresponsive state to HGG can also be investigated by the reconstitution of tolerant animals with normal spleen cells. Tolerance cannot be terminated in these recipients unless they are lethally irradiated immediately before reconstitution (92). The ability to terminate the unresponsive state in these tolerant recipients is also dependent on the time between the injection of tolerogen (DHGG) and cell transfer. Restoration of responsiveness with normal spleen cells does not occur until 45 days after tolerization and correlates with the spontaneous termination of unresponsiveness in spleen B cells which is shown in Fig. 2. Presumably the mechanisms that maintain the unresponsiveness in the splenic B cells of the tolerant recipient and induce unresponsiveness in the normal spleen transferred to tolerant recipients are similar.

As mentioned above, LPS can prevent the induction of unresponsiveness to serum proteins when injected soon after the tolerogen (76–79). In addition, the injection of LPS with the AHGG challenge results in the termination of the unresponsive state to HGG in mice only when the B cells are responsive (91). In contrast, no effect is observed when LPS and AHGG are administered at earlier times, when both the T and B cells are unresponsive. When challenged with antigen and LPS after 45 days, the response engendered in the splenic B cells gradually increases (Fig. 2), presumably reflecting the increasing numbers of responsive B cells in this organ as termination of the unresponsive state spontaneously progresses (92). The ability of LPS to substitute for the T cell helper function suggests that LPS may terminate tolerance by circumventing the need for specific T cells that are unresponsive and by stimulating the B cells either directly or through other nonspecific cell interactions.

The induction of a mild GVH reaction and establishment of an "allogeneic effect" inhibit the induction of unresponsiveness to DHGG (89) and DNP-D-GL (90), as mentioned above. Similarly, the injection of allogeneic cells and immunogen (AHGG) will terminate the unresponsive state to HGG in adult mice (94). This interference with the tolerant state can only be accomplished when B cells of the recipient are responsive; the GVH reaction is ineffective in terminating unresponsiveness when both T and B cells are unresponsive. Likewise, the injection of syngeneic cells and AHGG has no effect.

The termination of immunologic unresponsiveness with cross-reactive antigens is well established and has been shown in a number of different models of tolerance (reviewed in ref. 2). It appears, however, that such termination can only occur if tolerance exists in only the T cells while immunocompetent B cells are present. This mode of termination is probably best documented in the unresponsive state induced to BSA in neonatal rabbits. Rabbits injected soon after birth with BSA remain completely unresponsive to subsequent injections of BSA for at least six months. However, the injection of chemically altered preparations of BSA (95), or cross-reactive heterologous albumins (96), three months after tolerization, terminates the unresponsive state. The antibody directed to BSA in such rabbits is quantitatively and qualitatively identical to the antibody produced in normal rabbits (97), indicating a normal complement of B cells in the unresponsive animal. This is consistent with the assumption that termination of the unresponsive state by cross-reactive antigens entails the bypass of the specifically unresponsive T cells, the activation of T cells responsive to unrelated determinants on the cross-reacting albumins, and the stimulation of B cells competent both for BSA and for the unrelated determinants. Furthermore, the simultaneous injection of BSA and cross-reacting albumins inhibits the termination of the unresponsive state (98,99). It is most likely that the newly injected BSA reinduces an unresponsive state in the competent B cells before they are stimulated by antigen or activated T cells. Similarly, Benjamin and Hershey (100) have shown

Table 2. Termination of Immunologic Unresponsiveness to Bovine Serum Albumin (BSA) Using Immune Complexes Made with Heterologous Antibody[a]

Group	Challenge	No. of Animals	Indirect PFC/10^6 Lymph Node Cells (Range)
A	GPGG–anti-HSA[b] + BSA	8	296 (71–609)
B	BSA	8	6 (0–31)
C	GPGG	5	0

[a]Rabbits were tolerized to BSA three months prior to challenge. Plaque-forming cells (PFC) to BSA were enumerated eight days after challenge.

[b]Guinea pig gamma globulin (GPGG). Human serum albumin (HSA).

Source: Habicht, Chiller, and Weigle (101). Reprinted with permission.

that the tolerance induced by a fragment of BSA can be terminated by immunization with intact BSA.

Antigen-antibody complexes can also terminate unresponsiveness by circumventing the specificity of the unresponsive T cells in animals possessing responsive B cells (Table 2). When complexes are prepared from the antigen (BSA) to which the rabbit is unresponsive and heterologous (guinea pig) antibody to a cross-reacting antigen (HSA), the unrelated antigenic portion of the guinea pig gamma globulin activates T cells while allowing the free BSA determinants to stimulate competent B cells (101). The result is circulating antibody specific for BSA in the unresponsive animal.

TOLERANCE TO SELF-ANTIGENS

Thyroiditis

Despite the fact that individuals under normal conditions tolerate their own body components, possibly either by the elimination of self-reacting clones of lymphocytes during the perinatal period or by a sequestering of self-components, as hypothesized by Burnet and Fenner (1), autoimmune disease states occur in which immune reactivity can be detected against any of a variety of self-components. Since tolerance to serum proteins injected either neonatally or in adult life appears to represent a state of central tolerance, involving either elimination or inactivation of specific clones of lymphocytes (102), the mechanisms involved in the termination of tolerance have obvious applications for understanding the mechanisms of certain autoimmune states.

Autoimmune reactivity in Hashimoto's thyroiditis in humans is directed against self-components of the thyroid gland. The pathologic events in this disease are coincident with the production of antibody to thyroglobulin (Tg) and/or to a second colloid antigen (CA-2) and microsomal antigens (103) and infiltration of the gland by mononuclear lymphocytes with formation of germinal centers within the gland (104). These events are accompanied by destruction of epithelial cells and loss of colloid, while the late course of the disease is characterized by severe hypothyroidism. Experimentally induced forms of the disease in subprimates resemble Hashimoto's thyroiditis except that antibody is formed primarily to Tg, germinal centers are not usually apparent, and the disease is not usually progressive (103). A spontaneously arising thyroiditis has also been observed in chickens (105), rats (106), dogs (107), and monkeys (108). The pathology of spontaneous autoimmune thyroiditis strikingly resembles that of Hashimoto's thyroiditis. This similarity includes the appearance of germinal centers in the thyroid and the progressive nature of the disease (109,110). In this chapter, experimental forms of thyroiditis will be considered. The human disease will be described in Chapter 9.

The ability to terminate acquired immunologic tolerance to BSA in rabbits by injection of altered or cross-reacting albumins (see above, 95,96) led to the proposal that B cells capable of producing antibody to tolerated antigens could be present and that the tolerant state is maintained because of the inability of T cells to recognize the tolerated antigens (95). Since tolerance to native Tg was subsequently shown to be terminated by injection of cross-reacting or altered thyroglobulins, it was postulated that the same mechanism as that involved in terminating acquired tolerance to BSA might be responsible for at least some autoimmune diseases (111). Based upon the demonstration of a synergistic role of T and B cells in the AFC response to certain antigens (14), the kinetic and dose differences in the ability of these two cell types to be made tolerant (62,69), and the ability of B cells to be stimulated under certain conditions without the need for specific T cells (112), it was proposed that the development of autoimmune thyroiditis could occur as the result of the stimulation of competent B cells, even though T cells remained tolerant (113). This hypothesis is strengthened by the fact that in most, if not all, forms of thyroiditis the disease is characteristically mediated by antibody (114). However, secondary T cell involvement may occur in experimental, chronic thyroiditis (115).

That the response to thyroglobulin is a thymus-dependent response has been shown by reconstitution of the response to heterologous Tg in thymectomized, lethally irradiated mice either with a combination of bone marrow cells and thymocytes or with splenic cells, but not with bone marrow cells alone (116). Both thyroid lesions and splenic PFC to heterologous Tg are observed after reconstitution with bone marrow cells and thymocytes. The production of autoantibody and thyroid lesions following injection of syngeneic Tg in complete Freund's adjuvant (CFA) has similarly been shown to be adoptively transferred by a combination of T and B cells, but not by B cells alone (117). Furthermore, production of antibody to thyroglobulin and thyroid lesions cannot be detected following immunization of athymic mice (118).

Although originally Tg was thought to be a sequestered antigen, it has been shown to be present in low levels in the serum of normal humans and animals (119,120). Evidence demonstrates that this concentration is sufficient to maintain tolerance in rabbits to a heterologous thyroglobulin (121). Since the induction of tolerance at the T cell level to serum proteins in mice has been shown to require a significantly lower antigen concentration than the induction of unresponsiveness at the B cell level (62), it is possible that serum levels of Tg are sufficiently low to allow specific B cells to remain responsive to determinants on autologous Tg while tolerance to the same determinants would be induced and maintained at the T cell level.

The ability to induce thyroiditis experimentally was first established in the rabbit by injection of isologous Tg in CFA (122). Experimental, autoimmune thyroiditis (EAT) has since been produced in the mouse, rat, guinea pig, dog, chicken, and monkey (103). Attempts to induce thyroiditis by injection of native Tg incorporated into incomplete Freund's adjuvant (IFA) (without mycobacteria) have been uniformly unsuccessful, although occasionally low levels of antibody are formed (111). The role of mycobacteria may be either to stimulate T cells nonspecifically, as has been observed in the response to DNP-poly-L-lysine in nonresponder guinea pigs (123), or to induce an alteration of the thyroglobulin molecule in vivo. Support for the latter possibility has come from histologic and biochemical analysis of adjuvant-injected rabbit spleens (124). Neutrophils infiltrate areas of adjuvant deposits in the spleens of rabbits injected with CFA, but not with IFA. The resulting acidic environment, combined with the release of proteolytic enzymes from neutrophils, may create conditions for partial denaturation of thyroglobulin. The presence of a complement of T cells capable of recognizing these new determinants could then result in the stimulation of B cells that are competent to both foreign and native determinants.

The termination of tolerance to native Tg has also been achieved by injection of either altered or cross-reacting thyroglobulins (111,125). After tolerance has been terminated and the initial immune response has subsided, subsequent injection of soluble, native Tg results in a reappearance of antibody and thyroid lesions (126,127). However, continued injection of native Tg leads to a reinduction of the tolerant state (128). Thus, it would appear that memory cells to native determinants can be stimulated without any T cell help for a limited period of time. The T-independent stimulation of memory cells has in fact been observed in some experimental situations (78,129). The reappearance of the tolerant state following injection of several courses of native thyroglobulin may result from exhaustive differentiation of memory B cells (130) combined with the inability of virgin B cells to respond due to the lack of T cell help. Tolerance to soluble serum proteins has been induced in antigen-primed mice, although the competence of the different cell populations was not determined (131).

Another prediction is that thyroiditis should be induced by injection of native thyroglobulin complexed to antibody directed to cross-reacting thyroglobulins. Thus, injection of rabbit Tg complexed with guinea pig antibovine Tg in IFA results in the development of thyroid lesions and antibody reactive with native Tg in rabbits (101). Guinea pig antibovine Tg or rabbit Tg alone was incapable of producing thyroiditis. Thus, T cells reacting with determinants on guinea pig antibovine Tg allow stimulation of B cells reactive to determinants on rabbit Tg and on guinea pig gamma globulin.

Tolerance to thyroglobulin has also been abrogated by injection of lipopolysaccharide and soluble, homologous Tg, resulting in the formation of both thyroid lesions and antibody to Tg (132). Lipopolysaccharide has been shown to be a B cell mitogen in mice (133) and has been shown to bypass the need for T cell help (112,134). Although LPS does not appear to terminate tolerance to thyroglobulin in rabbits as readily as in mice, approximately 10% of rabbits injected with LPS and soluble, native thyroglobulin do develop thyroiditis (Table 3). The limited nature of the response may be due to the relative ineffectiveness of LPS as a mitogen for rabbit lymphocytes (135). Alternatively, termination of tolerance by LPS may require the involvement of low numbers of antigen-reactive T cells, which have been reported to be involved in B cell stimulation in other systems (136).

The ability to assay for lymphocytes bearing immunoglobulin receptors for a specific antigen has allowed further confirmation of the status of T and B cells. Antigen-binding cells specific for homologous Tg have been detected in normal humans (137,138), mice (116), and rats (139). The ABC appear to represent B, rather than T, lymphocytes since they are depleted after passage of the initial cell population over anti-immunoglobulin columns that remove essentially all the lymphocytes bearing surface immunoglobulin (137), or by pretreatment of the cells with anti-immunoglobulin sera (116,137,138). Furthermore, ABC for homologous thyroglobulin cannot be detected in the thymus of mice under conditions in which ABC for heterologous thyroglobulins can be detected (116). The relevance of these cells for the immune response to Tg has been demon-

Table 3. Effect of Bacterial Lipopolysaccharide (LPS) on Induction of Thyroiditis with Native Thyroglobulin (Tg)

Treatment	No. of Rabbits Showing Immune Elimination/Total	Eliminating Rabbits with Thyroid Lesions[a]
2 mg rabbit Tg + 10 μg LPS K235	3/13	1/3
2 mg rabbit Tg + 100 μg LPS K235	0/12	—
10 mg rabbit Tg + 10 μg LPS K235	1/9	1/1
10 mg rabbit Tg + 10 μg LPS 0111:B4	1/9	0/1
10 mg rabbit Tg + 100 μg LPS 0111:B4	3/27	2/3
10 mg rabbit Tg + 10 μg LPS 0111:B4 + 500 R day 1	2/10	1/2
Thyroidectomized rabbits 10 mg rabbit Tg + 10 μg LPS K235	1/6	1/1
TOTAL	11/86	6/11

[a]No lesions were observed in rabbits not showing immune elimination.

strated by functional inactivation (suicide) of cells binding syngeneic Tg radioiodinated to a high specific activity. Thus, the reconstitution of the splenic PFC response to heterologous Tg by adoptive transfer of T and B cells into irradiated recipients is suppressed over 80% by preincubation of the B cells with highly radiolabeled, syngeneic Tg (116). On the other hand, preincubation of only the T cells with radioiodinated Tg has little effect on the adoptively transferred response. The incidence of lesions in the thyroid gland is also markedly reduced by suicide of the B cells, but not the T cells. Furthermore, increased numbers of ABC are observed in patients with Hashimoto's thyroiditis compared to healthy individuals (138), and mice in which thyroiditis has been induced by injection of cross-reacting thyroglobulins similarly show increased numbers of ABC to syngeneic Tg (116).

Other evidence implicates a primary role for the B cell and its product in the production of thyroiditis. In confirmation of the initial observation in the rabbit (140), passive transfer of the disease with antibody has also been reported in mice (141). In the rabbit, sera obtained relatively late after immunization with native Tg in CFA are incapable of transferring the disease, whereas sera obtained early are effective (140). Recent experiments in mice have implicated antigen-antibody complexes in the passive transfer of thyroiditis with early antibody (142). Antigen-antibody complexes have previously been proposed as agents for the disease process in active forms of thyroiditis in the mouse (143). An alternate possibility is that a particular class or subclass of antibody with a short half-life may be necessary in initiating the lesions. Once injury is induced, the thyroid may then be susceptible to subsequent damage by late-appearing antibody (143).

Further evidence that a primary role is played by B cells in the development of thyroiditis has been obtained from a kinetic analysis of the appearance of PFC to Tg in the spleen and thyroid glands of rabbits and the appearance of circulating antibody and thyroid lesions following injection of bovine Tg (Fig. 3) (114). A marked association is noted between the appearance of PFC in the gland and infiltration of the gland by mononuclear cells. Significant lesions do not appear until PFC are detected in the gland, and the most severe lesions are observed shortly after peak numbers of PFC are observed in the gland. Circulating antibody also precedes the appearance of lesions. However, once lesions develop, antibody disappears from the circulation at an accelerated rate. Thus, the historical lack of correlation between circulating antibody levels and thyroid lesions could be due to antibody being absorbed from the circulation by the thyroid or by antigen released from a damaged gland. A similar appearance of circulating antibody prior to development of lesions is observed in mice injected with heterologous thyroglobulins (143). In these latter studies, immunoglobulin, C3, and Tg can be demonstrated by immunofluorescence in the interstitial space between the follicular basement membrane and follicular cells subsequent to the appearance of circulating antibody. Since extrathyroidal deposits of these complexes are not observed, it was postulated that they are formed in situ and result

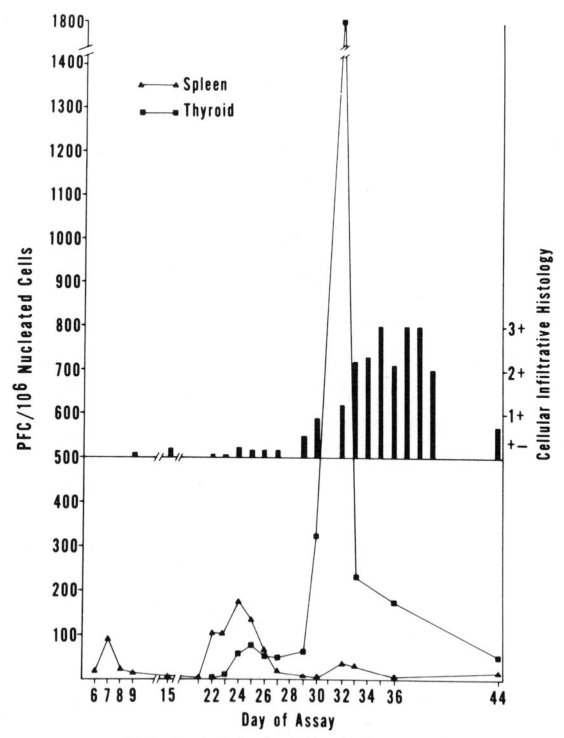

Figure 3. The PFC response to rabbit thyroglobulin of cells from the spleen and the thyroid gland. The degree of infiltration of mononuclear cells is shown by *solid bars*. From Clinton and Weigle (114). Reprinted with permission.

in tissue damage via infiltration of polymorphonuclear leukocytes by mechanisms similar to those of the Arthus reaction.

Antibody-mediated, rather than cell-mediated, immunity has also been implicated in the cytotoxic activity of lymphocytes against thyroid cells. Thus, normal lymphocytes are able to kill chicken erythrocytes coated with both Tg and anti-Tg antibody (144). Furthermore, normal lymphocytes can become similarly cytotoxic to Tg-coated erythrocytes after incubation with anti-Tg antibody (145). Cell-mediated hypersensitivity is often observed in thyroiditis (146,147), although such T cell involvement may be a manifestation of more chronic forms and may not play a role in the acute phase of the disease. Following limited courses of injection of bovine Tg, migration inhibition factor (MIF) is elicited from rabbit peritoneal cells with bovine Tg, but only subsequent to the infiltration of mononuclear cells into the gland (114). No MIF activity can be detected to rabbit Tg, confirming a lack of T cell involvement in disease production. In contrast, in experimentally induced thyroiditis in the rabbit, which is perpetuated by prolonged monthly injections of bovine Tg, cell-mediated hypersensitivity, as assayed by MIF activity to native thyroglobulin, developed (115). It was proposed that continued production of antibody to Tg might reduce the level of thyroglobulin in contact with lymphoid cells, resulting in a loss of tolerance in the T cells. In contrast to the thyroiditis produced after only a few courses of immunization with heterologous thyroglobulins, in which the tolerant state resumes after subsequent injection of soluble, native thyroglobulin, rabbits in which the disease has been perpetuated by prolonged injection of bovine thyroglobulin continue to respond to subsequent injections of native thyroglobulin, as would be expected if specific T cell help were available (115).

Experimental Allergic Encephalomyelitis (EAE)

EAE is an autoimmune disease resulting from the injection of laboratory animals with brain tissue incorporated into CFA (148–150). This neurologic disorder involves the central nervous system and is characterized by demyelinaton of nerve fibers, infiltration of inflammatory cells (reviewed in refs. 151,152), and deposition of fibrin in the brain (153). EAE is of special importance since it is thought to be the experimental counterpart of multiple sclerosis in humans. In addition to being induced with brain tissue, EAE has more recently been induced by immunization with CFA containing basic protein (BP) isolated from myelin (153), or encephalitogenic peptides either isolated from myelin (154–156) or synthesized in vitro (154). In contrast to experimental thyroiditis, EAE has been proposed to result from cell-mediated immunity rather than from humoral immunity, because the immunologic aspects of EAE are characterized by a number of parameters of cell-mediated hypersensitivity and because it is readily transferred with sensitized lymphocytes (157–159), but not with serum (reviewed in ref. 157). It is therefore not unexpected that the cellular events and subcellular mechanisms of EAE differ from those of experimental thyroiditis. This hypothesis has recently been tested by two different approaches involving (1) inactivation of T cells with antithymocyte serum (ATS) (160) and (2) elimination of specific cells by incubation with highly radiolabeled BP, which, when concentrated on specific cells by receptors, results in death (suicide) of the cell by irradiation (161). In both approaches, inbred Lewis rats are immunized with syngeneic BP isolated from spinal cord.

T cells have previously been implicated in the susceptibility of rats to EAE. After depletion of T cells by thoracic duct drainage, rats become unresponsive to the BP of myelin in that they fail to develop EAE when immunized with BP incorporated into CFA (162). These studies demonstrate that T cells are involved in EAE, but do not differentiate between a role as helper cells for humoral immunity or as effector cells involved in cell-mediated immunity. At best, these experiments merely define the thymus dependency of EAE. More recent experiments have established the role of the T cells as the effector cells responsible for both the histologic lesions and the clinical symptoms of EAE. As in the above experiment, the requirement for T cells in the induction of EAE in Lewis rats was demonstrated (161). Thymectomized (Tx), lethally irradiated rats were injected with normal spleen and lymph node cells from which the T cells were deleted by treatment with ATS and complement. These reconstituted rats, when injected with BP, do not develop antibody, histologic lesions, or clinical symptoms in comparison to rats reconstituted with untreated spleen and lymph node cells. Again, these experiments verify the need for T cells in the induction of EAE. On the other hand, Tx, lethally irradiated rats reconstituted with spleen and lymph nodes of syngeneic rats immunized nine days previously with BP develop both antibody and EAE without any further challenge with BP. Treatment of the immunized cells with ATS and complement, however, inhibits the development of EAE, but has no effect on the antibody response (Table 4). In the latter experiments, neither clinical symptoms nor perivascular infiltrates of the brain are detected. It is of special interest that sera from recipients receiving either treated or untreated cells contain similar levels of antibody to BP. Apparently, lymphocytes transferred nine days after sensitization are already committed to the production of antibodies to BP and need no further T cell help, since ATS treatment of these cells does not alter their capacity to produce antibody. Furthermore, in spite of the synthesis of antibody to BP, EAE does not develop, indicating that antibody to BP by itself is incapable of initiating EAE. This is in agreement with the failure to transfer EAE with serum antibody (157,163,164). It is evident from these data that induction of EAE is dependent on T effector cells and that cell-mediated immunity plays the major role.

From the above studies with both experimental thyroiditis and EAE, it would appear that the immune status of the T cells to BP and to thyroglobulin is different. The involvement of effector T cells and humoral antibody to BP in EAE suggests a degree of competence in both the T and B cells. This assumption is supported by the observation of specific receptors on both the T and B cells of normal Lewis rats as detected with ^{125}I-labeled BP and autoradiography (Table 5). Antigen-binding cells to BP are detected in the thymus and spleen cells of Lewis rats. Furthermore, the elimination of T cells from the spleen cell population by treatment with ATS and complement and the resulting diminution of the number of ABC indicate that ABC in the spleen consist of both T and B cells. Others have also been able to detect ABC in lymphoid tissues of normal guinea pigs (165). The finding in Lewis rats of both T and B cells capable of binding BP suggests that BP of myelin is effectively sequestered from the lymphoid system

Table 4. Effect of T Cells on Induction of Experimental Allergic Encephalomyelitis (EAE) in Thymectomized, Irradiated Rats Reconstituted with Primed Cells[a]

Experiment	No. of Animals	Treatment of Cells Transferred	EAE Clinically	EAE Histologically	Serum ABC[b]
1	10	None	7/10[c]	10/10	2.3 (2.0–2.6)
	10	ATS +C	0/10	0/10	2.3 (2.1–2.4)
	6	ATS (abs)[d] +C	5/6	6/6	N.D.
2	5	None	3/5	5/5	3.0 (2.9–3.3)
	5	ATS +C	0/5	0/5	2.8 (2.7–2.9)
	5	Normal rabbit serum +C	5/5	5/5	N.D.

[a]Lewis rats were thymectomized, irradiated (900 R), and reconstituted with 250 × 10⁶ lymph node cells and 350 × 10⁶ spleen cells from rats sensitized nine days before with basic protein in complete Freund's adjuvant (BP-CFA). The transferred cells were untreated, treated with antithymocyte serum (ATS), or treated with normal rabbit serum.
[b]Values for antigen-binding cells (ABC) represent the μg of BP bound per ml of serum. Mean of animals tested.
[c]Numerator = number of animals with indicated manifestations of EAE; denominator = number of rats under study.
[d]Absorbed with thymus cells to remove in vitro T cell cytotoxicity.
N.D. = not done.
Source: Ortiz-Ortiz, Nakamura, and Weigle (160). Reprinted with permission.

Table 5. Frequency of Antigen-Binding Lymphocytes (ABL) to Basic Protein (BP) in Spleen and Thymus of Normal Lewis and Brown Norway (BN) Rats

Amount of ^{125}I-BP (ng)	Source of Normal Lymphoid Cells	Rat Strain	ABL per 10^5 Cells
100	thymus	Lewis	8
100	thymus	BN	0
100	spleen	Lewis	17
100	spleen	BN	11

Source: Ortiz-Ortiz and Weigle (161). Reprinted with permission.

or that BP is not present in sufficient amounts in the body fluids to be capable of inducing and maintaining unresponsiveness in either the T or B lymphocytes.

The role of the T and B cells in the development of EAE was further established by selective elimination (suicide) of these cells with heavily ^{125}I-labeled BP (161). In these experiments, Tx, irradiated Lewis rats were reconstituted with a mixture of normal thymus and bone marrow cells so that they respond to injection of BP in CFA by developing clinical symptoms of EAE, typical lesions in the brain, and antibody to BP. On the other hand, clinical symptoms, lesions, and antibody are not produced when the thymus cells were specifically deprived of competent cells by incubation with heavily ^{125}I-labeled BP and transferred with normal bone marrow cells to Tx, irradiated Lewis rats that were subsequently challenged with BP in CFA. These results can be interpreted to mean that the specific elimination of competent T cells aborted cell-mediated immunity and that it is this parameter of the immune response that is responsible for the events associated with EAE. The specificity of such elimination of competent cells to BP is evidenced by the ability of ^{125}I-labeled BP-treated thymus cells to cooperate normally with bone marrow cells in response to burro red blood cells when transferred to Tx, irradiated recipients. However, more convincing evidence for cell-mediated immunity in EAE was obtained by elimination of specific B cells with heavily ^{125}I-labeled BP. When bone marrow cells are treated with ^{125}I-labeled BP and injected into Tx, irradiated recipients, together with normal thymus cells, the antibody response to BP is inhibited. However, the histologic lesions and clinical symptoms of EAE are the same as those observed in rats injected with untreated bone marrow and normal thymus cells. These data leave little question that thymus-derived cells are wholly responsible for both the histologic lesions and the clinical symptoms of EAE and that antibody plays no role in the induction of the disease.

The complexity of the cellular events that lead to autoimmunity is further evidenced by the comparative results obtained in Brown Norway (BN) rats and Lewis rats. Not only does the BN rat differ from the Lewis rat in that the BN is resistant to the induction of EAE by injection of BP in CFA (166–168), but the BN rat also lacks ABC in its thymus (Table 5) (161). However, ABC are present in the B cell population of the BN rat, suggesting a state of T cell tolerance and B cell competence; a situation identical to the immune status of T and B cells to thyroglobulin. This model of EAE in the BN rat is of particular interest since it should be possible to bypass specific T cell helper activity and induce the production of circulating antibody to BP by specifically responsive B cells without the development of disease. Knowledge of the effect of the prolonged production of such anti-BP antibody on the histology of central nervous tissue and clinical EAE would be of considerable help in correlating the cellular events in EAE and other autoimmune diseases.

CYCLIC PRODUCTION OF ANTIBODY

In addition to the relatively long-lasting effects on the immune response produced by those mechanisms responsible for tolerance, there are ongoing immune responses that may be continually subject to self-regulatory control, as manifested in some cases by continuous fluctuations in antibody production. The ability to control the immune response in such a manner may confer a selective advantage on the host since persisting antigens, such as microorganisms and possibly spontaneously arising tumors, might be prevented from overwhelming and exhausting potentially reactive cells. Such control might also function in limiting the extent of autoimmune disease processes. Experimental systems that offer conditions for studying this type of immune regulation include those in which fluctuations in the immune response are observed following a single injection of antigen (169). These fluctuations represent a phenomenon that is wide-

Table 6. Cyclical Systems in Immune Responses

Antigen	Species	Assay [a]	Investigator
Albumin, hen egg	hamster	PFC	Portis and Coe (170)
Gamma globulin			
bovine	mouse	PFC	Dresser (171)
human	rabbit	ABC	Romball and Weigle (172)
		Ab, PFC	Romball and Weigle (173)
rabbit	mouse	Ab, PFC	Segre and Segre (174)
Escherichia coli LPS [b]	mouse	Ab, PFC	Britton and Möller (175)
Flagellin	human	ABC	Dwyer and MacKay (176)
	marine toad	Ab	Azzolina (177)
H-2 antigens	mouse	Ab	Rubinstein (178)
			Stimpfling and Richardson (179)
		cytotoxicity	Britton (180)
			Denham et al. (181)
			Gillespie and Barth (182)
			Simpson and Beverley (183)
		tumor growth	Barrett and Hansen (184)
			Snell et al. (185)
NIP-POL [c]	mouse	PFC	Schlegal (186)
Polyglycerophosphate (teichoic acid)	rat	Ab, PFC	Bolton et al. (187)
Pneumococcal polysaccharide	rabbit	Ab	Chen et al. (188)
Rh factor	human	Ab	Rubinstein (189)
Salmonella O antigens	chicken	Ab	Nielsen and White (190)
Sheep erythrocytes	mouse	Ab	Eidinger and Pross (191)
			Stimpfling and Richardson (179)
		PFC	Eidinger and Pross (191)
			Sell et al. (192)
			Wortis et al. (193)

[a] PFC = plaque-forming cells, ABC = antigen-binding cells, Ab = antibody.
[b] LPS = bacterial lipopolysaccharide.
[c] NIP-POL = 4-hydroxy-3-iodo-5-nitrophenylacetic acid-polymerized flagellin.

spread, as evidenced by their occurrence in many species and to a variety of antigens (Table 6) (170–193). However, whether identical mechanisms control the fluctuations in all the systems is not known.

In the rabbit, a single, intravenous injection of AHGG induces a cyclic PFC response in the spleen (Fig. 4). The response has been followed for a period of 22 days and is characterized by an initial peak of PFC in the spleen on day 5, followed by two subsequent peaks on days 13 and 21 (173). Thus, succeeding peaks appear to be separated by well-defined, eight-day refractory periods. The refractoriness is antigen-specific, since a normal PFC response can be detected during this time to the non-cross-reacting antigen, aggregated turkey gamma globulin. A similar cyclic pattern is obtained when the response is assayed by quantitating the number of antigen-binding cells appearing in the spleen (172).

Reduction and alkylation of antibody secreted by PFC indicate that the successive peaks are composed of simultaneously appearing PFC secreting either IgM

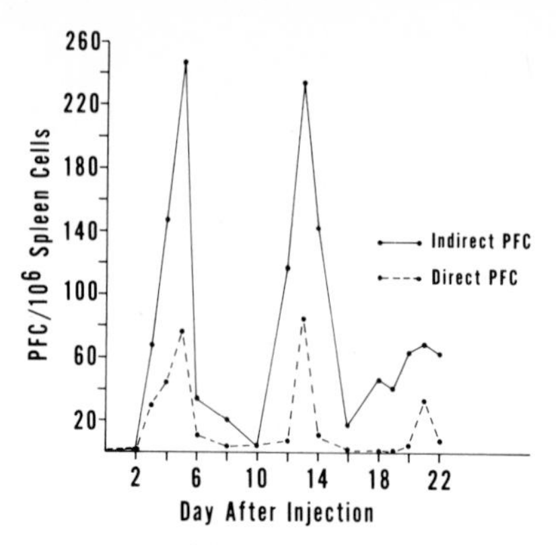

Figure 4. Kinetics of the appearance of PFC in spleens of rabbits after a single intravenous injection of 2 mg of aggregated HGG. From Romball and Weigle (173). Reprinted with permission.

or IgG antibodies (173). Circulating antibody levels rise and fall subsequent to the rise and fall of PFC, although differences are not as well-defined due to the relatively long half-life of the antibody.

After immunization with AHGG, plaque-forming cells appear in the peripheral blood of rabbits, with kinetics identical to their appearance in the spleen (173). Since antigen is not retained in the circulation, PFC in the blood are probably derived from cells stimulated in the spleen, as has been shown in other systems (194–196). Also, in rabbits injected with bovine Tg, a biphasic appearance of PFC occurs in the spleen. During the second phase, PFC also appear in the thyroid gland, apparently due to migration to the thyroid from the spleen (114). Furthermore, relatively little response is obtained in lymphoid organs other than the spleen in mice after primary challenge with SRBC, whereas peripheral and mesenteric lymph nodes, Peyer's patches, thymus, blood, and bone marrow cells respond well to secondary challenge in normal but not in splenectomized animals (196).

Although direct evidence is lacking, fluctuations in PFC levels would appear to be dependent on the presence of the antigen throughout the various response phases. LPS, SRBC (197), and HGG (173) have been shown to persist in a functionally active form for prolonged periods of time, and each of these antigens induces a cyclic response. In fact, the ability to produce a cycling response in lymphoid organs correlates with the half-life of the antigen in that organ as assayed by the quantity of radioactivity present after injection of radiolabeled antigen (173). Thus, only a single peak of PFC appears in mesenteric nodes of rabbits injected intravenously with 2 mg of AHGG, whereas two additional peaks of PFC are observed on days 13 and 21 in the spleen. Localization of antigen in both the spleen and lymph node occurs two days following injection of antigen, whereas only the spleen shows localization of antigen ten days after injection.

The cyclic fluctuations do not appear to be due to the sequential production of different classes or subclasses of antibody since the cyclic response to SRBC in spleens of mice involves the almost simultaneous appearance of PFC of the IgA,

IgG_1, IgG_{2a}, and IgG_{2b} classes (192). Furthermore, in rabbits immunized with AHGG, cyclic fluctuations in the IgG and IgM response occur concurrently (173).

Evidence that the response in the different phases may be directed towards different determinants or possibly to determinants formed as the result of in vivo alteration of the antigen has been obtained in mice immunized with SRBC (198). Isoelectric focusing of serum samples taken at the time of two different peaks of PFC shows differences in electrophoretic mobility of the serum immunoglobulin components. However, such differences show no correlation with cycles of PFC in the response in rabbits to pneumococcal polysaccharide (188). In addition, the response to a single determinant, polyglycerophosphate, is characterized by cycling in the rat (187). Finally, the inhibition of the appearance of the second peak of the response to LPS by injection of antibody formed during the first peak of the response in mice immunized with LPS is additional evidence against this possibility (175). Although varying responses to individual determinants may occur during the cyclic PFC fluctuations, response to different determinants would not appear to be the underlying mechanism.

Antibody is another possible mechanism of control for cycling. It has been shown that primary immune responses can be inhibited by injection of specific antibody (199) and that removal of circulating antibody results in the subsequent enhancement of antibody levels (200,201), presumably by covering antigenic determinants (202). On the basis of these studies, it was proposed that an equilibrium of antigen, antigen-antibody complexes, and antibody in the extravascular compartment functions in controlling the immune response (203). However, in the response to AHGG in rabbits, despite markedly different levels of antibody resulting from injection of varying doses of antigen or among individual animals injected with the same dose of antigen, the interval between peak PFC phases remains constant (173). Thus, antibody-mediated control via removal of antigenic stimulation would not appear to be the only controlling factor, unless such antibody is produced locally at the site of cellular interaction (173).

A more complex mechanism of control has been proposed by Jerne (204). This model suggests that the synthesis of antibody is followed by synthesis of anti-idiotypic antibody, which can cause a suppression of the response to the original antigen. In fact, injection of anti-idiotypic antibody has been shown to suppress production of antibody of that idiotype (205). Rabbits immunized with the *p*-azophenyltrimethyl ammonium group, and then immunized with their own antihapten antibody, produce anti-idiotypic antibody reactive with only their own antihapten antibody (206). Immunization with several antigens has been shown to result in antibody production followed by synthesis of anti-idiotypic antibody. Serum from BALB/c mice repeatedly immunized with phosphorylcholine (PC) has agglutinating activity to both PC and to the myeloma protein TEPC-15, which carries the idiotype of anti-PC antibodies (207). The appearance of anti-TEPC-15 activity in the sera coincides with a decrease in the splenic PFC response to PC. In another system, Lewis rats immunized to Brown Norway tumor cells initially show anti-BN antibodies which disappear on continued immunization with BN cells. At the time of cessation of anti-BN antibody production, the serum contains anti-idiotypic antibody to the anti-BN antisera (208). In rabbits immunized to SRBC, serum taken as early as seven days after antigen injection blocks the ability of that individual rabbit's previously isolated lymph node cells to form rosettes to SRBC, while not affecting lymph node cells from a second rabbit (209). The presence of antibody to the anti-SRBC idiotypes was implicated since this antirosetting activity could not be eliminated by exhaustive adsorption of the sera with antigen. The combination of antibody with receptors on cells (210) and activation of suppressor cells (211) have both been implicated as mechanisms by which anti-idiotypic suppression occurs. However, the role that anti-idiotypic antibody plays in cyclical responses remains to be elucidated.

The possible role of other immunoregulatory molecules in cyclic responses is also under investigation. For example, alpha fetoprotein (AFP) has been reported to be immunosuppressive for both cellular and humoral immunity (212,213). The levels of membrane-bound AFP on murine lymphocytes correlate inversely with the level of protein synthesis in those cells, implicating a possible feedback control by AFP on the immune response (214). Suppression of the immune response in splenic lymphocytes in association with increased levels of membrane-bound AFP occurs in animals showing normal serum AFP levels and normal lymph node responses. This indicates that regulation may be occurring via AFP produced locally in the lymphoid organ.

Recent experimental work has focused on the involvement of suppressor cells in immunoregulation (215). Results obtained in the cyclic response of rabbits to AHGG are consistent with the involvement of a specific suppressor cell in this response. In this system, the normal cyclic response observed after injection of antigen alone is disrupted by modifying the immunization procedure to include the simultaneous injection of concanavalin A and the immunogen (216). Under these conditions, the PFC response on day 5 is suppressed compared to rabbits injected with antigen alone, whereas PFC values on days 8 and 13 reflect a continued increase in the number of PFC. Neither simultaneous injection of lipopolysaccharide nor phytohemagglutinin affects the cyclic response, although these mitogens do enhance the response to AHGG (217). Since serum antibody levels in Con A-treated rabbits are as high as or higher than the levels in rabbits injected with antigen alone (216), these differences in response would not appear to be controlled by antibody. One interpretation of these results is that Con A activates suppressor cells nonspecifically, as has been observed in other systems (218), resulting in the suppressed PFC response on day 5. These suppressor cells, including those specifically reactive to HGG, may then become exhausted, thereby permitting a continued rise in PFC levels on days 8 and 13.

In the popliteal nodes of rabbits injected with 0.2 mg of AHGG, PFC increase in a linear manner after subcutaneous injection of the antigen (216). However, if 2 mg of AHGG is simultaneously injected intravenously, the number of PFC increases until day 5, remains constant between days 5 and 8, and then increases again between days 8 and 13 at approximately the same rate as in rabbits injected only subcutaneously. Thus, intravenous injection of antigen changes the linear response observed in the node after subcutaneous injection of antigen to a cyclic response corresponding to that observed in the spleen. Suppressor cell activity has been implicated in three other systems that also demonstrate the modulating effect of the splenic response on the popliteal node response in the rabbit. First, the adoptively transferred SRBC response in distal nodes of mice has been shown to be suppressed by spleen-seeking cells because the response in the node is enhanced if recipients are splenectomized three hours after injection of syngeneic spleen cells, but not of syngeneic node cells (219). Similarly, the suppressive effect of an intravenous injection of AHGG on the response in the popliteal lymph nodes of rabbits following subcutaneous injection of antigen is abolished by splenectomy prior to injection of the antigen (220). Second, DNA synthesis by node-localizing cells during a GVH reaction induced by injection of parental cells into F_1 recipients is enhanced by splenectomy within six hours of injection. This implies a suppressive role of spleen-seeking lymphocytes (221). Since the effect observed depends on the dose of parental cells injected, it was proposed that cells localizing in the spleen are able to exert a dual effect. They are suppressive in the presence of a high response (high dose of parental cells) and enhancing in the presence of a low response (low dose of parental cells). Third, splenectomy suppresses the development of a spontaneously arising tumor in hamsters, which normally develops until it kills the host despite the presence of cell-mediated immunity (222). These results suggest a suppressive role of the spleen in controlling the immune response to the tumor.

Thus, cyclic fluctuations in the immune response both in the spleen and in tors originating in the spleen. Other examples exist in which a central role is played by the spleen in regulating responses in other lymphoid organs. Skin graft survival has been shown to be significantly longer if cells are injected intravenously or if the graft is placed in an "immunologically privileged site" (223). Although these areas lack lymphatic drainage, the more significant feature appears to be that they are vascularized and antigen is able to stimulate the spleen. In confirmation, splenectomy abolishes the enhanced survival of grafts in these sites. It has been proposed that the phenomenon of antigenic competition involves splenic suppressor cells. This hypothesis is supported by the observations that such competition does not occur in splenectomized mice, nor is evident in the response to subcutaneously injected antigen in the distal lymph nodes of intact mice (224). However, the latter authors did observe antigenic competition in athymic mice reconstituted with either normal spleen or lymph node cells (224). Nevertheless, it has also been shown that in vitro suppressor activity can be elicited more readily from spleen cells than from lymph node cells (225).

T cell regulation may actually play a critical role in many situations in which antibody appears to be the regulatory molecule. It has been proposed that both specific and nonspecific suppressive effects result from activation of T cells by antigen-antibody complexes (226). T cells possess Fc receptors (227), and removal of the Fc fragment from antibody results in a loss of the suppressive effect of antibody (228). It is possible that T cells may be able to recognize the molar ratio of antibody to antigen in the complexes and amplify or suppress accordingly (229). In an experimental situation, antibody to the L-1210 line of tumor cells has been shown to suppress the immune response to the tumor that is caused by those cells (230). The presence of T cells, antibody, and tumor cells appears to be necessary for this suppressive effect.

In conclusion, self-regulatory control of ongoing immune responses appears to be mediated by a variety of mechanisms that may interact to produce fluctuations in the immune response. In the response to AHGG in the rabbit, the fluctuations are characterized by a constant periodicity and may be regulated by feedback mechanisms involving both antibody and suppressor cells, and the responding cells, once inhibited, may go through an obligate phase of inactivity before they can be restimulated (169).

SUMMARY

The cellular events involved in the induction, maintenance, and termination of immunologic tolerance in mice to HGG have been investigated. It appears that this model of tolerance is the result of a central unresponsive state and does not involve peripheral inhibition requiring regulatory mechanisms such as suppressor T cells, antigen blockade, or antibody feedback inhibition. The uniqueness of this model is that it appears to be identical to the unresponsive state to self-constituents present in the body fluid. Furthermore, conditions can be generated in which the acquired tolerance to HGG is a property only of T cells, while a normal complement of competent B cells is present. Such a situation can occur as a result of the temporal difference between the spontaneous termination of tolerance in B cells and T cells or as a result of a difference in the small dose of tolerogen required to induce tolerance in T cells in comparison to the large dose needed for B cell tolerance.

Of paramount interest to the maintenance of acquired tolerance both to exogenous antigen and to self-antigens is the immune status in which T cells are unresponsive while B cells are competent. It is this situation that readily lends itself to the termination of unresponsiveness by a variety of mechanisms that bypass the need for antigen-specific T cells in thymus-dependent responses. This immune status is of particular importance where self-antigens are at a concentration in the body fluids that is not sufficient to maintain tolerance in B cells, but that is sufficient to maintain unresponsiveness in the T cells. This type of regulation may play an important role in the control of certain autoimmune phenomena. In addition to control by the tolerant and responsive states of T and B cells, it has also been demonstrated that the mechanisms that control the immune response may be characterized by a precise cycling of antibody and antibody-forming cells.

Germane to the termination of unresponsiveness of acquired tolerance to foreign antigens are the cellular events responsible for thyroiditis, in which it has been shown that tolerance exists at the T cell, but not at the B cell, level. Furthermore, this experimental model has revealed a normal complement of specific antigen-binding B cells, whereas antigen-binding T cells are absent. Thus, it is not surprising that a bypass of T cell specificity by cross-reacting thyroglobulins results in experimental thyroiditis accompanied by antibody to autologous thyroglobulin. The available evidence presented shows that this disease is induced by humoral antibody caused by the circumvention of T tolerance and stimulation of competent B cells. This is in contrast with the cellular events that characterize experimental allergic encephalitis. In this latter disease, both the T and B cell populations contain specific binding cells for the basic protein of myelin. Treatment of lymphoid cells with antithymocyte serum and elimination of specific T cells has established that this disease results from pathologic changes caused by activated, effector T cells and that humoral antibody plays no significant role in its induction.

Although two different models of experimental autoimmunity have been presented to explain the respective diseases and although these models may be representative of a number of autoimmune phenomena in humans, a variety of mechanisms may be active in other autoimmune phenomena. The self-regulation of the immune response, involving a precise, cyclic production of antibody and the delicate balance between enhancing and suppressing factors, would certainly be expected to be involved in the control of autoimmune diseases. Furthermore, suppressor T cells have been demonstrated to be at least partially responsible for the spontaneous autoimmune phenomenon in New Zealand mice (231,232). However, it may be presumptuous to ascribe the control of most autoimmune diseases to active suppression. The main defense of suppressor cells against autoimmunity may be as a "fail safe" mechanism that regulates the autoimmune response once it has been induced.

REFERENCES

1. Burnet, F. M., and Fenner, F., *The Production of Antibodies,* Macmillan, Melbourne, 1949.
2. Weigle, W. O., *Adv. Immunol.* **16**, 61 (1973).
3. Howard, J. G., and Mitchison, N. A., *Prog. Allergy* **18**, 43 (1975).
4. Baker, P. J., Stashak, P. W., Amsbaugh, D. F., et al., *Immunology* **20**, 481 (1971).
5. Howard, J. G., *Transplant. Rev.* **8**, 50 (1972).
6. Schrader, J. W., and Nossal, G. J. V., *J. Exp. Med.* **139**, 1582 (1974).
7. Klaus, G. G. B., *Eur. J. Immunol.* **6**, 200 (1976).
8. Aldo-Benson, M., and Borel, Y., *J. Immunol.* **112**, 1793 (1974).
9. Aldo-Benson, M., and Borel, Y., *J. Immunol.* **116**, 223 (1976).
10. Scott, D. W., *Cell. Immunol.* **22**, 311 (1976).
11. Gronowicz, E., Coutinho, A., and Sjöberg, O., *Eur. J. Immunol.* **4**, 226 (1974).
12. Gronowicz, E., and Coutinho, A., *Eur. J. Immunol.* **5**, 413 (1975).
13. Möller, G., Gronowicz, E., Persson, U., et al., *J. Exp. Med.* **143**, 1429 (1976).
14. Claman, H. N., and Chaperon, E. A., *Transplant. Rev.* **1**, 92 (1969).
15. Miller, J. F. A. P., and Mitchell, G. F., *Transplant. Rev.* **1**, 3 (1969).
16. Horiuchi, A., and Waksman, B. H., *J. Immunol.* **101**, 1322 (1968).
17. Gershon, R. K., and Kondo, K., *Immunology* **21**, 903 (1971).
18. Gershon, R. K., *Transplant. Rev.* **26**, 170 (1975).
19. Droege, W., in *The Immune System: Genes, Receptors, Signals* (E. E. Sercarz, A. R. Williamson, and C. F. Fox, eds.), Proc. 1974 I.C.N.-U.C.L.A. Symp. on Mol. Biol., Academic Press, New York, 1974, p. 431.
20. Dutton, R. W., *Transplant. Rev.* **26**, 39 (1975).
21. Rich, R. R., and Pierce, C. W., *J. Exp. Med.* **137**, 649 (1973).
22. Dutton, R. W., *J. Exp. Med.* **138**, 1496 (1973).
23. Tse, H., and Dutton, R. W., *J. Exp. Med.* **143**, 1199 (1976).
24. Takatsu, K., and Ishizaka, K., *J. Immunol.* **116**, 125 (1976).
25. Tada, T., Taniguchi, M., and Takemori, T., *Transplant. Rev.* **26**, 107 (1975).
26. Nachtigal, D., Zan-Bar, I., and Feldman, M., *Transplant. Rev.* **26**, 87 (1975).
27. Kapp, J. A., Pierce, C. W., Schlossman, S., et al., *J. Exp. Med.* **140**, 648 (1974).
28. Phanuphak, P., Moorhead, J. W., and Claman, H. N., *J. Immunol.* **113**, 1230 (1974)
29. Asherson, G. L., and Zembala, M., *Curr. Top. Microbiol. Immunol.* **72**, 55 (1975).
30. Basten, A., in *Immunological Tolerance: Mechanisms and Potential Therapeutic Applications* (D. H., Katz, and B. Benacerraf, eds.), Academic Press, New York, 1974, p. 107.
31. Basten, A., Miller, J. F. A. P., and Johnson, P., *Transplant. Rev.* **26**, 130 (1975).
32. Benjamin, D., *J. Exp. Med.* **141** 635 (1975).
33. Weigle, W. O., Sieckmann, D. G., Doyle, M. V., et al., *Transplant. Rev.* **26**, 186 (1975).
34. Doyle, M. V., Parks, D. E., and Weigle, W. O., *J. Immunol.* **116**, 1640 (1976).
35. Doyle, M. V., Parks, D. E., and Weigle, W. O., *J. Immunol.* **117**, 1152 (1976).
36. Kapp, J. A., Pierce, C. W., De La Croix, F., et al., *J. Immunol.* **116**, 305 (1976).

37. Zembala, M., Asherson, G. L., Matthew, B., et al., *Nature* (London) **253**, 72 (1975).
38. Taniguchi, M., Hayakawa, K., and Tada, T., *J. Immunol.* **116**, 542 (1976).
39. Munro, A. J., Taussig, M. J., Campbell, R., et al., *J. Exp. Med.* **140**, 1579 (1974).
40. Burnet, F. M., *The Clonal Selection Theory of Acquired Immunity,* Cambridge University Press, London, 1959.
41. Nossal, G. J. V., and Pike, B.L., *J. Exp. Med.* **141**, 904 (1975).
42. Metcalf, E. S., and Klinman, N. R., *J. Immunol.* **143**, 1327 (1976).
43. Ada, G. L., Byrt, P., Mandel, T., et al., in *Developmental Aspects of Antibody Formation and Structure* (J. Sterzl and I. Riha, eds.), Academia, Prague, 1970, p. 503.
44. Cooper, H. G., Ada, G. L., and Longman, R. E., *Cell. Immunol.* **4**, 289 (1972).
45. Humphrey, J. H., and Keller, H. U., in *Developmental Aspects of Antibody Formation and Structure* (J. Sterzl and I. Riha, eds.), Academia, Prague, 1970, p. 485.
46. Naor, D., and Sulitzeanu, D., *Int. Arch. Allergy Appl. Immunol.* **36**, 112 (1969).
47. Katz, D.H., Davie, J. M., Paul, W. E., et al., *J. Exp. Med.* **134**, 201 (1971).
48. Louis, J., Chiller, J. M., and Weigle, W. O., *J. Exp. Med.* **137**, 461 (1973).
49. Golub, E. S., Mishell, R. I., Weigle, W. O., et al., *J. Immunol.* **100**, 133 (1968).
50. Jerne, N. K., and Nordin, A. A., *Science* **140**, 405 (1963).
51. Dresser, D. W., *Immunology* **5**, 378 (1962).
52. Dietrich, F. M., and Weigle, W. O., *J. Immunol.* **92**, 167 (1964).
53. Ruben, T. J., Chiller, J. M., and Weigle, W. O., *J. Immunol.* **111**, 805 (1973).
54. Chiller, J. M., Louis, J. A., Skidmore, B. J., et al., in *Immunological Tolerance: Mechanisms and Potential Therapeutic Applications* (D. H. Katz and B. Benacerraf, eds.), Academic Press, New York, 1974, p. 373.
55. Habicht, G. S., Chiller, J. M., and Weigle, W. O., in *Developmental Aspects of Antibody Formation and Structure* (J. Sterzl and I. Riha, eds.), Academia, Prague, 1970, p. 893.
56. Isakovic, K., Smith, S. B., and Waksman, B. H., *J. Exp. Med.* **122**, 1103 (1965).
57. Taylor, R. B., *Nature* (London) **220**, 611 (1968).
58. Playfair, J. H. L., *Nature* (London) **222**, 882 (1969).
59. Talal, N., Steinberg, A. D., Jacobs, M. E., et al., *J. Exp. Med.* **134**, 52*s* (1971).
60. Chiller, J. M., Habicht, G. S., and Weigle, W. O., *Proc. Natl. Acad. Sci.* (U.S.A.) **65**, 551 (1970).
61. Basten, A., Miller, J.F.A.P., Warner, N. L., et al., *Nature (New Biol.)* **231**, 104 (1971).
62. Chiller, J. M., Habicht, G. S., and Weigle, W. O., *Science* **171**, 813 (1971).
63. Chiller, J. M., and Weigle, W. O., *J. Immunol.* **110**, 1051 (1973).
64. Smith, R. T., and Bridges, R. A., *J. Exp. Med.* **108**, 227 (1958).
65. Eitzman, D. V., and Smith, R. T., *Proc. Soc. Exp. Biol. Med.* **102**, 529 (1959).
66. Golub, E. S., and Weigle, W. O., *J. Immunol.* **102**, 389 (1969).
67. Chiller, J. M., and Weigle, W. O., *Contemp. Top. Immunobiol.* **1**, 119 (1972).
68. Katsura, Y., Kawaguchi, S., and Muramatsu, S., *Immunology* **23**, 537 (1972).
69. Rajewsky, K., and Brenig, C., *Eur. J. Immunol.* **4**, 120 (1974).
70. Das, S., and Leskowitz, S., *J. Immunol.* **112**, 107 (1974).
71. Martin, W. J., *Aust. J. Exp. Biol. Med. Sci.* **44**, 605 (1966).
72. Chiller, J. M., Romball, C. G., and Weigle, W. O., *Cell. Immunol.* **8**, 28 (1973).
73. Lukic, M. L., Wortis, H. H., and Leskowitz, S., *Cell. Immunol.* **15**, 457 (1975)
74. Unanue, E. R., and Cerottini, J.-C., *Semin. Hematol.* **7**, 225 (1970).
75. Cowing, C., Miodrag, L., and Leskowitz, S., in *Immunological Tolerance: Mechanisms and Potential Therapeutic Applications* (D. H. Katz and B. Benacerraf, eds.), Academic Press, New York, 1974, p. 61.
76. Claman, H. N., *J. Immunol.* **91**, 833 (1963).
77. Golub, E. S., and Weigle, W. O., *J. Immunol.* **98**, 1241 (1967).
78. Louis, J. A., Chiller, J. M., and Weigle, W. O., *J. Exp. Med.* **138**, 1481 (1973).
79. Louis, J. A., Chiller, J. M., and Weigle, W. O., *Fed. Proc.* **33**, 723 (1974).
80. Schmidtke, J. R., Johnson, A. G., *J. Immunol.* **106**, 1191 (1971).
81. Capanna, S. L., and Kong, Y. M., *Immunology* **27**, 647 (1974).
82. Kong, Y. M., and Capanna, S. L., *Cell. Immunol.* **11**, 488 (1974).
83. Rey, O. A., and Azar, M. M., *Cell. Immunol.* **18**, 49 (1975).
84. Hamaoka, T., and Katz, D. H., *Cell. Immunol.* **7**, 246 (1973).
85. Cooper, N. R., *J. Exp. Med.* **137**, 451 (1973).
86. Azar, M. M., Yunis, E. J., Pickering, P. J., et al, *Lancet* **1**, 1279 (1968).

87. Morrison, D. C., Louis, J. A., and Weigle, W. O., *Immunology* **30**, 317 (1976).
88. Pepys, M. B., and Taussig, M. J., *Eur. J. Immunol.* **4**, 349 (1974).
89. Lankford, J. R., Blackstock, R., Szatalowicz, V., et al., *Cell. Immunol.* **14**, 163 (1974).
90. Osborne, D. P., and Katz, D. H., *J. Exp. Med.* **136**, 439 (1972).
91 Chiller, J. M., and Weigle, W. O., *J. Exp. Med.* **137**, 740 (1973).
92. Parks, D. E., Doyle, M. V., and Weigle, W. O., *Fed. Proc.* **35**, 789 (1976).
93. Weigle, W. O., Chiller, J. M., and Louis, J. A., *Transplant. Proc.* **4**, 373 (1972).
94. Weigle, W. O., Louis, J. A., Habicht, G. S., et al., in *Advances in the Biosciences 12, Schering Symp. on Immunopathol. Cavtat, Yugoslavia* (G. Raspe and S. Bernhard, eds.), Pergamon Press, Elmsford, N.Y., 1974, p. 93.
95. Weigle, W. O., *J. Exp. Med.* **116**, 913 (1962).
96. Weigle, W. O., *J. Exp. Med.* **114**, 111 (1961).
97. Benjamin, D. C., and Weigle, W. O., *J. Exp. Med.* **132**, 66 (1970).
98. Weigle, W. O., *Immunology* **7**, 239 (1964).
99. Benjamin, D. C., and Weigle, W. O., *J. Immunol.* **105**, 1231 (1970).
100 Benjamin, D. C., and Hershey, C. W., *J. Immunol.* **113**, 1593 (1974).
101. Habicht, G. S., Chiller, J. M., and Weigle, W. O., *J. Exp. Med.* **142**, 312 (1975).
102. Weigle, W. O., Chiller, J. M., and Louis, J. A., in *Progress in Immunology II*, vol. 3, Proc. Second Int. Cong. Immunol. (L. Brent and E. J. Holborow, eds.), North Holland, Amsterdam, 1975, p. 87.
103. Shulman, S., *Adv. Immunol.* **14**, 85 (1971).
104. Mellors, R. C., Brzosko, W. J., and Sonkin, L. S., *Am. J. Pathol.* **41**, 425 (1962).
105. Van Tienhoven, A., and Cole, R. K., *Anat. Rec.* **142**, 111 (1962).
106. Reuber, M. D., and Glover, E. L., *Proc. Soc. Exp. Biol. Med.* **129**, 509 (1968).
107. Fritz, T. E., Norris, W. P., and Kretz, N. D., *Proc. Soc. Exp. Biol. Med.* **134**, 450 (1970).
108. Levy, B. M., Hampton, S., Dreizen, S., et al., *J. Comp. Pathol.* **82**, 99 (1972).
109. Wick, G., Sundick, R. S., and Albini, B., *Clin. Immunol. Immunopathol.* **3**, 272 (1974).
110. Bigazzi, P. E., and Rose, N. R., *Prog. Allergy* **19**, 245 (1975).
111. Weigle, W. O., *J. Exp. Med.* **121**, 289 (1965).
112. Sjöberg, O., Andersson, J., and Möller, G., *Eur. J. Immunol.* **2**, 326 (1972).
113. Weigle, W. O., *Clin. Exp. Immunol.* **9**, 437 (1971).
114. Clinton, B. A., and Weigle, W. O., *J. Exp. Med.* **136**, 1605 (1972).
115. Weigle, W. O., and Romball, C. G., *Clin. Exp. Immunol.* **21**, 351 (1975).
116. Clagett, J. A., and Weigle, W. O., *J. Exp. Med.* **139**, 643 (1974).
117. Allison, A. C., in *Immunological Tolerance: Mechanisms and Potential Therapeutic Applications* (D. H. Katz, and B. Benacerraf, eds.), Academic Press, New York, 1974, p. 25.
118. Vladutiu, A. O., and Rose, N. R., *Fed. Proc.* **33**, 814 (1974).
119. Daniel, P. M., Pratt, O. E., Roitt, I. M., et al., *Immunology* **12**, 489 (1967).
120. Roitt, I. M., and Torrigiani, G., *Endocrinology* **81**, 421 (1967).
121. Nakamura, R. M., and Weigle, W. O., *J. Immunol.* **98**, 653 (1967).
122. Rose, N. R., and Witebsky, E., *J. Immunol.* **76**, 417 (1956).
123. Green, I., Benacerraf, B., and Stone, S. H., *J. Immunol.* **103**, 403 (1969).
124. Weigle, W. O., High, G. J., and Nakamura, R. M., *J. Exp. Med.* **130**, 243 (1969).
125. Anderson, C. L., and Rose, N. R., *J. Immunol.* **107**, 1341 (1971).
126. Weigle, W. O., *J. Exp. Med.* **122**, 1049 (1965).
127. Weigle, W. O., and Nakamura, R. M., *J. Immunol.* **99**, 223 (1967).
128. Weigle, W. O., *Immunology* **13**, 241 (1967).
129. Miller, J. F. A. P., Basten, A, Sprent, J., et al., *Cell. Immunol.* **2**, 469 (1971).
130. Byers, V. S., and Sercarz, E. E., *J. Exp. Med.* **127**, 307 (1968).
131. Von Felten, A., and Weigle, W. O., *Cell. Immunol.* **18**, 31 (1975).
132. Esquivel, P. S., Rose, N. R., and Kong, Y. M., *Fed. Proc.* **35**, 512 (1976).
133. Andersson, J., Möller, G., and Sjöberg, O., *Cell. Immunol.* **4**, 381 (1972).
134. Jones, J. M., and Kind, P. D., *J. Immunol.* **108**, 1453 (1972).
135. Shek, P. N., Chou, C.-T., Dubiski, S, et al., *Int. Arch. Allergy Appl. Immunol.* **46**, 753 (1974).
136. Shinohara, N., and Kern, M., *J. Immunol.* **116**, 1607 (1976).
137. Bankhurst, A. D., *Lancet* **1**, 226 (1973).
138. Roberts, I. M., Whittingham, S., and MacKay, I. R., *Lancet* **2**, 936 (1973).
139. Penhale, W. J., Farmer, A., Urbaniak, S. J., et al., *Clin. Exp. Immunol.* **19**, 179 (1975).

140. Nakamura, R. M., and Weigle, W. O., *J. Exp. Med.* **130**, 263 (1969).
141. Vladutiu, A. O., and Rose, N. R., *J. Immunol.* **106**, 1139 (1971).
142. Tomazic, V., and Rose, N. R., *Clin. Immunol. Immunopathol.* **4**, 511 (1975).
143. Clagett, J. A., Wilson, C. B., and Weigle, W. O., *J. Exp. Med.* **140**, 1439 (1974).
144. Calder, E. A., Penhale, W. J., Barnes, E. W., et al., *Clin. Exp. Immunol.* **14**, 19 (1973).
145. Calder, E. A., McLeman, D., and Irvine, W. J., *Clin. Exp. Immunol.* **15**, 467 (1973).
146. McMaster, P. R. B., and Lerner, E. M., *J. Immunol.* **99**, 208 (1967).
147. Söborg, M., and Halberg, P., *Acta Med. Scand.* **183**, 101 (1968).
148. Morgan, I. M., *J. Bacteriol.* **51**, 614 (1946).
149. Kabat, E. A., Wolf, A., and Bezer, A. E., *Science* **104**, 362 (1946).
150. Kabat, E. A., Wolf, A., and Bezer, A. E., *J. Exp. Med.* **85**, 117 (1947).
151. Paterson, P. Y., *Adv. Immunol.* **5**, 131 (1966).
152. Rauch, H. C., and Roboz-Einstein, E., *Rev. Neurosci.* **1**, 283 (1974).
153. Paterson, P. Y., *Fed. Proc.* **35**, 2428 (1976).
154. Eylar, E. H., *Proc. Natl. Acad. Sci.* (U.S.A.) **67**, 1425 (1970).
155. Carnegie, P. R., *Biochem. J.* **123**, 57 (1971).
156. Lamoreux, G., Thibault, G., Richer, G., et al., *Union Med. Can.* **101**, 674 (1972).
157. Paterson, P. Y., *J. Exp. Med.* **111**, 119 (1960).
158. Waksman, B. H., and Morrison, L. R., *J. Immunol.* **66**, 421 (1951).
159. Paterson, P. Y., Richardson, W. P., and Drobish, D. H., *Cell. Immunol.* **16**, 48 (1975).
160. Ortiz-Ortiz, L., Nakamura, R. M., and Weigle, W. O., *J. Immunol.* **117**, 576 (1976).
161. Ortiz-Ortiz, L., and Weigle, W. O., *J. Exp. Med.* **144**, 604 (1976).
162. Gonatas, N. K., and Howard, J. C., *Science* **186**, 839 (1974).
163. Kabat, E. A., Wolf, A., and Bezer, A. E., *J. Exp. Med.* **88**, 417 (1948).
164. Morgan, I. M., *J. Exp. Med.* **85**, 131 (1947).
165. Coates, A. S., and Lennon, V. A., *Immunology* **24**, 425 (1973).
166. Levine, S., and Sowinski, R., *J. Immunol.* **114**, 597 (1975).
167. Gasser, D. L., Newlin, C. M., Palm, J., et al, *Science* **181**, 872 (1973).
168. Williams, M. R., and Moore, M. J., *J. Exp. Med.* **138**, 775 (1973).
169. Weigle, W. O., *Adv. Immunol.* **21**, 87 (1975).
170. Portis, J. L., and Coe, J. E., *J. Immunol.* **117**, 835 (1976).
171. Dresser, D. W., in *Immunological Tolerance: Mechanisms and Potential Therapeutic Applications* (D. H. Katz and B. Benacerraf, eds.), Academic Press, New York, 1974, p. 3.
172. Romball, C. G., and Weigle, W. O., *Fed. Proc.* **35**, 862 (1976).
173. Romball, C. G., and Weigle, W. O., *J. Exp. Med.* **138**, 1426 (1973).
174. Segre, M., and Segre, D., *J. Immunol.* **99**, 867 (1967).
175. Britton, S., and Möller, G., *J. Immunol.* **100**, 1326 (1968).
176. Dwyer, J. M., and MacKay, I. R., *Lancet* **1**, 164 (1970).
177. Azzolina, L. S., *Eur. J. Immunol.* **6**, 227 (1976).
178. Rubinstein, P., *Transplantation* **2**, 695 (1964).
179. Stimpfling, J. H., and Richardson, A., *Transplantation* **5**, 1496 (1967).
180. Britton, S., in *Immunological Tolerance: Mechanisms and Potential Therapeutic Applications* (D. H. Katz and B. Benacerraf, eds.), Academic Press, New York, 1974, p. 319.
181. Denham, S., Grant, C. K., Hall, J. G., et al., *Transplantation* **9**, 366 (1970).
182. Gillespie, G. Y., and Barth, R. F., *Cell. Immunol.* **13**, 472 (1974).
183. Simpson, E., and Beverley, P. C. L., *Int. J. Cancer* **9**, 299 (1972).
184. Barrett, M. K., and Hansen, W. H., *J. Natl. Cancer Inst.* **18**, 57 (1957).
185. Snell, G. D., Winn, H. J., and Kandutsch, A. A., *J. Immunol.* **87**, 1 (1961).
186. Schlegal, R. A., *Aust. J. Exp. Biol. Med. Sci.* **52**, 99 (1974).
187. Bolton, R. W., Rozmiarek, H., and Chorpenning, F. W., *J. Immunol.* **118**, 1154 (1977).
188. Chen, F. W., Strosberg, A. D., and Haber, E., *J. Immunol.* **110**, 98 (1973).
189. Rubinstein, P., *Vox Sang.* **23**, 508 (1972).
190. Nielsen, K. H., and White, R. G., *Nature* (London) **250**, 234 (1974).
191. Eidinger, D., and Pross, H. F., *J. Exp. Med.* **126**, 15 (1967).
192. Sell, S., Park, A. B., and Nordin, A. A., *J. Immunol.* **104**, 483 (1970).
193. Wortis, H. H., Taylor, R.B., and Dresser, D.W., *Immunology* **11**, 603 (1966).
194. Hulliger, L., and Sorkin, E., *Immunology* **9**, 391 (1965).
195. Sorkin, E., and Landy, M., *Experientia* **21**, 677 (1965).

196. Benner, R., and van Oudenaren, A., *Cell. Immunol.* **19**, 167 (1975).
197. Britton, S., Wepsic, T., and Möller, G., *Immunology* **14**, 491 (1968).
198. Phillips, J. M., and Dresser, D. W., *Eur. J. Immunol.* **5**, 684 (1975).
199. Uhr, J. W., and Möller, G., *Adv. Immunol.* **8**, 81 (1968).
200. Graf, M. W., and Uhr, J. W., *J. Exp. Med.* **130**, 1175 (1969).
201. Bystryn, J.-C., Graf, M. W., and Uhr, J. W., *J. Exp. Med.* **132**, 1279 (1970).
202. Dixon, F. J., Jacot-Guillarmod, H., and McConahey, P. J., *J. Exp. Med.* **125**, 1119 (1967).
203. Bystryn, J.-C., Schenkein, I., and Uhr, J. W., in *Progress in Immunology* (B. Amos, ed.), Academic Press, New York, 1971, p. 627.
204. Jerne, N. K., *Ann. Immunol.* (Inst. Pasteur) **125C**, 873 (1974).
205. Hart, D. A., Wang, A., Pawlak, L. L., et al., *J. Exp. Med.* **135**, 712 (1974).
206. Rodkey, L. S., *J. Exp. Med.* **139**, 712 (1974).
207. Kluskens, L., and Köhler, H., *Proc. Natl. Acad. Sci.* (U.S.A.) **71**, 5083 (1974).
208. McKearn, T. J., Stuart, F. P., and Fitch, F. W., *J. Immunol.* **113**, 1876 (1974).
209. Bankert, R. B., and Pressman, D., *Fed. Proc.* **35**, 550 (1976).
210. Cosenza, H., and Köhler, H., *Proc. Natl. Acad. Sci.* (U.S.A.) **69**, 2701 (1972).
211. Eichmann, K., *Eur. J. Immunol.* **5**, 511 (1975).
212. Murgita, R. A., and Tomasi, T. B., Jr., *J. Exp. Med.* **141**, 440 (1975).
213. Murgita, R. A., and Tomasi, T. B., Jr., *J. Exp. Med.* **141**, 269 (1975).
214. Keller, R. H., and Tomasi, T. B., Jr., *J. Exp. Med.* **143**, 1140 (1976).
215. Gershon, R. K., *Contemp. Top. Immunobiol.* **3**, 1 (1974).
216. Romball, C. G., and Weigle, W. O., *J. Exp. Med.* **143**, 497 (1976).
217. Romball, C. G., and Weigle, W. O., *J. Immunol.* **115**, 556 (1975).
218. Pierce, C. W., and Kapp, J. A., *Contemp. Top. Immunobiol.* **5**, 91 (1976).
219. Wu, C.-Y., and Lance, E. M., *Cell. Immunol.* **13**, 1 (1974).
220. Romball, C. G., and Weigle, W. O., *Cell. Immunol.* **34**, 376 (1977).
221. Gershon, R. K., Lance, E. M., and Kondo, K., *J. Immunol.* **112**, 546 (1974).
222. Gershon, R. K., *Isr. J. Med. Sci.* **10**, 1012 (1974).
223. Kaplan, H. J., and Streilein, J. W., *Nature* (London) **251**, 553 (1974).
224. Monier, J. C., *J. Immunol.* **115**, 644 (1975).
225. Rich, S. S., and Rich, R. R., *J. Exp. Med.* **140**, 1588 (1974).
226. Gorczynski, R., Kontianen, S., Mitchison, N. A., et al., in *Cellular Selection and Regulation in the Immune Response* (G. M. Edelman, ed.), Raven Press, New York, 1974, p. 143.
227. Yoshida, T. O., and Andersson, B., *Scand. J. Immunol.* **1**, 401 (1972).
228. Chan, P. L., and Sinclair, N. R. S., *Immunology* **24**, 289 (1973).
229. Gershon, R. K., Orbach-Arbouys, S., and Calkins, C., in *Progress in Immunology II* vol. 2, Proc. Second Int. Cong. of Immunol. (L. Brent and E. J. Holborow, eds.), North Holland, Amsterdam, 1974, p. 123.
230. Gershon, R. K., Mokyr, M. B., and Mitchell, M. S., *Nature* (London) **250**, 594 (1974).
231. Barthold, D. R., Kysela, S., and Steinberg, A. D., *J. Immunol.* **112**, 9 (1974).
232. Allison, A. C., *Contemp. Top. Immunobiol.* **3**, 227 (1974).

Chapter Eight

General Aspects of Autoimmune Disease

NOEL R. ROSE
Department of Immunology and Microbiology, Wayne State University, Detroit, Michigan

The maturation of immunology as a distinct natural science entailed a widening definition of antigenicity. Initially, when immunology was concerned primarily with protection or treatment of infectious diseases, antigens were thought of only as pathogenic microorganisms or their products. Before long, however, it became apparent that all alien cells or cell products elicit a similar immunologic response marked by production of antibody to the parenterally injected antigen. Even harmless blood cells or serum of foreign species are fully antigenic. This broadening concept of antigenicity made even more impressive the often repeated observation that components of one's own body are usually not antigenic. The nonantigenicity of autologous molecules is not due to any peculiarity of their chemical structure or physical arrangement, since these same molecules are often strongly antigenic in other species (i.e., as xenoantigens) and sometimes even in other members of the same species (i.e., as alloantigens). What is operating, evidently, is a fundamental recognition mechanism for distinguishing self from nonself.

This self-nonself discrimination is marvelously precise; substances of similar stereochemical structure are unerringly distinguished. A striking example is provided by the blood group substances that differ only in one or two terminal monosaccharide substitutions. Similar statements can be made about other cell membrane antigens, such as the major histocompatibility antigens responsible for transplant rejection, although their chemical definition is not yet so far advanced. In approaching the subject of autoimmune disease, it is necessary to keep the general validity of self-nonself discrimination in mind. To induce autoimmunity, it becomes necessary to circumvent one of the basic properties of immunologic recognition. In fact, the study of autoimmunization sheds considerable light on the basis of normal immunologic function and regulation. As we shall see, there is considerable overlap between the concepts useful in understanding self-recognition and its breakdown and the concepts involved in those aspects of tolerance discussed in the previous chapter.

BASIS OF SELF-RECOGNITION

What are the possible mechanisms by which nonresponsiveness to self-antigens is normally maintained? In the days when inductive theories of antibody production held sway, the most reasonable explanation rested upon the continued presence in the body of large amounts of the particular self-antigen. The term "antigen sink" was used to describe the notion that antibodies can be formed regularly to self-constituents, but are taken up by the respective antigen as rapidly as they are synthesized. There may still be some validity to this concept in explaining the difficulty in finding high-affinity autoantibodies in the bloodstream.

This theory presages several predictions. One would expect that antigens that are isolated from the blood and lymphatic circulation would engender an antibody response more readily than accessible antigens. Certain examples of so-called sequestered autoantigens have been identified. The first instance, described many years ago by Uhlenhuth, was the lens of the eye (1). It is well shielded from the bloodstream and inaccessible to the antibody-forming cells. If rabbit lens crystallins are extracted and injected into a rabbit, antibody production results (2). Lens-specific antibodies that react in the test tube with lens of the immunized animal itself can be identified. These autoantibodies, however, do not harm the intact lens in the living animal. Spermatozoa behave in a similar manner. Injected even into the same animal from which they came, they elicit autoantibodies (3).

The brain also behaves as if it is sequestered, because brain suspensions obtained from foreign species elicit autoantibody production (4,5). However, brain suspensions of the same species do not elicit antibody production unless altered in some way. It is necessary to combine brain extract with foreign protein carrier (such as hog serum), culture brain cells with vaccinia virus, permit autolysis to occur, or combine the extract with complete Freund's adjuvant, a mixture of mineral oil and acid-fast bacteria (6–8). Under these conditions, the brain demonstrates its autoantigenic capabilities in the same animal.

With other tissues, demonstration of autoantigenic potential becomes more difficult. Thyroglobulin, the major protein of the thyroid antigen, was long thought to represent an anatomically isolated substance confined to the follicles of the gland. By itself, thyroglobulin is not antigenic in the same individual or members of the same species. However, injection of foreign thyroglobulins cross-reactive with autologous thyroglobulin elicits autoantibody formation (9,10). Moreover, thyroglobulin is antigenic to members of the same species if it is first enzymatically degraded (11,12). Chemically modified thyroglobulin prepared by insertion of sulfanilic or arsenilic groups is also autoantigenic (13). Finally, thyroglobulin combined with Freund's adjuvant is antigenic for members of the same species or for the same individual.

Like thyroglobulin, many other tissue proteins are not autoantigenic on their own, but acquire autoantigenic properties when combined with complete Freund's adjuvant. The best examples are antigens that are organ-specific, the ones that are confined to a single organ or cell type. The fact that they are not widely distributed throughout the body may be important to their autoantigenic capacity.

The observations described above require major revision of the original theory of the "antigen sink." It would seem that certain autologous antigens elicit antibody production when presented in a slightly modified form, even if the antigen is not naturally sequestered. Even greater reason to doubt the "antigen sink" concept, however, was provided by experiments using organ-specific antigens that can be eliminated from the body. Thyroglobulin provides a pertinent case in point. One would predict on the basis of the "antigen sink" hypothesis that completely thyroidectomized animals would respond readily to injections of their own thyroglobulin. Experimentally, this is not the case. Thyroidectomized rabbits do not produce thyroid autoantibodies after injections of unmodified rabbit thyroglobulin (14). The converse experiment was carried out by removing lymph nodes from normal rabbits (15,16). In a tissue culture environment containing no thyroglobulin, one might expect these cells spontaneously to produce thyroglobulin autoantibodies. This does not occur, showing that cells synthesizing antibody to thyroglobulin are not normally present in the body. However, such antibodies can be produced if the cells are first stimulated with thyroglobulin. Thus it has been shown that cells committed to production of autoantibodies are not normally active, although they are present and can be triggered into activity if appropriately challenged with antigen.

The difficulties in explaining self-recognition on the basis of inductive theories of antibody formation provided a major impetus toward development of Burnet's clonal selection theory (17). A corollary of the original clonal theory stated that precursors of lymphocytes reactive with self-antigens are eliminated during fetal and embryonic life. The basis of this elimination of self-reactive clones was not clearly stated, but it rests on the supposition that large amounts of antigen given prematurely may lead to functional abortion of the committed clones (18). The experiments of Medawar and his colleagues on artificially acquired immunologic tolerance were based largely on this hypothesis and lent it strong experimental support (19,20).

More recent information on cellular interactions in the immunologic response has provided alternate ways of visualizing clonal elimination. It is quite possible that only one of two (or more) populations of cells necessary for antibody production has been eliminated. Weigle and his colleagues demonstrated that smaller amounts of antigen inactivate T lymphocytes as compared with B lymphocytes (21). Small quantities of circulating self-antigen may lead in some manner to T cell elimination, leaving precursors only of self-reactive B cells (22). Supporting evidence for this hypothesis is provided by experiments showing that thyroglobulin-reactive B cells are present in the peripheral blood of normal animals and humans (23–25). These B cells can be triggered into action when suitable T cells are provided, either by activation of T cells with a cross-reactive antigen or by giving antigen with substances (adjuvants) that act as nonspecific T cell stimuli.

One explanation of clonal inactivation states that antigen impinging on only one of the two cooperating cells required for antibody production may result in unresponsiveness rather than a positive response (26). Since self-antigens are present at all times, they would be present whenever self-reactive lymphocytes arise by somatic mutation. Such single self-reactive lymphocytes would be easy prey to elimination, whereas foreign antigens would usually encounter two or more committed cells and therefore elicit a positive immunologic response.

The theories outlined above accord with the general notion of clonal elimination; that is, the view that self-reactive lymphocytes are inactivated when they arise during embryonic life or even in later life. However, they fail to account for the finding that self-reacting T cells, as well as B cells, can readily be induced to self-antigens like thyroglobulin. More recently, other theories of immunologic unresponsiveness have been put forward, based on principles of immunologic regulation. The immunologic response, like other physiologic reactions, has built-in homeostatic mechanisms; antibody production is normally limited in time and extent. Antibody levels reach a peak and gradually diminish, with kinetics depending upon the nature of the antigen, the route of injection, the form of antigen, and other factors. Even during a waning immunologic response, large numbers of competent cells are still present. If they are transferred to a new host, they will continue to elaborate antibody (27). There must, therefore, be mechanisms that actively suppress antibody production. One of these controls depends upon the antibody itself. Antibody to a particular antigen or antigen-antibody complexes diminishes production of more antibody (28). Likewise, antigen sometimes limits an immunologic response. An antigen given in excessive amounts, antigens that are poorly metabolized, such as pneumococcus polysaccharides, or dextrorotatory amino acid polymers, often induce long-standing immunologic unresponsiveness rather than antibody production (29).

There seem to be other ways in which the immunologic response is turned off under natural conditions. Antibody molecules contain unique configurations that are called idiotypes; they include the antigen-combining sites or receptors (30,31). This particular structure is found on variable portions of the immunoglobulin molecule and upon the lymphocyte responsible for its production (32). Antibody to this receptor site is capable of arresting production of more antibody with that combining site. Such antibodies, called antireceptor or anti-idiotype antibodies, are probably produced during all immunologic responses and serve as potent immunoregulators (33,34). In the case of autoimmune responses, the continuous presence of autoanti-idiotype antibodies may completely prevent production of autoantibody.

Another important regulatory mechanism involves interactions of lymphocytes. Positive production of an immunologic response generally depends upon the cooperation of T and B lymphocytes. Some T lymphocytes seem to interact with B lymphocytes (and other T lymphocytes) in a negative fashion so as to prevent or shut off an immunologic response. These lymphocytes represent a unique subset of T cells that bears special surface markers. The presence of suppressor T lymphocytes has been most convincingly demonstrated using purified basic protein, the autoantigen of brain (35).

At least partial compatibility of the major histocompatibility antigens is necessary for cellular cooperation to take place in the immunologic response. It seems that this complex of genes not only determines the strongest antigens involved in rejection of transplanted tissues but also encodes other surface receptors necessary for the cellular interactions of the immunologic response (36).

The number of lymphocytes committed to respond to major histocompatibility antigens of the same species seems to be significantly greater than the number of cells committed to respond to ordinary foreign antigens (37). It is reasonable to suppose that responsiveness to the major histocompatibility antigens is of high priority in the evolution of the immunologic response. Curiously, this closely linked group of genes is decisive in both sides of tissue rejection; it determines both the strength and the target of the immunologic response.

This critical role of the major histocompatibility complex in immunologic reactions brings up the question of its implication in self-recognition. The development of autoimmune reactions is sometimes correlated to the major histocompatibility antigens, as can be demonstrated by immunizing different inbred strains of mice with mouse thyroglobulin (38,39). It has also been demonstrated in the natural occurrence of autoimmune disease, such as a hereditary form of thyroiditis found in a strain of chickens, which is linked to the major histocompatibility locus of the chicken (40).

Regulation of the immunologic response is complex and depends upon several different mechanisms. The thymus is the central organ in immunologic regulation, through its ability to control both production of regulatory humoral antibodies (including anti-idiotypic antibodies) and production of suppressor T lymphocytes. Clinically, lesions of the thymus are frequently associated with autoimmune disorders (41). Not only are thymus lesions found in human diseases, but they are found in autoimmune diseases of animals (42). Autoimmune hemolytic anemia develops in the inbred New Zealand black (NZB) mouse, as will be discussed in more detail later; and its hybrid with New Zealand white (NZW) mice shows a high incidence of glomerulonephritis. Neonatal thymectomy increases the incidence of severity of autoimmune disease in the New Zealand mice (43). As another example, the presence of an intact, functional thymus seems to be critical in preventing abnormal autoimmune responses to thyroglobulin in otherwise normal mice. (44,45).

During aging, the thymus involutes and its function diminishes. As might be expected, therefore, the occurrence of autoimmune disease is more frequent in older persons, as well as in patients who have a demonstrable abnormality in their thymus glands (46,47).

The concept of autoimmunity as a defect in immunologic regulation brings autoimmune disease closer to other instances of dysfunction and deficiency of the immunologic system. Autoimmune diseases are relatively common (simultaneously or sequentially) in persons or family groups with immunodeficiency diseases and lymphocytic cancer, lymphomas, and leukemias. Patients with lymphoma are often troubled by production of antibodies to their own red blood cells, shown by positive antiglobulin tests, as a complication of their major disease. Conversely, the autoimmune disease, lupus erythematosus, is sometimes associated with a deficiency of IgA (48).

In the preceding section, an impressive list of mechanisms for avoiding immunologic reactions to constituents of one's own body was presented. Yet autoimmune responses occur frequently in animals and man, sometimes in association with disease. A study of these exceptions to the principle of self-recognition not only is valuable in understanding the mechanisms of immunopathology but provides additional evidence of the basis of immunologic recognition.

PRODUCTION OF AUTOANTIBODIES

The first authentic example of a human disorder associated with the abrogation of self-recognition came to light during the investigations by Donath and Landsteiner of the puzzling disease, paroxysmal cold hemoglobinuria (49), which used to be encountered mainly as a complication of syphilis. They found that many of the patients had antibodies to human red blood cells, reactive even with their own erythrocytes. Interestingly, these antibodies combined with red cells only at low temperatures. However, once combined with the erythrocyte, the antibodies could activate complement at 37°C, giving rise to hemolysis. The peculiar ability of these antibodies to react with the red cell antigens only at reduced temperatures represents a sort of protective device, preventing too great pathologic consequences of autoimmune reactivity.

The nature of the antigen to which the Donath-Landsteiner biphasic antibodies are directed has been elucidated only relatively recently. It belongs to the red cell alloantigens of the blood group P system (50). It seems significant for our later discussions that autoantibody production in this disease is stimulated by an alloantigen.

Following elucidation of the Donath-Landsteiner antibody, other autoantibodies to red blood cells and other circulating blood cells were demonstrated (49). In the human these antibodies can be an important cause of hemolytic anemias (51). Of course, the most significant antibodies clinically are the ones that can combine with their respective antigens at body temperature. Interestingly, the antigens of the red cell surface responsible for autoimmunity are often alloantigens, frequently members of the Rh constellation (52). Other autoantibodies to red blood cells combine with their antigens only in the cold. These cold-reactive hemagglutinins are generally less important in direct production of disease, but are often of value in diagnosis of a variety of infectious and malignant diseases. The cold hemagglutinins are frequently directed to the alloantigen, I (53). It must be pointed out, however, that the presence of low titers of cold hemagglutinins is virtually universal, since practically all humans and animals have low levels of antibodies capable of agglutinating their own red blood cells at reduced temperatures. Although the natural role of these antibodies is far from clear, some investigators have proposed that they are essentially physiologic, their function being that of removing damaged, effete blood cells by aiding their ingestion by the mononuclear phagocytes (54).

In addition to red cells, autoantibodies can be demonstrated to white blood cells and platelets (55,56). Sometimes these antibodies seem responsible for leukopenias and thrombocytopenias, respectively. Their production frequently follows upon viral infections or intake of certain drugs. Some drugs have the property of combining firmly with the white cell or platelet surface, thereby providing a complex antigen. Antibodies are produced to this complex antigen and result in cellular damage. These antibodies may be directed to the drug or virus itself (producing so-called "innocent bystander" damage to the cell); to a normal cell surface constituent combined with drug (i.e., "self plus X"); or to the altered cell (i.e., "altered self"). It is interesting that alloantigens are often the cell surface component involved in these reactions, even those initiated by drugs or infectious agents.

Soluble components of blood may also elicit autoantibody formation. These antibodies are generally produced to "hidden" determinants of serum proteins. For example, pepsin degradation of immunoglobulin exposes an antigen that reacts with serum of many normal and diseased individuals (57). These pepsin agglutinators are particularly conspicuous in diseases such as rheumatoid arthritis. Rarely, one finds evidence of autoantibodies to intact constituents of blood such as the gamma globulins (58).

Other autoantibodies are formed to determinants of serum constituents that are exposed during physiologic reactions. Combinations of antibody with antigen, or aggregation by other means, alter the configurations of the immunoglobulin molecule. Common examples are the rheumatoid factors found in the serum of patients with rheumatoid arthritis and related connective tissue diseases (59,60). They are normally directed to sites on IgG that become exposed after interaction with antigen or aggregation (61).

Antibody may be formed to split products of the third component of complement, especially during prolonged infection (62). The term "immunoconglutinin" is applied to these constituents. They have diagnostic value in certain long-standing infections and may even enhance the process of opsonization and immunologic resistance.

Autoantibodies can also be demonstrated to internal constituents of tissue cells. Presumably these constituents are normally inaccessible, so that the corresponding autoantibodies do no harm. The widely distributed glycoside, cardiolipin, is the basis for the most commonly used serologic tests for syphilis (63). If a sensitive enough technique is used, it seems likely that most humans will have some trace of antibody to this substance. Another intracellular constituent to which autoantibodies are commonly formed was described by Kidd and Friedewald many years ago (64). It is common to most cells of rabbits, and the corresponding antibodies are found in the serum of virtually all rabbits.

In addition to the widely distributed autoantigens of the Kidd-Friedewald type, more restricted tissue-specific natural autoantigens have been demonstrated. An interesting example of a tissue-specific autoantigen is found in the pancreas of rabbits (65). Antibodies to this constituent are found in sera of most rabbits. The antigen itself seems to be a typical example of an alloantigen, being found in tissues of some rabbits and not in others. A whole family of alloantigens has been discovered (66). By immunization, rabbits can be induced to produce elevated levels of antibodies to all the pancreas-specific alloantigens, except for the ones present in their own tissues (67). If pancreas extract is administered in an altered form, that is, by trichloracetic acid precipitation, rabbits can even be induced to form autoantibodies to their own pancreas-specific alloantigens (67). The pancreas of such autoimmunized rabbits seems to be normal in appearance.

INDUCTION OF AUTOIMMUNE DISEASE

The body has several ways of circumventing the potential pathogenetic effects of autoimmune responses. A striking example was first shown by Metalnikoff, who found that spermatozoa of the guinea pig induced autoantibody production in guinea pigs, as described above (3). However, the immunized guinea pig itself showed no ill effects of this immunization. Metalnikoff found that if he mixed the spermatozoa of an experimentally immunized guinea pig with normal serum as a source of complement in a test tube, immobilization resulted. He concluded, therefore, that although antibodies would penetrate the testicle and combine with the spermatozoa, no damage took place in the body because of the absence of effective levels of complement. This sample experiment illustrates the important balance of factors that is necessary to produce autoimmune disease.

The induction of an autoimmune disease is dependent upon administration of xenoantigen, alloantigen, or autoantigen by an appropriate method. Occasionally the simple process of purifying a protein is sufficient to bring out its autoantigenic potential. More often, however, it is necessary deliberately to alter the antigen in some way; proteolytic breakdown of the antigen is one effective way. Moreover, proteolytic breakdown may be analogous to natural processes going on in the body. Thyroglobulin is naturally cleaved into simple amino acids and released into the bloodstream. If thyroglobulin is partially degraded by proteolytic enzymes, the split products are antigenic for animals of the same species, whereas intact thyroglobulin is not (11). In the case of papain-generated fragments, intravenous injection elicits not only autoantibody production but lymphocytic infiltration of the animal's thyroid, i.e., thyroiditis (12).

An alternate mechanism for inducing autoantibody disease is introduction of the antigen in a related, cross-reactive form (68,10). For instance, foreign thyroglobulins will elicit the autoantibody production to thyroglobulin of the same species. Following repeated injections, lymphocytic infiltration of the thyroid gland of the immunized animal may take place. An analogous situation is found when antigens shared by bacteria and cells of the body are used for immunization. Beta hemolytic streptococci have surface antigens closely resembling sarcolemmal or subsarcolemmal components of the myocardium (69). Therefore, repeated injections of a streptococcal vaccine sometimes elicit autoantibodies to heart muscle. This mechanism has been postulated to explain the origin of rheumatic fever.

In other diseases it seems likely that self-antigens are altered through the agency of viruses or other infectious agents. In mice antibodies were generated during infection by lymphocytic chorimeningitis (LCM) virus which are cytotoxic for cells containing these viruses (70). It is not always certain what the specificity of these antibodies is; that is, whether they are directed to the virus, or to the host cell, or to a combination, but the outcome remains the same. The cell is destroyed by self-reactive antibodies or lymphocytes. This immunopathologic mechanism may prove to be important in persistent or "slow" virus infections, including some of the demyelinating diseases. Subacute sclerosing panencephalitis has been associated with previous measles infection (71). Prolonged viral infection has also been implicated in multiple sclerosis (72).

Many autoimmune responses seem to be due to changes in the immunologic apparatus itself, rather than to alteration of the antigen. In his original formulation of the clonal selection theory, Burnet proposed that "forbidden clones" of lymphocytes reactive to self-antigens are constantly arising by somatic mutation (17). If these clones escape elimination or suppression by one of the mechanisms described previously, they may produce autoantibodies. Such somatic mutations continue during life, so that production of autoantibodies is a statistically predictable, stochastic process.

In cases where autoimmunity arises because of a change in an antigen, one might expect that the autoimmune response is directed primarily to a single antigen. However, when the immunologic apparatus itself is at fault, a variety of different autoantibodies may be anticipated. In the case of the human disease, lupus erythematosus, one finds such a great variety of autoantibodies. The most conspicuous antibodies, and the ones of the greatest importance diagnostically, are directed to constituents of the nucleus, such as DNA or DNA-histone, as well as RNA and the nuclear membrane (73). However, autoantibodies may also be bound to surface antigens of the red blood cells, white blood cells, and platelets, and even to clotting factors, as well as to a great variety of tissue antigens (74). This disease, therefore, is the prototype for autoimmune disease related to a fundamental disturbance of immunologic regulation.

Although it is possible to produce organ-specific autoimmune diseases by experimental immunization, no such counterpart of the generalized autoimmune diseases has been developed. However, the naturally occurring diseases seen in the New Zealand mice serve as valuable models for the study of these diseases. In NZB mice hemolytic anemia consistently develops, starting at the age of approximately 3 months (75,76). By 9 months of age, essentially all members of this inbred population have severe anemia and splenomegaly; a few have other manifestations of autoimmune reactions, such as antinuclear antibodies. However, antinuclear antibodies are much more commonly seen in hybrid mice resulting from the cross between the NZB and apparently normal NZW lines. In the (NZB × NZW)F_1 hybrids, one sees many of the clinical and pathologic features of lupus erythematosus, including deposition of immunoglobulin and complement components in the kidneys, eventually leading to glomerulonephritis.

Analysis of the disease in NZB mice has brought to light several etiologic and pathogenic factors. One is the complex nature of genetic control in this disease. It would appear that disease susceptibility is polygenic with both dominant and recessive genetic characteristics (77). A second feature is the presence of leukemia viruses in the New Zealand stocks (78,79). These oncogenic viruses may be a necessary component of autoimmune disease. Another factor of the disease is the early development of antibodies damaging to thymic cells (80). A premature arrest of thymic functions and reduced levels of T cells appear in mice with this disorder (81). Finally, it should be noted that lymphomas often develop in the NZB mice at older ages; this suggests a connection between lymphoid cancer and autoimmunity.

Genetic control of autoimmune responses is an important feature not only in the generalized, multiple immune reactions of NZB mice but in organ-specific autoimmune diseases such as thyroiditis (82). As mentioned above, the immunologic response of mice to injections of thyroglobulin is dependent upon the strain used. The major genetic control of this immune response maps within the major histocompatibility complex of the mice. Possibly an immune response (Ir) gene codes for recognition of one or more determinants of the thyroglobulin molecule (83). However, the genetic control is clearly complex because of autoantibody production and can sometimes be dissociated from control of lesions in the thyroid.

As one might expect, it is possible by extensive breeding to develop colonies of animals in which a tendency towards a particular autoimmune response is so great that the reaction occurs spontaneously. This seems to have taken place in the development of the Obese strain (OS) of chicken (84). By selection of a few animals with clinical and biochemical evidence of hypothyroidism, a colony was developed in which thyroid failure develops spontaneously in more than 90% of the members (85). This disease was shown to be autoimmune in origin, since specific autoantibodies to thyroglobulin correlate with development of disease. For the study of organ-specific autoimmune maladies, the OS chicken represents the counterpart of the NZB mouse. This experimental model has provided several unexpected bits of evidence about the origin of autoimmune thyroiditis. One is that the disease is greatly reduced by bursectomy, which prevents antibody production (86). On the other hand, neonatal thymectomy, which reduces cell-mediated immunity, significantly increases the severity of the disease (87). This finding suggests that the pathologic changes of the disease are dependent upon bursa-derived cells or antibody, whereas the major role of the thymus is probably one of suppression. In inducing autoimmune thyroiditis experimentally, the role of adjuvants is crucial. Although it is not yet clear precisely what all the effects of these agents may be, the net result is that they replace in part the need for a genetic tendency to develop autoimmune disease. With complete Freund's adjuvant, virtually any animal can be induced to develop autoantibodies to thyroglobulin.

PATHOGENETIC MECHANISMS

Immune responses generally produce pathogenic effects by a variety of mechanisms that are dealt with in detail in other parts of this book. The most clearly recognized mechanisms include antibody-dependent, complement-mediated cytotoxicity; antibody-dependent, cell-mediated cytotoxicity; and immune complex deposition and direct cell-mediated cytotoxicity. All these mechanisms have been implicated in autoimmune diseases.

There are a few instances wherein autoantibodies and complement appear to have a cytotoxic effect. In some hematologic disorders, autoantibodies may be formed against elements of the blood, as described above. Fortunately for most patients, relatively few cases are encountered in which hemolysis occurs in vivo. Ehrlich first showed that intravascular hemolysis can be produced in cases of paroxysmal cold hemoglobinuria by immunizing the patient's finger in cold water and then allowing it to warm up (88). In other types of autoimmune hemolytic anemia, the conditions required for in vitro hemolysis are rarely found. It is necessary that the complement-fixing hemolysins be active at body temperature and be capable of reacting with erythrocytes that are not enzyme-treated. However, the survival time of red blood cells coated with antibody and complement is shortened, probably due to greater uptake by mononuclear phagocytes, either because of opsonization and phagocytosis of the red cells or because of adherence to monocytes by means of Fc receptors.

Knowledge about the pathogenic properties of thrombocyte antibodies is much less advanced due to technical difficulties in handling the platelets. They tend to stick to each other and to bind immunoglobulin nonspecifically. However, it has been shown that the plasma of patients with idiopathic thrombocytopenia induces thrombocytopenia in normal volunteers (89).

Autoantibodies to leukocytes are equally difficult to demonstrate reliably in cases of leukopenia (90), even though alloantibodies are rather easily detected in patients with multiple transfusions or pregnancies (91). By use of the antiglobulin consumption test, autoreactive immunoglobulins can be found in some patients with lupus associated with a positive lupus erythematosus test, in whom they may play a role in nuclear phagocytosis (92). Perhaps of more clinical importance are the autolymphotoxins found in the serum of some patients with lupus and other diseases characterized by abnormal immunologic responses (93). Similar antibodies to thymocytes have been described in NZB mice.

Antibodies combining with soluble antigens may also produce cellular damage. The role of antigen-antibody complexes has been well established in the pathogenesis of several autoimmune diseases. Complexes of antigen and antibody are frequently deposited in the kidney, and they may also be found in the lung and the skin. At these sites the immune complexes activate complement and induce an inflammatory reaction. The reactions are often caused by foreign antigens, but autologous antigens may also be responsible. These mechanisms of tissue damage are important in cases of human lupus erythematosus or in NZB/W mice in which nuclear antigens may induce immune complexes that produce severe and sometimes fatal glomerulonephritis (94,95). Complexes have been identified along the basement membrane of thyroid glands for cases of human chronic thyroiditis and experimentally induced thyroiditis (95,96). This may represent the product of a local antigen-antibody reaction. Such complexes, formed in vitro, seem to be capable of initiating an active process of autoimmune disease in genetically susceptible strains of mice (97). On the other hand, no evidence for immune complex deposition was found in the thyroids of BUF rats in which the spontaneous form of thyroiditis developed (98).

When one is dealing with autoantigens found in organized tissues, antibodies rarely seem to penetrate in concentrations sufficient to produce direct damage. In these cases the highly motile lymphocyte may serve as the pathogenic agent. Sometimes sensitized lymphocytes bear receptors reactive with tissue surface antigens and can produce direct cell damage (99). Specific T lymphocytes can be shown to attack allogeneic target cells both in vitro and in vivo without the participation of antibody, complement, or macrophages. Although extensive efforts have been made to demonstrate direct lymphocyte effects in autoimmune disease, they have always led to ambiguous results, primarily because stimulated lymphocytes nonspecifically injure susceptible epithelial target cells. For example, lymph node cells from rabbits immunized with rabbit thyroglobulin attack and prevent growth of rabbit thyroid cells. However, lymphoid cells from control rabbits injected with unrelated antigens do produce cell damage, although it is quantitatively somewhat less (100). Peripheral blood lymphocytes from patients with chronic thyroiditis were shown to lyse mastocytoma cells coated with thyroglobulin, although it was not clearly established that T cells were responsible (101).

In other cases, normal lymphocytes can cooperate with antibody to produce cytotoxic effects on target cells (102,103,104). This antibody-dependent, cell-mediated cytotoxic reaction depends for specificity upon the antibody, but the damaging effects are due to the lymphocyte. The lymphocyte population involved in killing has not yet been fully characterized, but in most species it lacks the typical surface markers of either T cells and B cells, so that the tentative designation of "null" cells has been applied (105).

Although the in vitro reaction does not require complement, IgG activates the effector cells by interaction with the Fc receptor. In the presence of antibody, nonsensitized lymphocytes from peripheral blood, spleen, and lymph nodes lyse chicken red blood cells coated with antigen. Cells capable of mediating antibody-dependent cytotoxicity have been demonstrated in the infiltrates of animals with experimental thyroiditis (106). In addition, nonsensitized lymphocytes from peripheral blood cooperate with antibody, or with antigen-antibody complexes, to damage target cells coated with human thyroglobulin (107). Lymphoid cells of normal as well as immunized experimental animals act with immune sera to injure living thyroid epithelial cells (108).

Cell-mediated reactions are certainly of importance in producing tissue damage in connection with autoimmune disease. The final destruction is the result of a long series of specific and nonspecific reactions that are difficult to analyze. The interplay of humoral factors with lymphocytes and macrophages, which act as the major effectors of tissue damage, will probably be a subject of continued investigation for many years to come.

REFERENCES

1. Uhlenhuth, P. T., in *Festschrift zum 60 Geburtstag Robert Koch,* Gustav Fischer, Jena, 1903.
2. Hektoen, L., *J. Infect. Dis.* **31**, 72 (1922).
3. Metalnikoff, S., *Ann. Inst. Pasteur* (Paris) **14**, 577 (1900).
4. Brandt, R., Guth, H., and Müller, R., *Klin. Wochenschr.* **5**, 655 (1926).
5. Witebsky, E., and Steinfeld, J., *Z. Immunitätsforsch.* **58**, 271 (1928).
6. Rivers, T. M., and Schwentker, F. F., *J. Exp. Med.* **61**, 689 (1935).
7. Rivers, T. M., Sprunt, D. H., and Berry, G. P., *J. Exp. Med.* **58**, 39 (1933).
8. Kabat, E. A., Wolf, A., and Bezer, A. E., *J. Exp. Med.* **85**, 117 (1948).
9. Witebsky, E., and Rose, N. R., *J. Immunol.* **83**, 41 (1959).
10. Weigle, W. O., *J. Exp. Med.* **121**, 289 (1965).
11. Stylos, W. A., and Rose, N. R., *Clin. Exp. Immunol.* **5**, 285 (1969).
12. Anderson, C. L., and Rose, N. R., *J. Immunol.* **107**, 1341 (1971).
13. Weigle, W. O., *J. Exp. Med.* **122**, 1049 (1965).
14. Rose, N. R., and Witebsky, E., *J. Immunol.* **76**, 408 (1956).
15. Doebbler, T. K., Kite, J. H., Jr., and Rose, N. R., *Fed. Proc.* **21**, 43 (1962).
16. Rose, N. R., Kite, J. H., Jr., Doebbler, T. K., et al., in *International Symposium on Injury, Inflamma-*

tion and Immunity (L. Thomas, J. W. Uhr, and L. Grant, eds.), Williams and Wilkins, Baltimore, 1964, p. 135.
17. Burnet, F. M., *The Clonal Selection Theory of Acquired Immunity,* Cambridge University Press, Cambridge, 1969.
18. Nossal, G. J. V., and Pike, B. L., *J. Exp. Med.* **141**, 904 (1975).
19. Billingham, R. E., Brent, L., and Medawar, P. B., *Proc. R. Soc. Lond. B.* **143**, 43 (1954).
20. Billingham, R. E., Brent, L., and Medawar, P. B., *Proc. R. Soc. Lond. B.* **143**, 58 (1954).
21. Weigle, W. O., *Clin. Exp. Immunol.* **9**, 437 (1971).
22. Allison, A. C., *Lancet* **2**, 1401 (1971).
23. Bankhurst, A. D., Torrigiani, G., and Allison, A. C., *Lancet* **1**, 226 (1973).
24. Allison, A. C., *Ann. Rheum. Dis.* **32**, 283 (1973).
25. Louis, J., Chiller, J., and Weigle, W. O., *J. Exp. Med.* **137**, 461 (1973).
26. Bretscher, P., and Cohn, M., *Science* **169**, 1042 (1970).
27. Wakefield, J. D., and Rose, N. R., *Transplantation* **6**, 91 (1968).
28. Uhr, J. W., and Möller, G., *Adv. Immunol.* **8**, 81 (1968).
29. Felton, L. D., Prescott, B., Kauffman, G., et al., *J. Immunol.* **74**, 205 (1955).
30. Ramseier, H., *Immunol. Commun.* **5**, 827 (1976).
31. Ramseier, H., and Lindenman, J., *Transplant. Rev.* **10**, 59 (1972).
32. Binz, H., and Wigsell, H., *J. Exp. Med.* **142**, 197 (1975).
33. McKearn, T. J., *Science* **183**, 94 (1974).
34. Rose, N. R., *Transplantation* **20**, 248 (1975).
35. Swanborg, R. H., *Clin. Exp. Immunol.* **26**, 597 (1976).
36. Shreffler, D. C., and David, C. S., *Adv. Immunol.* **20**, 125 (1975).
37. Ford, W. L., Simmonds, S. J., and Atkins, R. C., *J. Exp. Med.* **141**, 681 (1975).
38. Vladutiu, A. O., and Rose, N. R., *Science* **174**, 1137 (1971).
39. Tomazic, V., Rose, N. R., and Shreffler, D. C., *J. Immunol.* **112**, 965 (1974).
40. Rose, N. R., Bacon, L. D., and Sundick, R. S., *Transplant. Rev.* **31**, 264 (1976).
41. Halperin, I. C., Minogue, W. F., and Komninos, Z. D., *N. Engl. J. Med.* **275**, 663 (1966).
42. Burnet, F. M., and Holmes, M. C., *Australas. Ann. Med.* **14**, 185 (1965).
43. Talal, N., and Steinberg, A. D., *Curr. Top. Microbiol. Immunol.* **64**, 79 (1974).
44. Kojima, A., Tanaka, Y., Kojima, T., et al., *Lab. Invest.* **34**, 550 (1976).
45. Kojima, A., Tanaka, Y., Kojima, T., et al., *Lab. Invest.* **34**, 601 (1976).
46. Roitt, I. M., and Doniach, D., *Br. Med. Bull.* **23**, 67 (1967).
47. Irvine, W. J., *Scot. Med. J.* **5**, 511 (1960).
48. Amann, A. J., and Hong, R., *Medicine* **50**, 223 (1971).
49. Donath, J., and Landsteiner, K., *München. Med. Wochenschr.* **51**, 1590 (1904).
50. Levine, P., Celano, B. S., and Falkowski, F., *Transfusion* **3**, 278 (1963).
51. Wiener, A. S., Unger, L. J., Cohen, L., et al., *Ann. Intern. Med.* **44**, 221 (1956).
52. Dacie, J. V., *The Haemolytic Anemias, Congenital and Acquired, Part II: The Auto-immune Haemolytic Anemias,* Grune and Stratton, New York, 1962.
53. Weiner, W., and Vos, G. H., *Blood* **42**, 445 (1973).
54. Boyden, S., *Nature* **201**, 200 (1964).
55. Moeschlin, S., and Wagner, K., *Acta Haematol.* **8**, 29 (1952).
56. Ackroyd, J. F., *Proc. R. Soc. Med.* **55**, 30 (1962).
57. Osterland, C. K., Harboe, M., and Kunkel, H. G., *Vox Sang.* **8**, 133 (1963).
58. Franklin, E. C., Holman, H. R., Müller-Eberhard, H. J., et al., *J. Exp. Med.* **105**, 425 (1957).
59. Waaler, E., *Acta Pathol. Microbiol. Scand.* **17**, 172 (1940).
60. Rose, H. M., Ragan, C., Pearce, E., et al., *Proc. Soc. Exp. Biol. Med.* **68**, 1 (1948).
61. Christian, C. L., *J. Exp. Med.* **108**, 139 (1958).
62. Coombs, R. R. A., Coombs, A. M., and Ingram, D. G., *The Serology of Coagulation and Its Relation to Disease,* Charles C Thomas, Springfield, Ill. 1961.
63. Pangborn, M. C., *J. Biol. Chem.* **161**, 71 (1945).
64. Kidd, J. G., and Friedewald, W. F., *J. Exp. Med.* **76**, 543 (1942).
65. Brinckerhoff, C. E., and Rose, N. R., *J. Immunol.* **102**, 1208 (1969).
66. Rose, N. R., Metzger, R. S., and Witebsky, E., *J. Immunol.* **85**, 575 (1960).
67. Rose N. R., in *Immunopathology, Fourth International Symposium,* (P. Grabar and P. A. Miescher, eds.), Grune and Stratton, New York, 1965.
68. Terplan, K. L., Witebsky, E., Rose, N. R., et al., *Am. J. Pathol.* **36**, 213 (1960).

69. Kaplan, M. H., *Ann. N. Y. Acad. Sci.* **124**, 904 (1965).
70. Oldstone, M. B. A., and Dixon, F. J., in *Textbook of Immunopathology,* 2d ed. (P. A. Miescher and H. J. Müller-Eberhard, eds.), Grune and Stratton, New York, 1976.
71. Adams, J. M., Baird, C., and Filloy, L., *J.A.M.A.* **195**, 150 (1966).
72. Dick, G. W. A., McKeown, F., and Wilson, D. C., *Br. Med. J.* **1,** 7 (1958).
73. Rothfield, N. F., in *Manual of Clinical Immunology* (N. R. Rose and H. Friedman, eds.), American Society for Microbiology, Washington, D.C., 1976, p. 647.
74. Miescher, P. A., Paronetta, F., and Lambert, P. H., in *Textbook of Immunopathology,* 2d ed. (P. A. Miescher and H. J. Müller-Eberhard, eds.), Grune and Stratton, New York, 1976.
75. Holmes, M. C., *Aust. J. Exp. Biol. Med. Sci.* **43**, 399 (1965).
76. Howie, J. B., and Helyer, B. J., *Adv. Immunol.* **9**, 215 (1968).
77. Playfair, J. H. L., *Immunology* **21**, 1037 (1971).
78. Mellors, R. C., *J. Infect. Dis.* **120**, 480 (1969).
79. Dixon, F. J., Oldstone, M. B. A., and Tonietti, G., *J. Exp. Med.* **134**, 655 (1971).
80. Shirai, T., and Mellors, R. C., *Proc. Nat. Acad. Sci.* **68**, 1412 (1971).
81. Talal, N., *Transplant. Rev.* **31**, 240 (1976).
82. De Groot, L. J., Hall, R., McDermott, W. V., et al., *N. Engl. J. Med.* **267** (1962).
83. Tomazic, V., Rose, N. R., and Shreffler, D. C., *J. Immunol.* **112**, 965 (1974).
84. Bigazzi, P., and Rose, N. R., *Prog. Allergy* **19**, 245 (1974).
85. Cole, R. K., Kite, J. H., Jr., Wick, G., et al., *Poult. Sci.* **49**, 839 (1970).
86. Wick, G., Kite, J. H., Jr., Cole, R. K., et al., *J. Immunol.* **104**, 45 (1970).
87. Welch, P., Rose, N. R., and Kite, J. H., Jr., *J. Immunol.* **110**, 575 (1973).
88. Ehrlich, P., and Morgenroth, J., *Berlin Klin. Wochenschr.* **37**, 453 (1900).
89. Harrington, W. J., Minnich, V., Hollingsworth, J. W., et al., *J. Lab. Clin. Med.* **38**, 1 (1951).
90. Dausset, J., and Nenna, A., *C. R. Soc. Biol.* (Paris) **146**, 1539 (1952).
91. van Loghem, J. J., *Vox Sang.* **3**, 303 (1958).
92. Meischer, P. A., Barker, L., Vanio, I., et al., in *International Symposium on Injury, Inflammation and Immunity* (L. Thomas, J. W. Uhr, and L. Grant, eds.), Williams and Wilkins, Baltimore, 1963, p. 346.
93. Koffler, D., *Pathobiol. Annu.* **5**, 221 (1972).
94. Lambert, P. H., and Dixon, F. J., *J. Exp. Med.* **127**, 50 (1968).
95. Kalderon, A. E., Bogaars, H. A., and Diamond, A., *Clin. Immunol. Immunopathol.* **4**, 101 (1975).
96. Clagett, J. A., Wilson, C. B., and Weigle, W. O., *J. Exp. Med.* **140**, 1439 (1974).
97. Tomazic, V., and Rose, N. R., *Clin. Immunol. Immunopathol.* **4**, 511 (1975).
98. Noble B., Bigazzi, P., and Rose, N. R., *Fed. Proc.* **34**, 835 (1975).
99. Cerottini, J. C., and Brunner, K. T., *Adv. Immunol.* **18**, 67 (1974).
100. Rose, N. R., in *Cell-Bound Immunity,* Wistar Institute Press, Philadelphia, 1963, p. 19.
101. Podleski, U., and Podleski, W. K., *J. Lab. Clin. Med.* **84**, 459 (1974).
102. Perlmann, P., and Holm, G., *Adv. Immunol.* **11**, 117 (1969).
103. Henney, C. S., *Transplant. Rev.* **17**, 37 (1973).
104. MacLennon, I. C. M., Loewi, G., and Howard, A., *Immunology* **17**, 897 (1969).
105. Greenberg, A. H., Shen, L., Walker, L., et al., *Eur. J. Immunol.* **5**, 474 (1975).
106. Paget, S. A., McMaster, P. R. B., and vox Boxel, J. A., *J. Immunol.* **117**, 2267 (1976).
107. Calder, E. A., Penhale, W. J., McCleman, D., et al., *Clin. Exp. Immunol.* **14**, 153 (1973).
108. Biörklund, A., *Lab. Invest.* **13,** 120 (1964).

Chapter Nine

Thyroiditis as a Model of Autoimmune Disorders in Man

PIERLUIGI E. BIGAZZI

University of Connecticut Health Center, Farmington, Connecticut

Autoimmune diseases are of interest from both a practical and a theoretical point of view. The study of autoimmunity has provided the basis for diagnostic and therapeutic advances in clinical medicine, and progress is still being made in many areas. In addition, investigations of autoimmunity have great theoretical importance, as they may help in the solution of the intriguing puzzle of immunologic tolerance.

Autoimmune diseases can be defined as those conditions in which structural or functional damage is produced by a humoral or cell-mediated immune reaction with normal components of the body. The antigens normally present and characteristic of the human being or animal involved in this response are defined as "autoantigens," and the antibodies capable of reacting with them are termed "autoantibodies." Autoimmune diseases may be classified as "organ-specific" or "tissue-specific" and "generalized" or "non-organ-specific." The former, such as thyroiditis, adrenalitis, pernicious anemia, pemphigus vulgaris, etc., are characterized by autoimmune reactions to organ- or tissue-specific antigens, i.e., antigens present in only one particular organ or tissue. Generalized or non-organ-specific autoimmune diseases, such as systemic lupus erythematosus, are distinguished by an autoimmune response to antigens common to various organs and tissues, e.g., nuclear antigens.

In a few disorders, autoimmune reactions to both organ- and non-organ-specific antigens regularly occur, as is observed in Sjögren's disease and pemphigus erythematosus. Similarly, autoantibodies to nuclear antigens may be observed in some patients with organ-specific autoimmune diseases, such as thyroiditis, pernicious anemia, etc.

The concept of autoimmunity originated at the turn of the century, when Ehrlich first suggested that normally the body avoids making antibodies that might damage its own tissues and introduced the suggestive term "horror autotoxicus," the living body's fear of destroying itself (1). However, he also acknowledged the possibility that under particular circumstances this biologic principle might fail and autoantibodies might be produced. This possibility was indeed confirmed at the same time by Metalnikoff (2), who described an "autospermatoxin," a substance produced in the serum of guinea pigs after injection with guinea pig spermatozoa and capable of destroying not only spermatozoa of other guinea pigs but also those of the immunized animals. Autoimmune responses were also observed in hemolytic anemias (3) and experimental encephalomyelitis (4), but in spite of these findings the concept of autoimmunity did not gain a wide acceptance until 1955, when the results of a full-scale investigation of organ-specific antigens of the thyroid were published (5).

It is to the credit of Ernest Witebsky and his associates to have demonstrated the production of thyroid antibodies in experimental animals of different species and to have been the first to raise the issue of thyroid autoantibody formation (6). In June of the following year two additional papers, which have since become classics in the field of autoimmunity, described the formation of rabbit autoantibodies to thyroid antigens and the histopathologic changes observed in the thyroids of rabbits with an autoimmune response (7,8). In a few months, these publications were followed by a preliminary communication from the group of Doniach and Roitt (9), who reported the presence of precipitating antibodies to thyroglobulin in the sera of 7 patients with Hashimoto's thyroiditis. These findings, followed in rapid sequence by additional confirmatory evidence (10–14), raised the interest of immunologists all over the world and opened the floodgates for publications on autoimmunity.

It has since become evident that although several conditions may have as an underlying mechanism an autoimmune reaction, a large number of diseases of unknown etiology and pathogenesis have been very summarily labeled as "autoimmune," especially when an autoimmune response of some sort can be demonstrated. The following criteria, a slightly modernized version of Witebsky's original postulates (13), may help in the distinction of autoimmune diseases from those conditions that are merely accompanied by autoimmune reactions and are not caused by them.

Circulating autoantibodies and/or delayed hypersensitivity reactions to autoantigens should be demonstrated in patients suffering from the disease. The autoantigen(s) involved should be recognized and if possible isolated and characterized. An autoimmune response to a similar autoantigen should be produced experimentally or found to occur spontaneously in laboratory animals. Pathologic changes, similar to those seen in the human disease, should appear in the corresponding tissues of experimental animals with an autoimmune response to the autoantigen in question.

These rather restrictive criteria are met in only a few of the many disorders labeled as autoimmune, the best examples being chronic lymphocytic thyroiditis, systemic lupus erythematosus, and, more recently, myasthenia gravis (Table 1).

Table 1. Some Human Diseases with Autoimmune Responses

Disease	Autoimmune Responses[a]	Autoantigens[b]	Animal Models[c]
Chronic lymphocytic thyroiditis	Humoral and cell-mediated (CMI)	Organ-specific of thyroid (thyroglobulin and microsomal)	Experimental (rabbits, rats, mice, etc.) and spontaneous (chickens, rats, and dogs)
Primary hypo-parathyroidism	Humoral	Organ-specific of parathyroid	No model
Addison's disease	Humoral and CMI	Organ-specific of adrenal cortex (microsomal)	Experimental
Diabetes mellitus	Humoral	Organ-specific of pancreas	No model
Pernicious anemia	Humoral and CMI	Organ-specific of stomach (intrinsic factor and microsomal)	Experimental
Inflammatory bowel disease	Humoral and CMI	Organ-specific of colon	No model
Goodpasture's syndrome	Humoral	Organ-specific of kidney and lung	Experimental
Myasthenia gravis	Humoral and CMI	Tissue-specific of striated muscle (acetylcholine receptors)	Experimental
Pemphigus vulgaris	Humoral	Tissue-specific of skin	No model
Bullous pemphigoid	Humoral	Tissue-specific of skin	No model

Continued on next page.

Table 1. Some Human Diseases with Autoimmune Responses *(continued)*

Disease	Autoimmune Responses [a]	Autoantigens [b]	Animal Models [c]
Systemic lupus erythematosus	Humoral	Non-organ-specific (nuclear antigens)	Experimental and spontaneous ((NZB/NZW) and Swan mice, dogs)
Rheumatoid arthritis	Humoral	Non-organ-specific (IgG)	Experimental
Scleroderma	Humoral	Non-organ-specific (nucleolar and nuclear antigens)	No model
Sjögren's disease	Humoral	Both organ-specific of salivary gland and non-organ-specific (nuclear antigens)	Spontaneous ((NZB/NZW) mice)
Pemphigus erythematosus	Humoral	Both tissue-specific of skin and non-organ-specific (nuclear antigens)	No model
Chronic active hepatitis	Humoral and CMI	Both tissue-specific of smooth muscle and non-organ-specific (nuclear antigens)	No model
Primary biliary cirrhosis	Humoral & CMI	Both non-organ-specific (mitochondria) and tissue-specific of smooth muscle	No model

[a] Most commonly reported to date.
[b] Only those autoantigens that have been isolated and well characterized are listed.
[c] Only those models that have been consistently reproducible are listed.

It is through the study of these disorders and their animal models that some progress has been made in the understanding of self-tolerance and its loss.

Since a full discussion of all the available literature on autoimmune diseases is practically impossible, in this presentation I will deal almost exclusively with autoimmune thyroiditis, one of the most closely studied examples of organ-specific autoimmune disease. This will serve as a model to illustrate many of the mechanisms and principles described in the preceding two chapters.

HUMORAL AND CELL-MEDIATED RESPONSE IN AUTOIMMUNE THYROIDITIS

Also termed chronic lymphocytic thyroiditis, Hashimoto's thyroiditis, struma lymphomatosa, and lymphadenoid goiter, autoimmune thyroiditis is a condition that was first described in 1912; but until 20 years ago there was no understanding of its pathogenetic mechanisms. It was only after the early studies of Witebsky and Rose (7) that a large body of evidence became available, pointing to the autoimmune nature of this condition, now generally defined as "autoimmune thyroiditis." The disease is characterized by an immune response, both humoral and cell-mediated, to thyroid-specific antigens and by inflammatory infiltration and tissue damage of the thyroid gland.

Thyroid-Specific Antigens

Organ-specific antigens of the thyroid that cause autoimmune responses are thyroglobulin, a second antigen localized in the thyroid colloid but different from thyroglobulin, an antigen localized in the cytoplasm of the follicular cells, and cell surface antigens.

Thyroglobulin, the main iodoprotein of the thyroid gland, is the storage form of the thyroid hormones and their immediate precursors. It is synthesized in the endoplasmic reticulum of the follicular cells, moves to their apical region, and is finally stored in the thyroid colloid. Early experiments performed by hemagglutination inhibition and radioimmunoassay demonstrated the presence of a thyroglobulin-like substance in a proportion of normal human sera (15–17). More recently, radioimmunoassay tests have shown that thyroglobulin is indeed present in small amounts in the circulation. In one study, detectable values were found in 54% of men and 70% of women, with values ranging between 10 and 150 ng/ml. Higher values were found in patients with colloid goiters and with Graves' disease (18,19). In another study, thyroglobulin was detected in the sera of 74% of normal subjects, with a mean concentration of 5.1 ng/ml. It was also detected in 90% of sera from pregnant women, with a mean concentration of 10.1 ng/ml. Higher levels were found in the sera of newborn infants, with a mean concentration of 29.3 ng/ml, and thyrotoxic individuals, with a mean concentration of 344 ng/ml (20).

Thyroglobulin is a glycoprotein, containing iodine, with a sedimentation coefficient of 19S, a molecular weight of approximately 700,000, and an electrophoretic mobility at pH 8.6, which resembles that of a serum alpha globulin.

Only certain portions of the thyroglobulin molecule may be capable of causing an autoimmune response. It has been estimated that each thyroglobulin molecule possesses approximately 50 antigenic determinants, 6 of which may be autoantigenic (21). It has also been suggested that autoantigenic determinants are formed by the folding of the secondary and tertiary structure of thyroglobulin and are masked by sialic acid (22).

A second antigen that causes autoimmune reactions is also localized in the colloid, but is different from thyroglobulin and thus was defined as "colloid antigen second" or CA2. The nature of CA2 is still unclear. Balfour et al. (23) hypothesized that it might be one of the thyroid proteases, but this was later excluded by further investigations (24). It is not known whether CA2, like thyroglobulin, is present in the circulation. Recently, the existence of CA2 as a separate antigen has been questioned, and it has been suggested that antibodies to CA2 "are probably complexes of thyroglobulin and thyroglobulin antibodies which have free antibody combining sites" (25).

A third organ-specific antigen of the thyroid is localized in the cytoplasm of the follicular cells. It was termed "microsomal" because it was separated by ultracentrifugation in the microsomal fraction, distinct from the mitochondrial and nuclear components. The nature and distribution of the thyroid "microsomal" antigen have been studied by the group of Doniach, who found it intimately associated with the lipoproteins of microvesicles with smooth profiles, which are particularly abundant at the apical margin of the thyroid cells and represent newly synthesized thyroglobulin droplets originating from the Golgi complex (24). It is not known whether the microsomal antigen, like thyroglobulin, is present in the circulation.

Very little is known about the organ-specific cell surface antigens of the thyroid. They have been identified by mixed hemadsorption and indirect immunofluorescence and have been found to be distributed in discrete areas over the cell surface (26,27).

Humoral and cell-mediated immune responses to one or more of these thyroid-specific antigens are detected in patients with autoimmune thyroiditis.

Humoral Autoimmune Responses

The sera of the great majority of patients with autoimmune thyroiditis contain autoantibodies capable of reacting in vitro with thyroglobulin, CA2, and the microsomal antigen.

Antibodies to thyroglobulin can be detected by a variety of procedures, such as precipitation in agar, indirect immunofluorescence, passive hemagglutination, and radioimmunoassay. However, most of the data reported in the literature have been obtained using the tanned cell passive hemagglutination procedure. The percentages of positive results obtained with this method vary from laboratory to laboratory and obviously reflect differences in the sensitivity of the technique, as well as variability in the patients' populations.

Antibodies to thyroglobulin have been detected in the sera of 60 to 90% of patients with autoimmune thyroiditis (28). Sera from histologically proved cases may be negative by the passive hemagglutination procedure; thus, a negative result does not exclude the diagnosis of autoimmune thyroiditis. In such cases, indirect immunofluorescence for CA2 and microsomal antibodies may be useful. Antibodies to thyroglobulin are detected in the sera of 63 to 82% of patients with primary myxedema; and when these patients have been staged on a clinical basis, antibodies were found in 47% of patients with subclinical hypothyroidism, 74% of patients with mild hypothyroidism, and 43% of patients with overt hypothyroidism (29). Thyroglobulin antibodies are also detected in 33 to 86% of patients with thyrotoxicosis, 28 to 65% of patients with thyroid carcinomas, 28 to 50% of patients with pernicious anemia, and 8% of subjects without overt thyroid disorders. When the incidence of thyroglobulin antibodies in normal subjects is analyzed in relation to age and sex, it is found that normal women between the ages of 21 and 70 have a higher incidence of such antibodies than men. Titers of thyroglobulin antibodies detected by tanned cell hemagglutination are extremely high in the fibrotic variant of thyroiditis and tend to be lower in most of the other patients with positive reactions. Antibodies to thyroglobulin can also be detected by chromic chloride passive hemagglutination, with a sensitivity higher than that of the commercially available tanned cell hemagglutination procedure (30), and by indirect immunofluorescence on cryostat sections of thyroid, a less sensitive method (31). The pattern of staining obtained by indirect immunofluorescence is characteristic and localized in the thyroid colloid, which assumes a three-dimensional appearance, with floccules having bright edges and dark centers.

Additional tests for the detection of antibodies to thyroglobulin have recently been suggested, but are not yet in routine diagnostic use. An immunoelectroosmophoretic method has proved to be a quick, inexpensive, and rather sensitive test (32). Antibodies to thyroglobulin have been also determined using the "defined antigen substrate spheres" (DASS) system. Agarose particles coated with human thyroglobulin were incubated with patients' sera, then with rhodamine-conjugated antiserum to human immunoglobulins, and finally the intensity of fluorescence was measured with a microfluorimeter system (33). Results obtained were comparable to those obtained by the tanned cell hemagglutination procedure.

Radioimmunoassay methods for antibodies to thyroglobulin have obviously proved more sensitive than all other methods (34–37). From 86 to 100% of patients with chronic lymphocytic thyroiditis, as well as 87 to 89% with untreated Graves' disease, 57% with treated Graves' disease, and 67 to 94% with primary myxedema, were found to have circulating antibodies to thyroglobulin detectable by radioimmunoassay (34,36). Antibodies to thyroglobulin were also detected in 15% of sera from patients with other autoimmune disorders, 8% of sera from patients with thyroid conditions not of an autoimmune nature, and 4% of sera from normal subjects. Antibodies to thyroglobulin are mostly IgG, with up to 20% IgA and less than 1% IgM (38,39). They are predominantly IgG_1, with lower amounts of IgG_2 and very small amounts of IgG_3 and IgG_4; thus, over 70% of the antigen-binding capacity is in subclasses that fix complement (40). The reason for the poor complement fixation observed in this system is most likely dependent on the fact that human autoantibodies can react with a maximum of four determinants on the thyroglobulin molecule. Since close proximity of bound IgG molecules is necessary for binding C1q, this limited number of autoantigenic sites on the thyroglobulin molecule may explain the lack of complement fixation.

Using a hemagglutination inhibition technique with cells coated with highly purified rabbit antibody to human thyroglobulin, Hjort (41) found that antibodies to thyroglobulin in sera from patients with autoimmune thyroiditis and myxedema had high avidity, whereas those in sera from Graves' disease patients have lower avidity.

The affinity constants and binding capacities of antibodies to thyroglobulin have been recently investigated by radioimmunoassay (42). Two populations of antibodies were detected in the sera of approximately 50% of the patients with Hashimoto's thyroiditis and Graves' disease. The first population of thyroglobulin antibodies had a high affinity and a low binding capacity, and the second population had lower affinity but a much higher binding capacity. In the remaining half of the patients only one population of thyroglobulin antibodies was detected, similar to the second population of the previous group, i.e., with a low affinity constant and a very high binding capacity. Circulating thyroglobulin antibodies observed in patients with Hashimoto's thyroiditis and Graves' disease were similar in their affinity constants and binding capacities.

Antibodies to the "colloid antigen second" or CA2 are detectable only by indirect immunofluorescence on cryostat sections of thyroid, with a characteristic bright green, uniform staining pattern of the entire colloid ("ground glass" pattern) (23). They were observed in 5 to 8% of sera negative by other tests for thyroiditis, 41% in patients with thyrotoxicosis, 16% in patients with primary myxedema, 30% in relatives of Hashimoto's thyroiditis patients, and 3% in controls. These findings have been confirmed by other investigators, but in smaller percentages of patients (43,44). Antibodies to CA2 belong to the IgG or IgA, but not the IgM, class (24).

Antibodies to the "microsomal" antigen of the follicular cells of the thyroid can be detected by complement fixation, indirect immunofluorescence, and passive hemagglutination. The most commonly used method is indirect immunofluorescence, by which these antibodies have been detected in 85 to 100% of patients with autoimmune thyroiditis, 57% with primary hypothyroidism, 37 to 66% with thyrotoxicosis, 26 to 67% with pernicious anemia, and 2 to 7% of normal controls (28). Less sensitive is complement fixation, which has given positive results in 55 to 73% of sera positive by immunofluorescence (45).

A hemagglutination method for thyroid microsomal antibodies, first developed in Japan, seems more sensitive than complement fixation and may be as sensitive as indirect immunofluorescence (45,46). By this procedure, antibodies to the microsomal antigen have been detected in 85 to 95% of patients with Hashimoto's thyroiditis and 66 to 86% with Graves' disease (47,48).

A radioimmunoassay for antibodies to the microsomal antigen has been developed, with positive results obtained in 95% of patients with thyroiditis, 98% with untreated Graves' disease, 75% with primary hypothyroidism, and 10% of hospitalized controls (34).

When patients with primary hypothyroidism have been staged on a clinical basis, antibodies to the microsomal antigen have been detected in 65% of patients with subclinical hypothyroidism, 75% of those with mild hypothyroidism, and 83% of those with overt hypothyroidism (29). From this point of view, it is interesting to note a recently reported case of transient hypothyroidism during the course of autoimmune thyroiditis that was associated with a concomitant increase of antibodies to the microsomal antigen, but not of antibodies to thyroglobulin (49).

A cytotoxic antibody is present in the serum of most patients with autoimmune thyroiditis (50,51,24). This antibody is effective in the presence of complement against cells obtained from thyrotoxic and normal thyroids dispersed with trypsin. It also acts against normal monkey thyroid cells. Cells obtained from the same thyroids by dispersion with collagenase are less affected, and thyroid cell explants are not affected at all by the same antisera. Cytotoxic antibodies are thought to be identical with microsomal antibodies, even though in some cases cytotoxic activity has been found to be dissociated from complement-fixing activity.

Antibodies to thyroid cell surface antigens have been demonstrated by mixed hemadsorption and indirect immunofluorescence in 98% of sera from patients with autoimmune thyroiditis, 76% with thyrotoxicosis, 34% with nontoxic goiter, and 45% with connective tissue diseases (26,27).

Cell-Mediated Responses

Delayed hypersensitivity reactions to thyroid autoantigens are observed in most patients with autoimmune thyroiditis. A few of these observations have been derived from studies performed in vivo, but the great majority are from in vitro studies that have shown lymphocyte stimulation and production of lymphokines.

Positive skin reactions were noted by Buchanan et al. (52) in 9 of 11 patients with Hashimoto's thyroiditis 24 hours after the intradermal injection of human thyroid extract. Strongly positive skin reactions characterized by both erythema and induration were seen only in patients with precipitating thyroid antibodies. The biopsy specimen of a strongly positive reaction showed edema and hemorrhage into the dermis and subcutis, with marked emigration of neutrophils and a few eosinophils. Weakly positive and negative skin reactions were much less extensive, but qualitatively similar to the strongly positive reactions. At that time, the skin reactions observed were interpreted as manifestations of a local antigen-antibody reaction, i.e., as an Arthus phenomenon. Saarma (53) also obtained positive skin tests with thyroid extract in 29 of 30 patients with goiter characterized by mononuclear cell infiltration. In addition, 27 of 54 patients with goiters and no infiltration were also positive by skin test.

Skin window experiments have shown that after injection of thyroid extract an increased percentage of basophilic leukocytes is found in the exudate of patients with thyroiditis. On the second day after injection, basophils reached a maximum of 4.2% of cells of the exudate, and eosinophils were 2.8%. No significant increases of neutrophils and macrophages were noted. These findings were interpreted as consistent with a delayed-type hypersensitivity reaction and as evidence of the involvement of basophils in autoimmune reactions. It is unfortunate that even in the recent renaissance of the basophil fostered by Dvorak

(55), not much attention has been paid to the role of these cells in autoimmune thyroiditis.

In vitro tests used by most investigators have shown lymphocyte stimulation and leukocyte migration inhibition. DeGroot and Jaksina (56) did not observe blast transformation or increased thymidine incorporation when lymphocytes from patients with Hashimoto's thyroiditis or Graves' disease were incubated with thyroid antigens. However, other investigators have since shown that circulating lymphocytes from such patients can indeed be stimulated by thyroid antigens (53,57–60). Lymphocytes from all patients with autoimmune thyroiditis are specifically stimulated to transform by human thyroglobulin or thyroid extract. There is a correlation between this phenomenon and the presence of thyroglobulin antibodies (60).

Another in vitro test detects the production of leukocyte inhibitory factor by patients' lymphocytes stimulated with thyroid antigens. Søborg and Halberg (61) demonstrated that the addition of crude thyroid extract to culture chambers containing peripheral leukocytes in capillary tubes caused the inhibition of migration of leukocytes from 6 to 15 patients with autoimmune thyroiditis. No correlation was observed between inhibition of migration and titers of thyroid antibodies. These results were later confirmed by other investigators, who reported inhibition of leukocyte migration in 63 to 86% of patients with autoimmune thyroiditis (62–65). The percentages of thyroiditis patients found positive by this procedure vary according to the antigens used for lymphocyte stimulation. Calder et al. (63), using crude thyroid extract, observed inhibition of migration in 66% of patients vs. 40% when purified thyroglobulin was used and 27% when "microsomal" antigen was used.

In a study by the group of Roitt and Doniach (66), leukocyte migration inhibition after incubation with thyroid microsomal antigen was obtained in all patients with autoimmune thyroiditis. Interestingly, none of these patients showed any inhibition when their leukocytes were incubated with thyroglobulin. The most intense inhibition with microsomal antigen was observed in patients with the "hypercellular" variant of thyroiditis, which has a mild clinical course, low or absent antibodies to thyroglobulin, and moderate titers of microsomal antibodies. Surprisingly, a very high percentage of the patients investigated in many of these studies also showed inhibition of leukocyte migration with mitochondria of thyroid, kidney, and liver (62,63,67).

Finally, a direct cytotoxic effect of lymphocytes from patients with autoimmune thyroiditis has also been noted. Initial studies, using thyroid cell monolayers, failed to demonstrate any cytotoxic activity of lymphocytes (68), but further investigations showed that mouse mastocytoma cells coated with purified human thyroglobulin were lysed by lymphocytes from six of eleven patients with Hashimoto's thyroiditis, while similar target cells coated with microsomal fractions from human thyrotoxic glands were destroyed by lymphocytes of seven of the same patients (69). With the exception of one case, lymphocytes reacted against both thyroglobulin and microsomal antigens. There was no apparent correlation between antibody titers and cytotoxic activity of lymphocytes; that is, in some patients thyroid antibodies were present in the absence of cytotoxic activity, and vice versa.

It was later reported that peripheral blood leukocytes from patients with autoimmune thyroiditis could destroy human thyroid cells in monolayer cultures when incubated together for five to six days (70). This effect was not mediated by thyroid antibodies released into the medium, but by a direct leukocyte-thyroid cell interaction.

Finally, lymphocyte-mediated cytotoxicity induced by thyroid antigens was observed using mouse fibroblasts as nonspecific target cells and concentrated supernatants from antigen-stimulated lymphocytes of patients with autoimmune thyroiditis (71).

Antibody-Dependent Cellular Cytotoxicity (ADCC)

An immunologic phenomenon that combines both humoral and cellular aspects, antibody-dependent cellular cytotoxicty (ADCC), is caused by antibodies capable of inducing lymphocyte-mediated target cell lysis in the absence of complement (72). The specificity of the reaction is determined by the IgG antibody moiety, and effector cells involved are nonsensitized lymphocytes bearing receptors for the Fc portion of the IgG molecules. Such lymphocytes do not seem to belong to either the mature B or T lymphocyte populations and have been termed "killer cells" or K cells. ADCC reactions have been observed in patients with autoimmune thyroiditis (73–75). When sera from these patients were incubated with thyroglobulin-coated chicken erythrocytes and normal human lymphocytes, lysis of the target cells, as estimated by radioactive chromium release, was observed in 66 to 74% of cases. In one study there was a correlation with the titer of IgG antibodies to thyroglobulin (73), whereas in another no such correlation was found (74).

Calder et al. (75) found that the ADCC of lymphoid cells from patients with Hashimoto's thyroiditis, primary hypothyroidism, and Graves' disease is significantly elevated above normal control values. An interaction between lymphocytes, antibodies, and thyroid antigens has also been demonstrated using cryostat sections of human thyroids preincubated with sera from patients with autoimmune thyroiditis and then incubated with nonimmune lymphocytes, which adhered to the sections (76,77).

Peripheral Lymphocytes and Antigen-Binding Cells

There has been some controversy about the number of T lymphocytes present in the peripheral blood of patients with autoimmune thyroiditis, but at present the consensus seems to be that there is no difference as compared to normal subjects. In a first report by Farid et al. (78), the percentage of peripheral T lymphocytes was 98% in Hashimoto's thyroiditis and 63% in controls. A correlation was observed between the percentage of T lymphocytes and production of migration inhibitory factor after stimulation of lymphocytes with thyroid antigens. No correlation was observed with titers of thyroid antibodies. Evidence for an increased sensitization of T lymphocytes in Hashimoto's thyroiditis, based on the inhibition of T rosette formation by antihuman thymocyte globulin, was also reported by the same group (79). However, these observations were found to be not reproducible and were later retracted (80). On the other hand, Urbaniak and Penhale (81,82) reported that the numbers of peripheral T lymphocytes were lower in patients with autoimmune thyroiditis than in controls, and then in a later study did not find any significant differences between normal subjects and patients (83).

More rewarding have been the investigations on antigen-binding lymphocytes (ABL) reacting with thyroid antigens. Rosette formation between red cells coated with human thyroglobulin and lymphocytes was observed in almost all patients with autoimmune thyroiditis (84,85). Autoradiographic techniques have demonstrated the presence of lymphocytes binding human thyroglobulin labeled with radioactive iodine both in normal subjects and in patients with autoimmune thyroiditis. In one study, thyroglobulin-binding lymphocytes were seen in nine out of eleven normal subjects, with an average number of 216 per 10^6 lymphocytes (86). Passage through a column of antihuman immunoglobulin-coated beads removed most of the thyroglobulin-binding cells, which were thus identified as B cells.

In another study it was found that ABL to human thyroglobulin were present in all of 23 thymuses from normal fetuses and children (87). ABL numbers were higher in early fetal thymus, with a maximum of 20 per 1,000 thymocytes, and decreased progressively with age to 5 per 1,000 in adolescence. Thyroglobulin-binding cells were also found to be present in the peripheral blood of all subjects, with mean counts of less than 4 per 1,000 lymphocytes in normal subjects, 23.1 in patients with thyroiditis, and 13.3 in patients with Graves' disease.

As far as the thyroid microsomal antigen is concerned, ABL were present in healthy subjects as well as patients with various types of thyroid disease (88). Patients with antibodies to thyroid cytoplasmic antigen had 11.21 ± 0.60 per 10^4 lymphocytes, whereas patients without antibodies had 3.49 ± 0.14 per 10^4 lymphocytes, a figure similar to that observed in normal subjects, or 3.26 ± 0.18 per 10^4 lymphocytes. Thus, patients with antibodies had three times more ABL than normal controls.

HISTOPATHOLOGY

In chronic lymphocytic thyroiditis, there is diffuse enlargement of the thyroid gland, with parenchymal hyperplasia and focal damage, changes at the level of the follicular basement membrane, and inflammatory infiltration (89–93). The parenchymal damage is focal, with follicles undergoing changes from normal to necrotic. The epithelial cells of the thyroid follicles are hyperplastic and especially in more advanced stages, swollen and oxyphilic. When the so-called "oxyphil cells" (also termed oncocytes, Hürthle's cells, and Askanazy's cells) are observed by electron microscopy, they are found to contain larger numbers of mitochondria, which also are increased in size. In even more advanced stages, there is cell lysis with destruction of the follicles, which eventually are replaced by connective tissue. Frequently there is slight to moderate thickening of the interlobular septa and irregular focal fibrosis.

The follicular basement membrane shows gaps and is focally and irregularly thickened, assuming a multilayered aspect. Irregular globoid electron-opaque deposits have been observed near the basement membrane and especially close to plasma cells (94).

The inflammatory infiltrate is composed of lymphocytes, plasma cells, and macrophages. There is a close association of lymphocytes with the cells of the thyroid follicular epithelium, and lymphocytes are observed crossing into the follicles, between epithelial cells or within damaged cells. Many follicles contain intraluminal lymphocytes, macrophages, and plasma cells. Approximately 50 to 60% of intrafollicular cells have been found to be plasma cells. There are characteristic lymphoid follicles with distinct germinal centers.

Approximately 10 to 13% of patients show extensive replacement of the thyroid parenchyma with broad bands of connective tissue separating zones of degenerating thyroid follicles. In all these cases, changes compatible with chronic lymphocytic thyroiditis, i.e., lymphocytic infiltration, epithelial oxyphilia, etc., are also seen. This pattern has been defined as a fibrous variant of Hashimoto's thyroiditis (95).

Over the years, there has been a certain amount of confusion and controversy with regard to definition and nomenclature of different forms of lymphocytic thyroiditis (89). This confusion not only is due to the love that some pathologists have for new classifications and nomenclatures of disease but is in part fostered because of the pronounced variation in morphologic changes observed in different patients. In the early literature three variants were described, a lymphoid variant in which lymphoid tissue predominates, a fibrous variant characterized by abundant fibrous tissue, and a fibrolymphoid variant, with a balanced increase in both lymphoid and fibrous tissues (96). Woolner (97) made an attempt to include under the same heading all cases of thyroiditis in which lymphocytic infiltration was a prominent feature. Great morphologic variation was found within this group, and thus an arbitrary classification was adopted, which distinguished diffuse thyroiditis from focal thyroiditis and thyroiditis with "hyperplastic" epithelium.

In another attempt to classify together those forms of thyroiditis with a basic similarity, both histopathologic and immunologic, a somewhat similar classification has been suggested, in which diffuse and focal thyroiditis are the two major groups, and then diffuse thyroiditis is subdivided into goitrous and nongoitrous, on the basis of the presence or absence of thyroid enlargement (98). The goitrous form can be divided into a hypercellular and a fibrous variant, the hypercellular in its turn divided into a primarily oxyphilic form, that is, the classic Hashimoto's disease, and a primarily nonoxyphilic or mild goitrous thyroiditis. The nongoitrous form is also divided into a severe atrophic form (myxedema) and a mild asymptomatic form.

Like all classifications, these divisions may be useful only if the great amount of overlapping between the various groups is understood, as well as the fact that one area of the thyroid may present one kind of lesion, whereas another area may present a different kind. The focal nature of the different changes observed in autoimmune thyroiditis should never be forgotten.

The immunopathologic correlations available in the literature are rather scarce. Senhauser (98) reported that sera from patients with the hypercellular variant of thyroiditis in general contain low titers of antibodies to thyroglobulin, only 16% having high titers; and that 88% of sera from patients with the fibrous variant have high titers. High titers of antibodies to the microsomal antigen are detected in both forms of thyroiditis. In patients with mild, hypercellular, nonoxyphilic thyroiditis, antibodies to thyroglobulin are rarely present, and low titers of antibodies to microsomal antigen are detected by complement fixation. In patients with focal thyroiditis, thyroid antibodies were observed in 65% of those with slight focal lesions and in all those with extensive focal lesions.

These studies are at best incomplete, since no attempt was made to correlate histopathology with both thyroid antibodies and delayed hypersensitivity to thyroid antigens. Furthermore, there are no studies in which the autoimmune response, both humoral and cell-mediated, is correlated with the stage of the disease. This is regrettable, because such investigations might help in clarifying the pathogenesis of autoimmune thyroiditis and determining whether the numerous variants of thyroiditis are separate entities or form a continuum of disease. The latter question is especially important because of the failure in correlating autoimmune thyroiditis with a specific HLA type.

IMMUNOHISTOPATHOLOGY

In earlier studies it was shown that immunoglobulins were bound to colloid material within the thyroid follicles and in the interstitial spaces, and that cells containing antibodies to thyroglobulin were abundant in the inflammatory infiltrate (99,100). It was also demonstrated that complement, as well as immunoglobulins, was bound to the thyroid colloid and that elution with acid buffers removed both immunoglobulins and complement (101). In more recent investigations, deposits of IgG, IgM, IgE, C1q, and C3 were found in focal areas of the stroma in 14 thyroid glands from patients with Graves' disease, and such deposits were also noted at the level of the follicular basement membrane in 10 of these thyroids (102). Similarly, heavy granular deposits of IgG, IgA, and C3 were observed at the follicular membrane level in one case of Hashimoto's thyroiditis clinically associated with systemic lupus erythematosus (94); and deposits of thyroglobulin, IgG, C3, and rarely IgM were demonstrated at the same level in a thyroid with unilateral multifocal carcinoma associated with chronic lymphocytic thyroiditis (103).

The structural and functional properties of immunoglobulins obtained from the thyroid of a patient with autoimmune thyroiditis have been investigated (104). Immunoglobulin concentration was ten times higher than in normal thyroids, and approximately 50% of it contained antithyroglobulin antibodies of the IgG class. There is some evidence that thyroid immunoglobulins in cases of autoimmune thyroiditis are not just derived from the serum, but may be synthesized in situ by thyroid lymphocytes (105).

The examination of biopsy specimens from patients with autoimmune thyroiditis has also provided some interesting information on the composition of the infiltrate. An increase in T lymphocytes per gram of thyroid tissue has been reported (106). In addition, a 100-fold excess of thyroglobulin-binding lymphocytes was noted in one thyroid biopsy specimen, as compared to the peripheral lymphocytes of the same patient (82). On the other hand, no microsomal antigen-binding lymphocytes were found in the cells obtained from the thyroid of another patient, who had high levels of microsomal antigen-binding lymphocytes in the peripheral blood (88).

Since at least one thyroid antigen, thyroglobulin, is known to be present in the circulation, immune complex formation may occur in patients with circulating thyroid antibodies. Indirect evidence of the presence of such complexes in the sera of patients with autoimmune thyroiditis, as indicated by marked inhibition of antibody-dependent cellular cytotoxicity, has been reported (107). If immune complexes are formed, they may cause glomerulonephritis, and indeed there have been a few isolated reports of such an occurrence. Antibodies reactive with thyroid colloid were found in the eluate from the kidneys of a patient with severe subacute glomerulonephritis (108). More recently, the occurrence of membranous glomerulonephritis has been observed in a patient with Hashimoto's thyroiditis (109). The kidney biopsy specimen contained granular deposits of IgG, C3, C4, thyroglobulin, and thyroid microsomal antigen. It is surprising that immune complex-mediated kidney disease has not been noted in larger numbers of patients with autoimmune thyroiditis. It is possible that immune complexes formed by antibodies to thyroglobulin and thyroglobulin do not bind C1q and thus are unable to initiate complement-mediated damage in this fashion. However, this explanation does not consider the possibility that complement could still be bound through some alternative mechanism. In addition, complexes formed by antibodies to the microsomal antigen should be fully capable of binding complement.

ASSOCIATION WITH OTHER AUTOIMMUNE DISEASES

A number of reports have suggested that autoimmune thyroiditis is associated with various other disorders that are possibly of an autoimmune nature (110,111).

Approximately 30% of patients with autoimmune thyroiditis have gastric antibodies. Conversely, thyroid antibodies are found with increased frequency in patients with pernicious anemia (up to 80%). Thyroiditis and Addison's disease can occur in the same patient, a condition defined as "Schmidt's syndrome," and thyroid antibodies are found in approximately 40% of patients with Addison's disease. On the other hand, patients with thyroiditis alone have no significant increase in adrenal antibodies. The possible association with myasthenia gravis, idiopathic hypoparathyroidism, diabetes mellitus, and non-organ-specific autoimmune diseases, such as systemic lupus erythematosus and rheumatoid arthritis, has also been suggested.

These suggestions have not been confirmed by one epidemiologic study, which revealed only a possible association with rheumatoid arthritis, an equivocal association with systemic lupus erythematosus, and no associations with Addison's disease, pernicious anemia, and myasthenia gravis (112). However, one is still left with the feeling that patients with autoimmune disorders such as thyroiditis have a tendency to be more prone to other disorders of an autoimmune nature and that more extensive studies are needed to prove this association.

IMMUNOGENETICS OF AUTOIMMUNE THYROIDITIS

The role of genetic factors in autoimmune thyroiditis is an interesting area of investigation, as evidenced by an increasing number of publications on this subject (113–117).

Several instances of autoimmune thyroiditis in identical twins have been reported (118). However, no definite conclusions about genetic influences can be drawn from these observations, because of the possible effects of environmental factors such as virus exposure, and the statistical bias associated with the ascertainment and reporting of data on individual twin pairs (114).

An increased incidence of thyroiditis, as well as circulating antibodies to thyroid antigens, has been observed in families of patients with autoimmune thyroiditis (119). Early studies showed that clinically evident thyroid disease was found in 33% of the siblings of patients with autoimmune thyroiditis and that thyroid antibodies were present in the sera of 56%, with incidence and titers much higher than in the normal population (120). Thyroid antibodies were also found in the parents of most children with autoimmune thyroiditis, a finding that was interpreted as compatible with dominant transmission with incomplete penetrance.

These and other similar studies were criticized on epidemiologic grounds, because the probands were selected from specialized hospital clinics, a method of selection that leads to overrepresentation in the sample of families with more than one affected member (121). Additional biases are introduced by the fact that patients from families with affected relatives are more aware of the disease and thus more likely to seek medical attention, and also by the fact that patients with an association of autoimmune diseases have a greater chance of being hospitalized and referred to specialized clinics.

Clear confirmation of previous evidence for a familial aggregation of thyroid antibodies was provided by Roitt and Doniach (122), who corrected for the bias in the selection of probands by considering only families wherein the proband had uncomplicated thyroiditis and was the sole clinically affected member. The incidence of thyroid antibodies in first-degree relatives of both sexes was 36%, compared to 14% in matched controls. When individual antibodies were analyzed, the sharpest difference between relatives and controls was observed in the incidence of antibodies to thyroglobulin and microsomal antigen, with an increase of five- and fourfold, respectively.

In conclusion, there is abundant evidence in favor of a family aggregation of thyroid autoimmunity, but family studies have been unable to evaluate the relative contribution of genetic and environmental factors and to clarify the genetic mechanisms involved.

A more recent approach to this problem is based on the identification of HLA antigens in patients with autoimmune thyroiditis. An association between major histocompatibility antigens and various human diseases has been demonstrated by several investigators (see reviews in refs. 123–129). In particular, it has been shown that some autoimmune diseases (systemic lupus erythematosus and rheumatoid arthritis) and other disorders with a possible autoimmune pathogenesis (pemphigus, Addison's disease, diabetes mellitus, etc.) are associated with specific HLA genotypes. However, to date the search for a correlation between histocompatibility genes and autoimmune thyroiditis has been fruitless.

Bode and Dorf (130) studied HLA antigens in 13 members of four families with Hashimoto's thyroiditis and could not establish any close linkage with HLA or any blood and serum groups. Negative results were also obtained by four other groups of investigators (65,131–133). Better results might have been expected from similar studies performed in a geographically defined population. As an example, Newfoundland has favorable demographic characteristics for immunogenetic studies, because it has a population of convenient size, immigration is limited, and there is considerable consanguinity, with a high rate of HLA homozygosity (134). In spite of these advantages, although initial observations suggested a weak association between HLA-B8 and Hashimoto's thyroiditis (135), further studies on a larger patient group failed to show any association with HLA antigens (136).

These negative results are difficult to explain, especially in view of the demonstration by some investigators of an association between HLA-B8 and Graves' disease, a condition that appears in familial aggregates together with Hashimoto's thyroiditis, is characterized by autoimmune responses to thyroid antigens similar to those observed in thyroiditis, and is often included in the group, "primary autoimmune thyroid disease" (24). One possible explanation is that, in spite of the apparent similarities in autoimmune responses, "autoimmune thyroiditis" may be rather heterogeneous from a clinical and histopathologic point of view, which could account for the difficulty in detecting correlations with histocompatibility antigens. A difference between autoimmune responses and histopathology has been observed in experimental thyroiditis induced in inbred strains of rats, in which immune responsiveness in terms of antibody formation does not appear to be linked to serologically demonstrable histocompatibility antigens, whereas the capacity to develop thyroid lesions may be (137). Another possibility is that autoimmune thyroiditis is not associated with the serum-defined antigens of the major histocompatibility system, but may be associated with lymphocyte-defined antigens. As an example, a strong association of the LD-8a determinant with juvenile diabetes mellitus and idiopathic Addison's disease has been recently reported (138). This association is stronger than the association of HLA-B8 with the same diseases, and it has been suggested that an LD-8-associated Ir gene may be the common denominator for the group of organ-specific autoimmune diseases.

PATHOGENESIS OF AUTOIMMUNE THYROIDITIS

In spite of more than 20 years of research, it is not yet clear whether thyroid damage is caused by autoantibodies, sensitized lymphocytes, both mechanisms, or neither.

As described in the section on humoral autoimmune responses, circulating autoantibodies to thyroid antigens are present in most patients with autoimmune thyroiditis and might cause damage directly or indirectly. Cytotoxic antibodies might directly damage the epithelial cells of the thyroid, even though in in vitro experiments they are capable of cytotoxic activity only against cells that have been previously altered by enzyme pretreatment. Antibodies directed against surface components of thyroid cells might also have cytotoxic activity, but very little is known at present about this type of antibody. The presence and titers of circulating antibodies to thyroglobulin and microsomal antigen do not correlate well with the severity of the disease, but they might still cause damage indirectly, through the in situ formation of immune complexes in the thyroid. Immune complexes with thyroglobulin as the antigen have indeed been observed both within the follicles and at the level of the follicular basement membrane. Attractive though this mechanism may be, such findings have been noted in a very limited number of instances.

Autoantibodies may also cause damage when associated with lymphocytes, as is the case in antibody-dependent cell cytotoxicity. This is another attractive possibility, but again the evidence at present available is very scarce.

Sensitized lymphocytes might mediate thyroid damage through the release of lymphokines. A number of these mediators, from migration inhibition factor (MIF) (or leukocyte inhibiting factor, LIF) to lymphotoxin have been demonstrated in autoimmune thyroiditis. MIF (or LIF) might cause thyroid infiltration and damage by the stimulation and immobilization of macrophages within the thyroid, while lymphotoxin might have a direct toxic effect on the thyroid epithelial cells themselves. However, as in the case of thyroid autoantibodies, no correlation has been established between lymphokines and course and severity of the disease.

Thus, when one peruses the literature on autoimmune thyroiditis, one finds that no definite links have been established between one or more pathogenetic mechanisms and this disease. What seems to be missing are studies that, within the limits of clinical investigation, correlate thyroid antibodies, antibody-dependent cell cytotoxicity, lymphokines, immunopathology, and histopathology, in an attempt to determine whether there is any association between these immunologic parameters and stage and type of thyroiditis.

ETIOLOGY OF AUTOIMMUNE THYROIDITIS

At present, we have no understanding of the cause of autoimmune thyroiditis. As in many other conditions of uncertain origin, autoimmune or not, one can suspect viral infections and/or genetic factors as initiators of the disease. However, there are no definite data in favor of any etiologic agent.

A possible association with mumps virus infection was suggested by early clinical reports, but has not been confirmed; similarly, an association between parainfluenza and adenovirus infections and antibodies to thyroglobulin has been suggested, but not confirmed. Recently, a few cases of congenital rubella and autoimmune thyroiditis have been reported in children. In one of these, rubella virus antigen was detected in the germinal centers of the lymphoid follicles in the thyroid (139). However, in spite of these suggestive case reports, conclusive evidence for a viral etiology of autoimmune thyroiditis is still missing.

Equally uncertain is the role of genetic factors. As discussed in the section on immunogenetics, a familiarity of autoimmune thyroiditis has been demonstrated, but no clear-cut genetic mechanism of transmission has been defined. To date, there is also no evidence for an association with a serologically defined major histocompatibility genotype, and the issue may be solved only by further studies on lymphocyte-defined antigens.

In any case, there is no doubt that the normally present immunologic unresponsiveness to self-antigens (self-tolerance) is broken in chronic lymphocytic thyroiditis and that the criteria used to define autoimmune diseases are met in this condition. Circulating autoantibodies and delayed hypersensitivity reactions to thyroid antigens can be demonstrated in patients suffering from the disease. The autoantigens involved, i.e., thyroglobulin, microsomal antigen, "colloid antigen second," and surface antigens, have been recognized and in the case of thyroglobulin isolated and characterized. Autoimmune responses to thyroid antigens have been experimentally induced in a variety of animal species and found to occur spontaneously in chickens, rats, and dogs (118). Thyroid damage similar to that observed in human thyroiditis has been noted both in the experimental and in spontaneous animal models. Thus, chronic lymphocytic thyroiditis can indeed be defined as "autoimmune thyroiditis."

Unfortunately, none of the many theories suggested to explain the loss of self-tolerance to thyroid antigens is completely satisfactory. The autoimmune reactions observed in autoimmune thyroiditis might be considered as a normal response to thyroid self-antigens, thyroglobulin, or others, normally "sequestered" or unavailable to the lymphoid system and released into the circulation because of trauma, infections, or other events. This simple explanation is no longer felt to be valid, especially in the case of thyroglobulin, which, as we have previously discussed, is continuously present in the circulation. Alternatively, autoimmune responses to thyroid antigens might be considered as normal immune responses to self-antigens modified by bacteria or viruses or to extrinsic antigens that cross-react with thyroid antigens. Again, there is no evidence in favor of either possibility.

On the other hand, we could be dealing with abnormal immunologic responses to self-antigens. The clonal selection theory of immune response implies that specific clones of lymphocytes capable of responding to autoantigens are eliminated or inactivated early in life and that autoimmune responses are due to the emergence of "forbidden" clones because of random somatic mutation (140). This does not seem to happen in the case of autoimmune thyroiditis. Lymphocytes bearing receptors for thyroglobulin and the microsomal antigen are normally present in the circulation, and thus they are not "forbidden" clones.

However, it has been hypothesized that self-tolerance to thyroglobulin may result from a state of tolerance present only in the T cell population and produced by the continuous presence in the circulation of low levels of thyroglobulin (141,142). B cells bearing receptors specific for this autoantigen may be present but unable to mount an immune response against it because of T cell unresponsiveness. This phenomenon may be due to the absence of a positive influence of T cells on B cells, but could also be interpreted as specific suppression by T cells. Self-tolerance to thyroid antigens might be terminated in the presence of T cell activity sufficiently strong to trigger B cells to respond to antigenic determinants that otherwise would be ignored. Alternatively, it might result from elimination of T suppressor cells. Such a stimulation or elimination of T cells might occur because of an infectious disease or another potent exogenous agent.

An additional explanation might be that some persons carry immune response genes capable of making their T cells highly responsive to certain autoantigens such as thyroid antigens. As previously discussed in the section on immunogenetics, even though a familial clustering of thyroiditis has been observed in man, at present the role of genetic factors is not clear. A correlation between response to thyroid antigens and histocompatibility (H-2) type has been demonstrated in some inbred strains of mice (143), and spontaneous thyroiditis occurs in one inbred strain of rats (144). On the other hand, autoimmune responses to thyroglobulin and sperm antigens in rats do not seem to be linked to major histocompatibility antigens (137,145).

At present, there is no definitive evidence supporting any of these theories. It is not altogether impossible that a number of mechanisms are operative in the initiation of autoimmune reactions to thyroid antigens, as well as all autoantigens in general.

CONCLUSION

In the last 20 years the immunologic community has changed from the blind acceptance of the "horror autotoxicus" hypothesis to a rather overenthusiastic following of the "autoimmune disease" concept. Many pathologic conditions have been defined as "autoimmune" for no other reason than the presence of circulating autoantibodies of one kind or another. Since autoimmune responses are observed in perfectly normal individuals, and may be of a transient and completely harmless nature, caution should be exercised before labeling a disease as "autoimmune." With these provisos in mind and considering chronic lymphocytic thyroiditis and systemic lupus erythematosus as the best examples of autoimmune diseases, one can evaluate from this point of view several other conditions that may be of an autoimmune nature.

An autoimmune response, both humoral and cellular, to acetylcholine receptors has been detected in patients with myasthenia gravis (146). Experimental models of this disease have been induced in several animal species by the injection of acetylcholine receptors (147–153). Thus, the advances in the isolation of acetylcholine receptors have provided the necessary tools to collect solid evidence showing that myasthenia gravis may indeed be an autoimmune disease.

Less novel is the demonstration of autoimmune responses to a variety of self-antigens in several disorders, such as Addison's disease (154), pernicious anemia (155), pemphigus vulgaris (156), and many others. Experimental animal models have been established for some of these disorders, but in general the evidence available at present is not as complete as in the case of systemic lupus erythematosus, autoimmune thyroiditis, and myasthenia gravis.

Finally, recent findings point to the possible involvement of autoimmune mechanisms in the pathogenesis of diabetes mellitus. This hypothesis is not new, and for many years several investigators have studied, without much success, the role of autoimmunity in this pathologic condition. However, circulating autoantibodies against antigens of the cells of the islets of Langerhans have lately been detected in patients with juvenile diabetes or diabetes associated with other endocrinopathies, as well as in older diabetics (157,158). This recent development has provided additional stimulus for more extensive investigations, and further progress can be expected in the near future.

In conclusion, even though the published evidence is staggering, much research remains to be done in the field of autoimmunity. From the early work with crude organ extracts, we have now progressed to experiments with isolated receptors of tissues, and from simple family studies to more sophisticated immunogenetic investigations. Thus, the study of organ-specific autoimmunity, which in the past has provided insight into the pathogenetic and etiologic mechanisms of human disease, continues to be an exciting area of immunology.

REFERENCES

1. Ehrlich, P., and Morgenroth, J., in *Collected Studies on Immunity* (P. Ehrlich, ed.), John Wiley, New York, 1906, p. 23.
2. Metalnikoff, S., *Ann. Inst. Pasteur* **14,** 577 (1900).
3. Miescher, P. A., and Dayer, J. M., in *Textbook of Immunopathology* (P. A. Miescher and H. J. Müller-Eberhard, eds.), Grune and Stratton, New York, 1976, p. 649.
4. Paterson, P. Y., in *Textbook of Immunopathology* (P. A. Miescher and H. J. Müller-Eberhard, eds.), Grune and Stratton, New York, 1976, p. 179.
5. Witebsky, E., and Rose, N. R., *J. Immunol.* **75,** 269 (1955).
6. Rose, N. R., and Witebsky, E., *J. Immunol.* **75,** 282 (1955).
7. Witebsky, E., and Rose, N. R., *J. Immunol.* **76,** 408 (1956).
8. Rose, N. R., and Witebsky, E., *J. Immunology* **76,** 417 (1956).
9. Roitt, I. M., Doniach, D., Campbell, P. N., et al., *Lancet* **2,** 820 (1956).
10. Doniach, D., and Roitt, I. M., *J. Clin. Endocrinol.* **17,** 1293 (1957).
11. Goudie, R. B., Anderson, J. R., Gray, K. G., et al., *Lancet* **2,** 976 (1957).
12. Paine, J. R., Terplan, K., Rose, N. R., et al., *Surgery* **42,** 799 (1957).
13. Witebsky, E., Rose, N. R., Terplan, K. L., et al., *J.A.M.A.* **164,** 1439 (1957).
14. Roitt, I. M., and Doniach, D., *Lancet* **2,** 1027 (1958).
15. Hjort, T., *Lancet* **1,** 1262 (1961).
16. Hjort, T., *Acta Med. Scand.* **174,** 137 (1963).
17. Assem, E. S. K., and Trotter, W. R., *Immunology* **9,** 21 (1965).
18. Roitt, I. M., and Torrigiani, G., *Endocrinology* **81,** 421 (1967).
19. Torrigiani, G., and Doniach, D., *J. Clin. Endocrinol.* **209,** 305 (1969).
20. Van Herle, A. J., Uller, R. P., Matthews, N. L., et al., *J. Clin. Invest.* **52,** 1320 (1973).
21. Shulman, S., *Time Specificity and Autoimmunity,* Springer-Verlag, New York, 1974.
22. Salabe, G. B., *Acta Endocrinol.* **79,** suppl. 196 (1975).
23. Balfour, B. M., Doniach, D., Roitt, I. M., et al., *Br. J. Exp. Pathol.* **42,** 307 (1961).
24. Doniach, D., and Roitt, I. M., in *Textbook of Immunopathology* (P. A. Miescher and H. J. Müller-Eberhard, eds.), Grune and Stratton, New York, 1976, p. 715.
25. Beutner, E. H., Hale, W. L., Nisengard, R. J., et al., in *Immunopathology of the Skin* (E. H. Beutner, T. P. Chorzelski, et al., eds.), Dowden, Hutchinson and Ross, Stroudsburg, Pa., 1973.
26. Jansson, J., and Fagraeus, A., *Clin. Exp. Immunol.* **3,** 287 (1968).
27. Fagraeus, A., and Jansson, J., *Immunology* **18,** 413 (1970).
28. Rose, N. R., and Bigazzi, P. E., in *Handbook of Microbiology,* vol. IV (in press).
29. Evered, D. C., Ormston, B. J., Smith P. A., et al., *Br. Med. J.* **1,** 675 (1973).
30. Aho, K., and Virkola, P., *Acta Endocrinol.* **68,** 196 (1971).
31. Bigazzi, P. E., and Rose, N. R., in *Manual of Clinical Immunology* (N. R. Rose and H. Friedman, eds.), American Society for Microbiology, Washington, D.C., 1976.
32. McElborough, D. J., *Med. Lab. Tech.* **31,** 221 (1974).
33. Knapp, W., Ludwig, H., Schernthaner, G., et al., *Z. Immunitätsforsch.* **151,** 61 (1976).
34. Mori, T., and Kriss, J. P., *J. Clin. Endocrinol.* **33,** 688 (1971).
35. Salabe, G. B., and Fontana, S., *Hormones* **3,** 1 (1972).
36. Peake, R. L., Willis, D. B., Asimakis, G. K., et al., *J. Lab. Clin. Med.* **86,** 907 (1974).

37. Rallison, M. L., Dobyns, B. J., Keating, F. R., et al., *J. Pediatr.* **86,** 675 (1975).
38. Torrigiani, G., and Roitt, I. M., *Clin. Exp. Immunol.* **3,** 621 (1968).
39. Torrigiani, G., and Roitt, I. M., *J. Immunol.* **102,** 492 (1969).
40. Hay, F. C., and Torrigiani, G., *Clin. Exp. Immunol.* **16,** 517 (1974).
41. Hjort, T., *Clin. Exp. Immunol.* **5,** 43 (1969).
42. Dussault, J. H., and Guay, D., *C.M.A.J.* **111,** 319 (1974).
43. Hjort, T., *Acta Med. Scand.* **174,** 147 (1963).
44. Tung, K. S. K., and Ramos, C. V., *Am. J. Clin. Pathol.* **61,** 549 (1974).
45. Bird, T., and Stephenson, J., *J. Clin, Pathol.* **26,** 623 (1973).
46. Perrin, J., and Bubel, M. A., *Med. Lab. Tech.* **31,** 205 (1974).
47. Aoki, N., Wakisaka, G., Higashi, T., et al., *Endocrinol. Japon.* **22,** 89 (1975).
48. Amino, N., Hagen, S. R., Yamada, N., et al., *Clin. Endocrinol.* **5,** 115 (1976).
49. Amino, N., Miyai, K., Fukuchi, M., et al., *Endocrinol. Japon.* **22,** 141 (1975).
50. Forbes, I. J., Roitt, I. M., Doniach, D., et al., *J. Clin. Invest.* **41,** 996 (1962).
51. Kite, J. H., Rose, N. R., Kano, K., et al., *Ann. N.Y. Acad. Sci.* **124,** 626 (1965).
52. Buchanan, W. W., Anderson, J. R., Goudie, R. B., et al., *Lancet* **1,** 928 (1958).
53. Saarma, V., *EndoKrinologic* **57,** 237 (1971).
54. Wolf-Jürgensen, P., and Halberg, P., *Acta Allergol.* **20,** 438 (1965).
55. Dvorak, H. F., and Dvorak, A. M., in *Progress in Immunology* II, vol. 3 (L. Brent and J. Holborow, eds.), North Holland, Amsterdam, 1974.
56. DeGroot, L. J., and Jaksina, S., *J. Clin. Endocrinol.* **29,** 207 (1969).
57. Ehrenfeld, E. N., and Klein, E., *J. Clin. Endocrinol.* **32,** 115 (1971).
58. Jäger, L., Schnabel, I., Wenz, W., et al., *Allergie Immunol.* **17,** 327 (1971).
59. Reinert, P., Deville Chabrolle, A., Bribet-Forette, F., et al., *Presse Med.* **79,** 1279 (1971).
60. Delespess, G., Duchateau, J., Collet, H., et al., *Clin. Exp. Immunol.* **12,** 439 (1972).
61. Søborg, M., and Halberg, P., *Acta Med. Scand.* **183,** 101 (1968).
62. Brostoff, J., *Proc. R. Soc. Med.* **63,** 905 (1970).
63. Calder, E. A., McLeman, D., Barnes, E. W., et al., *Clin. Exp. Immunol.* **12,** 429 (1972).
64. Lamki, L., and Row, V. V., *J. Clin. Endocrinol.* **36,** 358 (1973).
65. Whittingham, S., Youngchaiyud, U., MacKay, I. R., et al., *Clin. Exp. Immunol.* **19,** 289 (1975).
66. Wartenberg, J., Doniach, D., Brostoff, J., et al., *Int. Arch. Allergy* **44,** 396 (1973).
67. Wartenberg, J., Doniach, D., Brostoff, J., et al., *Clin. Exp. Immunol.* **14,** 203 (1973).
68. Ling, N. R., Acton, A. B., Roitt, I. M., et al., *Br. J. Exp. Pathol.* **46,** 348 (1965).
69. Podleski, W. K., *Clin. Exp. Immunol.* **11,** 543 (1972).
70. Laryea, E., and Row, V. V., *Clin. Endocrinol.* **2,** 23 (1973).
71. Amino, N., and DeGroot, L. J., *Cell. Immunol.* **11,** 188 (1974).
72. Perlmann, P., Perlmann, H., Larsson, A., et al., *J. Reticuloendothel. Soc.* **17,** 241 (1975).
73. Calder, E. A., Penhale, W. J., McLeman, D., et al., *Clin. Exp. Immunol.* **14,** 153 (1973).
74. Wasserman, J., von Stedingk, L. V., Perlmann, P., et al., *Int. Arch. Allergy* **47,** 473 (1974).
75. Calder, E. A., Irvine, W. J., Davidson, N. M., et al., *Clin. Exp. Immunol.* **25,** 17 (1976).
76. Fakhri, O., and Hobbs, Jr., *Lancet* **2,** 403 (1972).
77. Pinedo, C., and Mul, N. A. J., *Clin. Immunol. Immunopathol.* **5,** 6 (1976).
78. Farid, N. R., Munro, R. E., Row, V. V., et al., *N. Engl. J. Med.* **288,** 1313 (1973).
79. Farid, N. R., Munro, R. E., Row, V. V., et al., *N. Engl. J. Med.* **289,** 1111 (1973).
80. Volpe, R., and Row, V. V., *N. Engl. J. Med.* **293,** 44 (1975).
81. Urbaniak, S. J., and Penhale, W. J., *Lancet* **2,** 452 (1973).
82. Urbaniak, S. J., and Penhale, W. J., *Clin. Exp. Immunol.* **15,** 345 (1973).
83. Urbaniak, S. J., and Penhale, W. J., *Clin. Exp. Immunol.* **18,** 449 (1974).
84. Perrudet-Badoux, A., and Frei, P. C., *Clin. Exp. Immunol.* **5,** 117 (1969).
85. Delespesse, G., Duchateau, J., Kennes, B., et al., *Biomedicine* **21,** 251 (1974).
86. Bankhurst, A. D., and Torrigiani, G., *Lancet* **1,** 226 (1973).
87. Roberts, I. M., and Whittingham, S., *Lancet* **2,** 936 (1973).
88. Khalid, B. A. K., and Hamilton, N. T., *Clin. Exp. Immunol.* **23,** 28 (1976).
89. Woolner, L. B., and McConahey, W. M., *J. Clin. Endocrinol.* **19,** 53 (1959).
90. Irvine, W. J., and Muir, A. R., *Q. J. Exp. Phynol.* **48,** 13 (1963).
91. Lupulescu, A., and Petrovici, A., *Ultrastructure of the Thyroid Gland,* Williams and Wilkins, Baltimore, 1968, p. 74.

92. Neve, P., and Ermans, A. M., in *Thyroiditis and Thyroid Function* (P. A. Bastenic and A. M. Ermans, eds.), Pergamon Press, Elmsford, N.Y., 1972, p. 109.
93. Reidbord, H. E., and Fisher, E. R., *Am. J. Pathol.* **59,** 327 (1973).
94. Kalderon, A. E., and Bogaars, H. A., *Am. J. Med.* **55,** 485 (1973).
95. Katz, S. M., and Vickery, A. L. J., *Hum. Pathol.* **5,** 161 (1974).
96. Hazard, J. B., *Am. J. Clin. Pathol.* **25,** 399 (1955).
97. Woolner, L. B., in *The Thyroid* (J. B. Hazard and D. E. Smith, eds.), Williams and Wilkins, Baltimore, 1964, p. 123.
98. Senhauser, D., in *The Thyroid* (J. B. Hazard and D. E. Smith, eds.), Williams and Wilkins, Baltimore, 1964, p. 167.
99. White, R. G., *Exp. Cell Res.* (suppl.) **7,** 263 (1959).
100. Mellors, R. C., and Brzosko, W. J., *Am. J. Pathol.* **41,** 425 (1962).
101. Koffler, D., and Friedman, A. H., *Lab. Invest.* **13,** 239 (1964).
102. Werner, S. C., Wegelius, O., Fierer, J. A., et al., *N. Engl. J. Med.* **287,** 421 (1972).
103. Kalderon, A. E., and Bogaars, H. A., *Clin. Immunol. Immunopathol.* **4,** 101 (1975).
104. Salabe, G. B., and Davoli, C., *Int. Arch. Allergy* **47,** 63 (1974).
105. Davoli, C., and Salabe, G. B., *Clin. Exp. Immunol.* **23,** 242 (1976).
106. Farid, N. R., and Row, V. V., *Clin. Res.* **21,** 1025 (1973).
107. Barkas, T., Al-Khateeb, S. F., Irvine, W. J., et al., *Clin. Exp. Immunol.* **25,** 270 (1976).
108. Koffler, D., and Sandson, J., *J. Clin. Invest.* **47, 55a** (1968).
109. O'Reagan, S., Fong, J. S. C., Kaplan, B. S., et al., *Clin. Immunol. Immunopathol.* **6,** 341 (1976).
110. Anderson, J. R., and Buchanan, W. W., *Autoimmunity.* Charles C Thomas, Springfield, Ill., 1967.
111. Fisher, D. A., and Beall, G. N., *Pharmac. Ther. C.* **1,** 445 (1976).
112. Mulhern, L. M., and Masi, A. T., *Lancet* **2,** 508 (1966).
113. DeGroot, L. J., Hall, R., McDermott, W. V., et al., *N. Engl. J. Med.* **267,** 267 (1962).
114. Fialkow, P. J., *Prog. Med. Genet.* **6,** 117 (1969).
115. Weinstein, I. B., and Kitchin, F. D., in *The Thyroid* (S. C. Werner and S. H. Ingbar, eds.), Harper and Row, New York, 1971, p. 400.
116. DeGroot, L. J., and Stanbury, J. B., *The Thyroid and Its Diseases,* John Wiley, New York, 1975, p. 587.
117. VanHaelst, L., Bonnyns, M., Ermans, A. M., et al., in *Thyroiditis and Thyroid Function* (P. A. Bastenic and A. M. Ermans, eds.), Pergamon Press, Elmsford, N.Y., 1972, p. 303.
118. Bigazzi, P. E., and Rose, N. R., *Prog. Allergy* **19,** 245 (1975).
119. Goldsmith, R. D., McAdams, A. J., Larsen, P. R., et al., *J. Clin. Endocrinol.* **37,** 265 (1973).
120. Hall, R., and Owen, S. G., *Lancet* **2,** 187 (1960).
121. Masi, A. T., and Hartmann, W. H., *J. Chron. Dis.* **18,** 1 (1965).
122. Roitt, I. M., and Doniach, D., *Clin. Exp. Immunol.* **2,** 727 (1967).
123. McDevitt, H. O., and Bodmer, W. F., *Lancet* **1,** 1269 (1974).
124. Svejgaard, A., Jersild, C., Nielsen, L. S., et al., *Tissue Antigens* **4,** 95 (1974).
125. Dausset, J., and Degos, L., *Clin. Immunol. Immunopathol.* **3,** 127 (1974).
126. Vladutiu, A. O., and Rose, N. R., *Immunogenetics* **1,** 305 (1974).
127. Kissmeyer-Nielsen, F., Kjerbye, K. E., Andersen, E., et al., *Transplant. Rev.* **22,** 164 (1975).
128. Svejgaard, A., Platz, P., Ryder, L. P., et al., *Transplant. Rev.* **22,** 3 (1975).
129. Terasaki, P. I., and Mickey, M. R., *Transplant. Rev.* **22,** 105 (1975).
130. Bode, H. H., and Dorf, M. E., *J. Clin. Endocrinol.* **37,** 692 (1973).
131. Richiardi, P., Salabe, B. G., Lucertini, L., et al., *Tissue Antigens* **5,** 213 (1975).
132. VanRood, J. J., and Van Hoof, J. P., *Transplant. Rev.* **22,** 75 (1975).
133. Chopra, I. J., Solomon, D. H., Chopra, U., et al., *J. Clin. Endocrinol.* **45,** 45 (1977).
134. Larsen, B., Barnard, J. M., Buehler, S. K., et al., *Tissue Antigens* **8,** 207 (1976).
135. Farid, N. R., Barnard, J. M., Kutas, C., et al., *Int. Arch. Allergy* **49,** 837 (1975).
136. Farid, N. R., and Barnard, J. M., *Tissue Antigens* **8,** 181 (1976).
137. Rose, N. R., *Cell. Immunol.* **18,** 360 (1975).
138. Thomsen, M., Platz, P., Ortved, X., et al., *Transplant. Rev.* **22,** 125 (1975).
139. Ziring, P. R., Gallo, G., Finegold, M., et al., *J. Pediatr.* **20,** 419 (1977).
140. Burnet, M., *Auto-immunity and Auto-immune Disease,* Davis Co., Philadelphia, 1972.
141. Weigle, W. O., *Adv. Immunol.* **16,** 61 (1973).

142. Allison, A. C., *N. Engl. J. Med.* **295,** 821 (1976).
143. Vladutiu, A. O., and Rose, N. R., *Science* **174,** 1137 (1971).
144. Noble, B., Yoshida, T., Rose, N. R., et al., *J. Immunol.* **117,** 1447 (1976).
145. Bigazzi, P. E., and Kosuda, L. L., *Science* **197,** 1282 (1977).
146. Lennon, V. A., *Immunol. Commun.* **5,** 323 (1976).
147. Patrick, J., and Lindstrom, J., *Science* **180,** 871 (1973).
148. Lennon, V. A., and Lindstrom, J. M., *J. Exp. Med.* **141,** 1365 (1975).
149. Heilbronn, E., Mattsson, C., Stalberg, E., et al., *J. Neurol. Sci.* **24,** 59 (1975).
150. Tarrab-Hazdi, R., Aharonov, A., Abramsky, O., et al., *J. Exp. Med.* **142,** 785 (1975).
151. Lindstrom, J. M., Einarson, B., Lennon, V. A., et al., *J. Exp. Med.* **144,** 726 (1976).
152. Lindstrom, J. M., Engel, A. G., Seybold, M. E., et al., *J. Exp. Med.* **144,** 739 (1976).
153. Sanders, D. B., Johns, T. R., Eldefrawi, M. E., et al., *Arch. Neurol.* **34,** 75 (1977).
154. Milgrom, F., and Bigazzi, P., in *Textbook of Immunopathology,* 2d ed. (P. A. Miescher and H. J. Müller-Eberhard, eds.), Grune and Stratton, New York, 1976, p. 831.
155. Roitt, I. M., and Doniach, D., in *Textbook of Immunopathology,* 2d ed. (P. A. Miescher and H. J. Müller-Eberhard, eds.), Grune and Stratton, New York, 1976, p. 737.
156. Beutner, E. H., and Jordan, R. E., in *Textbook of Immunopathology,* 2d ed. (P. A. Miescher and H. J. Müller-Eberhard, eds.), Grune and Stratton, New York, 1976, p. 931.
157. Bottazzo, G. F., and Florin-Christensen, A., *Lancet* **2,** 1279 (1974).
158. Irvine, W. J., McCallum, C. J., Gray, R. S., et al., *Diabetes* **26,** 138 (1977).

Chapter Ten

Immunopathology of Anti-Basement Membrane Antibodies

CURTIS B. WILSON

Department of Immunopathology, Scripps Clinic and Research Foundation, La Jolla, California

Antibodies can initiate tissue injury in at least two ways. One involves the formation of antibodies reactive with antigens present at the site of eventual injury. The other involves passive entrapment of circulating antigen-antibody complexes in vascular structures. The latter antigen-antibody reaction has no specificity for the site of injury. Nevertheless, both mechanisms result in the accumulation of phlogogenic antigen-antibody immune reactants in tissue, bringing into play a variety of immunologic mediator pathways leading to tissue damage. Antibodies that react specifically with basement membrane antigens and initiate injury are one of the best examples of the first mechanism, and are the subject of this chapter. Other chapters deal with immune complex mechanisms in tissue injury.

The historical and experimental features of anti-basement membrane antibody-induced nephritis have been the subject of recent review (1,2). The nephritogenic potential of antikidney antisera (later to be known as anti-basement membrane antisera) was first demonstrated by Lindemann in 1900, when he induced proteinuria and uremia in rabbits, using guinea pig antirabbit kidney antisera. In the 1930s, Masugi studied the nephrotoxic model of ne-

This is publication No. 1310 from the Department of Immunopathology, Scripps Clinic and Research Foundation, La Jolla, California. This work was supported in part by U.S. Public Health Service Contract AI 42505 and U.S. Public Health Service Grants AI 07007, AM 18626, AM 20043, and BRS Grant RRO-5514.

phritis extensively, and the disease is still sometimes referred to as "Masugi nephritis." During the 1940s, Kay demonstrated that nephrotoxic nephritis occurred in two phases: the first, or heterologous, phase produced by the direct toxicity of the heterologous antisera; and a second, or autologous, phase, beginning when antibody to the foreign immunoglobulin formed in the host, bound to its glomerular basement membrane (GBM), and compounded the injury. In the 1950s, Krakower and Greenspon demonstrated that the GBM was the source of the nephritogenic antigen, with similar cross-reactive antigens in other vascular tissues (3). At that time, the term "nephrotoxic sera" was properly superseded by the term "anti-GBM antibody-induced nephritis." Anti-GBM nephritis can also be induced by immunization with basement membrane material that incites the production of autologous anti-basement membrane antibodies (4). The injury induced by either heterologously or autologously produced anti-basement membrane antibodies appears to be mediated, in part at least, by the activation of complement and the subsequent participation of polymorphonuclear leukocytes (PMNs) (5,6).

Although anti-GBM nephritis is the major disease induced by anti-basement membrane antibody, it is only part of the spectrum of similar reactions. Anti-basement membrane activity has been recognized in many tissues, including the alveoli, renal tubules, choroid plexus, skin, and perhaps intestine (2).

EXPERIMENTAL ANTI-BASEMENT MEMBRANE ANTIBODY-INDUCED DISEASE

Heterologous Anti-GBM Antibody Injury

Heterologous Phase. A test animal enters the heterologous or immediate phase of nephrotoxic nephritis only when sufficient amounts of antibody have been administered. Intravenous administration of antibody is most efficacious, since vascular basement membranes in tissue can absorb portions of antibody after intramuscular or intraperitoneal injection. Amounts of anti-GBM antisera necessary to induce acute heterologous phase injury have been quantitated in several species. Studies such as this showed that 75, 5, and 15 μg, respectively, of kidney-fixing antibody per gram are necessary to induce acute heterologous phase injury in rats, sheep, and rabbits (7,8,9). Unanue and Dixon calculated that acute proteinuria was induced in the rat when 1.2×10^{10} molecules of antibody per glomerulus were fixed, or 1 antibody molecule for every 20 $m\mu^2$ of glomerular capillary filtering surface area (7). Depending on the steric factors involved, they estimated that roughly one-half of the filtering surface would be covered by antibody molecules in this situation. After intravenous injection, the majority of antikidney antibodies in nephrotoxic serum bind rapidly to the kidney, with maximum binding at one hour, and 65 to 85% of the maximum bound within ten minutes (7). Most heterologous anti-basement membrane antibodies contain a mixture of antibodies with differing specificities and affinities, which accounts for differences in binding and turnover rates in the kidney and other visceral organs.

Antigenically, the GBM is a complex structure of collagen and noncollagenous proteins, some of which appear to be unique to the GBM, whereas others are shared with other basement membranes (2). The latter cross-reactivity is clearly shown by the ability of many vascular organs, such as the lung, spleen, and placenta, to induce nephrotoxic anti-basement membrane antisera upon injection into a heterologous species. Heterologous anti-basement membrane antibodies have a variable, but generally widespread, reactivity with basement membranes throughout the body when studied in vitro. Their fixation following in vivo injection, however, may be quite different and is apparently partly related to the accessibility of the basement membrane to the circulating antibody. The GBM, which is in close contact with the circulation via its fenestrated endothelial lining, then, is an easy target for such antisera.

The nephrotoxic antigens appear to be largely confined to the noncollagenous protein portion of the basement membrane (2), as evidenced by the lack of nephritogenicity of antibodies raised specifically to collagen. Also, anti-GBM antibodies are not absorbed well by prior reaction with collagen. Antisera made against collagen-free fragments of basement membrane remaining after collagenase digestion appear to be nephritogenic.

Once sufficient quantities of anti-basement membrane antibody have bound to the GBM, injury proceeds through at least two pathways, one dependent upon complement activation and subsequent PMN participation, and the other apparently independent of complement (5,6). In complement-dependent injury, the activated complement serves apparently in large part as a chemotactic agent responsible for PMN accumulation and subsequent enzymatic injury (10). The complement-independent mechanisms are not well understood, but appear to be responsible for the acute damage produced by avian nephrotoxic antisera, which do not normally activate mammalian complement, and certain mammalian antisera, which are active in animals experimentally depleted of complement and/or PMNs. Certain mammalian antisera contain different populations of antibodies that fix to the GBM; some induce injury independent of complement and PMNs, some are dependent upon them, and some do not produce injury at all (11). Apparently, more molecules of the complement-independent than of the complement-dependent antibodies are needed to produce injury. Antisera utilizing the complement- and PMN-dependent pathways may also be more destructive. In considering this area, then, one must realize that although antisera to basement membranes are similar in a general way, they differ somewhat from one another, which could influence experimental results.

Autologous Phase. Induction of the autologous phase of nephrotoxic nephritis depends upon the host's immune response to the heterologous antibody bound to its basement membrane. Autologous phase injury appears as a delayed event, dependent upon the host's immune response, and can augment injury of the heterologous phase, or, in animals receiving insufficient antibody to cause heterologous phase injury, may be the initial presentation of disease. Small amounts of antibody, identifiable by immunofluorescence (2 to 5 μg/gm of kidney) but insufficient to cause heterologous phase injury, are easily capable of inducing injury during the autologous phase (12). There is no evidence of production of autoantibodies to the kidney during the autologous phase of injury. This is most clearly demonstrated by studies in which clamping of a renal artery during antibody administration prevented fixation of heterologous antibody and subsequent damage in the clamped kidney.

Clinical, Morphologic, and Pathophysiologic Features of Heterologous Anti-GBM Antibodies. The nature and severity of nephrotoxic nephritis depend, in part, upon the species and are somewhat influenced by age, sex, and strain (1). Rats tend to have more progressive glomerulonephritis than other species, and mice seem to have a delayed onset of disease with little correlation detectable between the amounts of nephrotoxic serum injected and the appearance of proteinuria. Dogs, rabbits, and monkeys are good experimental subjects for this work, and sheep appear to be particularly susceptible to injury with nephrotoxic antibodies (2).

Complement-fixing nephrotoxic antisera produce a rapid influx of PMNs, reaching a peak two to four hours after injection of sufficient amounts of nephrotoxic serum to induce heterologous phase injury (5) (Figs. 1 and 2). The PMN infiltration declines as mononuclear cells accumulate (13). Proliferative changes ensue, often with striking extracapillary proliferation, leading to crescent formation (Fig. 2). Gaps or disruptions of the GBM have been observed, and urinary excretion of basement membrane-like materials increases (14,15). Some biochemical and enzymatic abnormalities of the basement membrane have also been reported subsequent to anti-GBM antibody administration (2).

Immunohistochemically, the glomerular lesion is typified by smooth, continuous linear deposits of heterologous immunoglobulin along the GBM (Fig. 3).

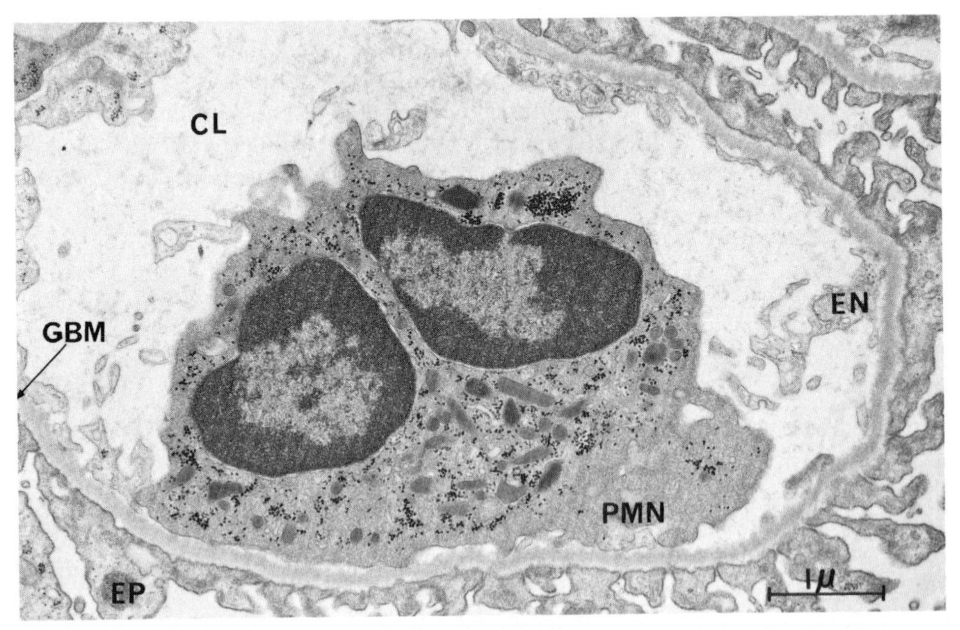

Figure 1. A polymorphonuclear leukocyte (PMN) has displaced the endothelial cell (EN) and approximated itself along the basement membrane of a rat glomerulus (GBM) one hour after administration of heterologous anti-GBM antibody. The epithelial cell (EP) foot processes are still well maintained, and the capillary lumen (CL) is patent. (Magnification × 19,000.)

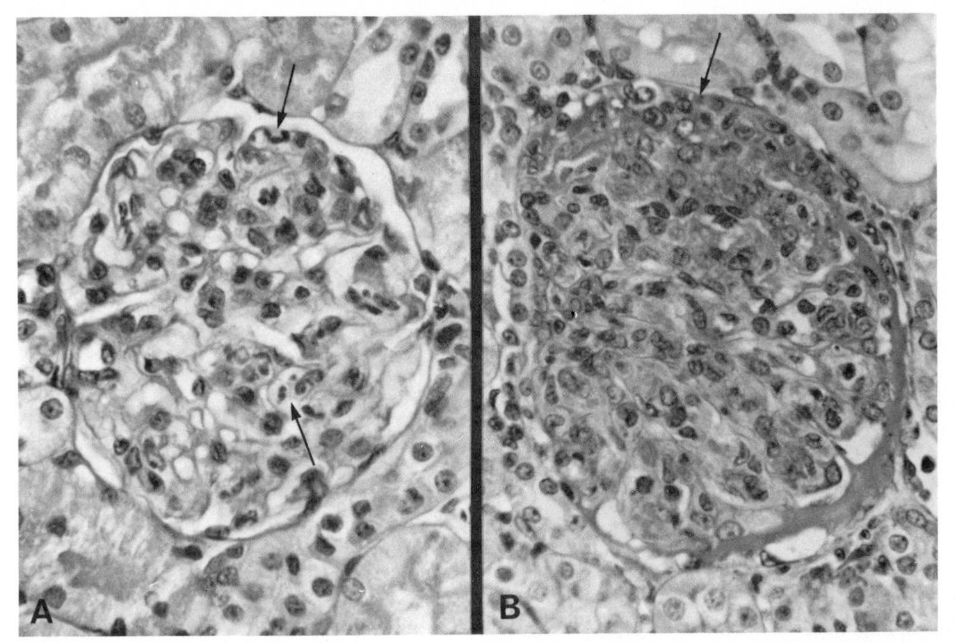

Figure 2. Histologic changes in heterologous anti-GBM antibody-induced glomerulonephritis are shown. In *A*, the initial PMN (*arrows*) infiltrate found in the first few hours of administration of the anti-GBM antibody is seen in a rat glomerulus. In *B*, the acute, proliferative, crescent-forming (*arrow*) glomerular response of a rabbit seven days after administration of anti-GBM antibody is shown. (Periodic acid Schiff stain, original magnification × 500.)

Early in the disease, the deposits are characteristically smooth, then irregularity increases, conforming to progressive disruption of the GBM architecture from the inflammatory response. Complement is visible in the same pattern as immunoglobulin when antisera capable of fixing complement are used. With the onset of the autologous phase of injury, host immunoglobulin deposits can be identified conforming to the distribution of the heterologous antibody, as described above. Electron-microscopic studies using electron-dense markers confirm the localization of antibody within the basement membrane structure itself. Studies late in the course of the disease have revealed subepithelial dense deposits similar to those described in immune complex forms of glomerular injury (16). The exact nature of these dense deposits is not known.

From a physiologic viewpoint, proteinuria starts soon after the administration of nephrotoxic sera. Micropuncture physiology studies reveal an almost immediate decrease in glomerular filtration rate, secondary to alterations in renal blood flow, and a decreased permeability of the basement membrane for water and small molecules (17). Later in the disease process, if the glomerular filtration rate is maintained, it is thought to be due to a compensating effect of increased transcapillary hydrostatic pressure (18). Considerable heterogeneity of nephron function is observed as the disease progresses; however, almost complete glomerular/tubular balance is maintained despite the markedly different filtration rates of single nephrons (19). These functional changes correlate well with the degree of glomerular hypercellularity and overall architectural derange-

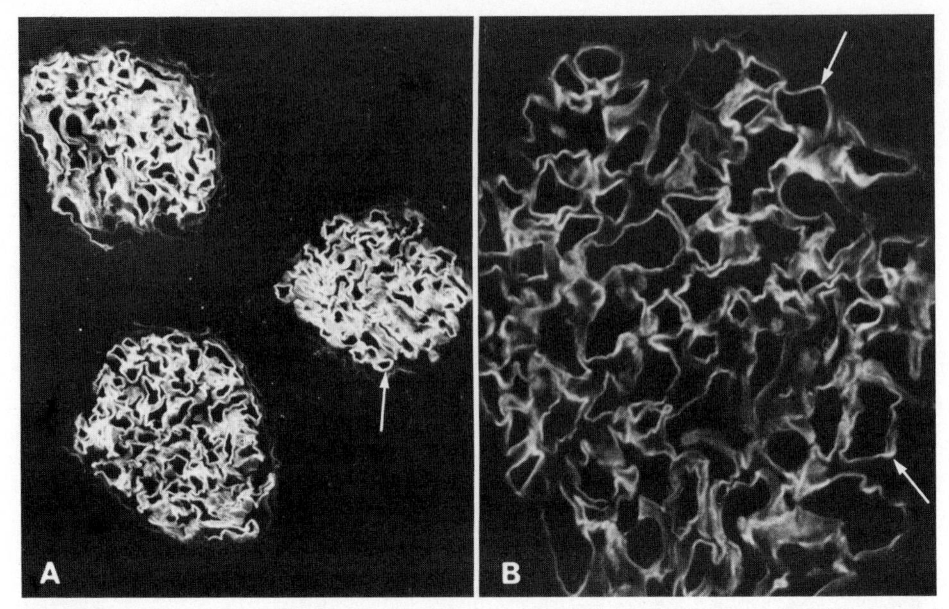

Figure 3. The typical linear deposit (*arrow*) of immunoglobulin from a heterologous anti-GBM serum is seen in three glomeruli from a rat two hours after antibody administration in *A*. In *B*, at higher magnification the smooth, continuous nature of the deposit can be better appreciated. (Fluorescein-isothiocyanate conjugated antirabbit IgG, original magnification *A*, × 250; *B*, × 630.)

ment. The cause of increased urinary protein loss, despite the decreased glomerular filtration of small molecules, may be due, at least partially, to changes in the charge characteristics of the glomerular capillary wall, which normally retard filtration of albumin (20,21).

The effects of heterologous antikidney sera in vivo are largely confined to glomeruli, in spite of the often widespread anti-basement membrane activity they possess in vitro. Injected into animals, some antikidney sera do fix to tubular basement membranes causing tubulointerstitial injury. In some experiments, sufficient fixation to pulmonary basement membranes has been observed to result in pulmonary edema and hemorrhage (22). Heterologous antilung sera, in addition to producing pulmonary hemorrhage, can induce glomerulonephritis (23,24).

Induction of Autoimmune Anti-GBM Nephritis

In 1962, Steblay reported the induction of nephritis in sheep after immunization with heterologous or homologous GBM in adjuvant (4,25). The glomerular lesion was severe and rapidly progressed to renal failure. The lesion was typified histochemically by linear deposition of IgG and complement along the GBM. Subsequent studies revealed the presence of circulating anti-GBM antibodies which, when isolated and injected, were capable of transferring the lesion to unilaterally nephrectomized lambs (8). Several other species immunized with various basement membrane preparations develop anti-GBM antibodies; however, the subsequent renal lesion is generally less severe than in sheep (2). There has been recent interest in autoimmune anti-GBM nephritis in guinea pigs, which may occur in the absence of detectable complement fixation (26). This interest is based on the observation that about one-third of human anti-GBM antibody-induced nephritides occur in the absence of detectable glomerular complement localization, suggesting that noncomplement, but as yet unidentified, pathways are involved (27).

Basement membrane-like materials in the urine of normal individuals can induce anti-GBM responses when isolated and injected with complete Freund's adjuvant. Indeed, anti-basement membrane antibodies and nephritis (28) develop in about one-third of rabbits immunized with basement membrane-rich fractions from their own urine. Similar cross-reactive basement membrane materials that have been identified in the serum increase following nephrectomy (24,29). This suggests that the potentially nephritogenic basement membrane material in serum and urine is part of normal basement membrane turnover and excretion, and that under certain, as yet undefined, circumstances it could induce anti-basement membrane responses. However, normally the material probably serves as a tolerogen, maintaining the body's usual unresponsive state to its own basement membrane antigens.

To date, the only report of spontaneous anti-GBM antibody production in mammals other than man has been in the horse (30). In this instance, the identification of anti-basement membrane antibodies was confirmed by dissociating the antibody from the kidney by elution, with subsequent in vitro study.

Experimental Anti-Tubular Basement Membrane Antibody-Induced Injury

The renal tubular basement membrane (TBM) has unique antigenic determinants apparently not shared by the GBM. At least three slightly different models of anti-TBM antibody-induced tubulointerstitial nephritis have been described, and all involve the production of antibodies to TBM antigens.

In guinea pigs, immunization with heterologous renal basement membrane preparations induces the development of anti-TBM antibodies, tubulointerstitial nephritis, and renal tubular dysfunction (31). Some anti-GBM reactivity is noted as well, but little glomerular histologic change occurs. Absorption studies have shown that the anti-GBM antibodies are directed largely toward collagen-related determinants, which probably explains the lack of nephritogenicity (32). The anti-TBM antibodies, on the other hand, are reactive with the noncollagenous TBM proteins and are nephritogenic.

When Brown Norway rats are immunized with rat kidney in complete Freund's adjuvant containing pertussis vaccine, anti-TBM antibodies develop and subsequently tubulointerstitial nephritis (33). This model is complicated by the eventual formation of immune complex-induced glomerular lesions of the type originally described by Heymann, and later shown by Edgington et al. to be immune complex-mediated and to contain a renal tubular brush border antigen (34). The nephritogenicity of the anti-TBM antibody in this model, as well as in the guinea pig model, was shown by using TBM antibodies harvested from the circulation of affected animals and passively administered to normal recipients (33,35).

A third model of anti-TBM antibody-induced tubulointerstitial nephritis has been reported in Brown Norway rats immunized with bovine TBM in complete Freund's adjuvant containing pertussis vaccine (36). In this model, anti-TBM antibodies without anti-GBM reactivity develop, making it a less complicated model of tubulointerstitial nephritis (Fig. 4). Interesting strain differences in TBM antigenicity have been noted in this model. In the Lewis rat, for example, anti-TBM antibodies develop after immunization with bovine basement membrane, but the rat lacks the necessary antigen in its TBM to react with the antibody and therefore the antibody does not localize in its kidney, nor does disease develop. When Lewis rats are transplanted with Brown Norway/Lewis F_1 hybrid kidneys containing the nephritogenic TBM antigen, antibodies form that are reactive with the TBM of the transplanted kidney, but not with their own TBM antigen-negative kidneys (37). The antibodies presumably contribute to the inflammatory response noted in the rejecting transplant, although the extent to which they are responsible for the damage is difficult to quantitate.

In the Brown Norway rat, tubulointerstitial nephritis induced with bovine basement membrane involves a lesion that appears to be mediated by complement (36). In this model, antibody begins to accumulate on the TBM six to seven days after immunization. By day 10, complement begins to deposit and PMNs accumulate in the interstitial tissue (Fig. 5). The PMN phase is transient, lasting

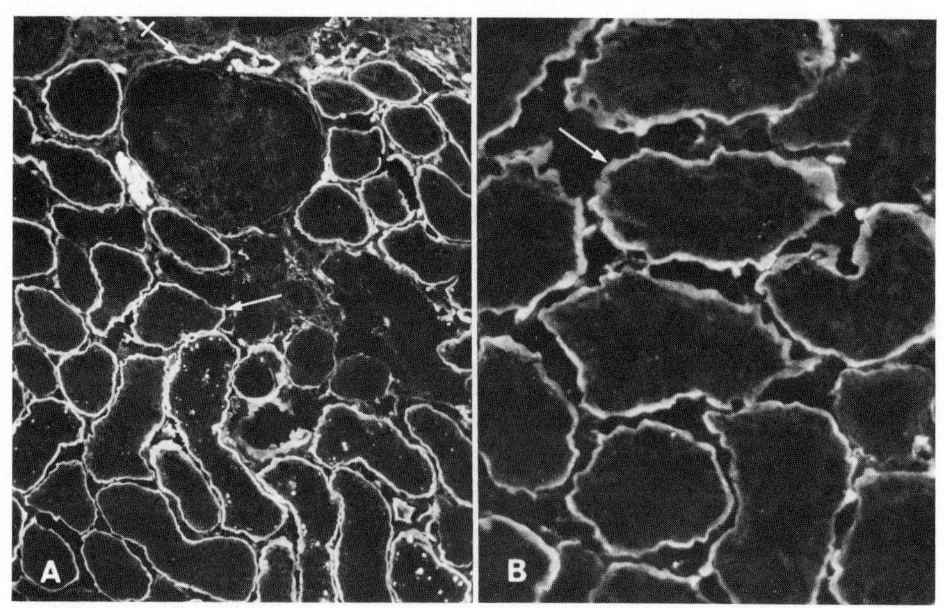

Figure 4. Linear deposits of rat IgG are present along the TBM (*arrow*) of a Brown Norway rat kidney ten days following immunization with bovine renal basement membrane in complete Freund's adjuvant containing pertussis vaccine. In *A*, the abrupt demarcation of staining can be seen where the TBM of the proximal renal tubule joins Bowman's capsule (*hatched arrow*). Note also that there is no fixation of antibody to the GBM. In *B*, at high magnification, the smooth, continuous nature of the deposit can be appreciated. (Fluorescein-isothiocyanate conjugated antirat IgG, original magnification *A*, × 250; *B*, × 630.)

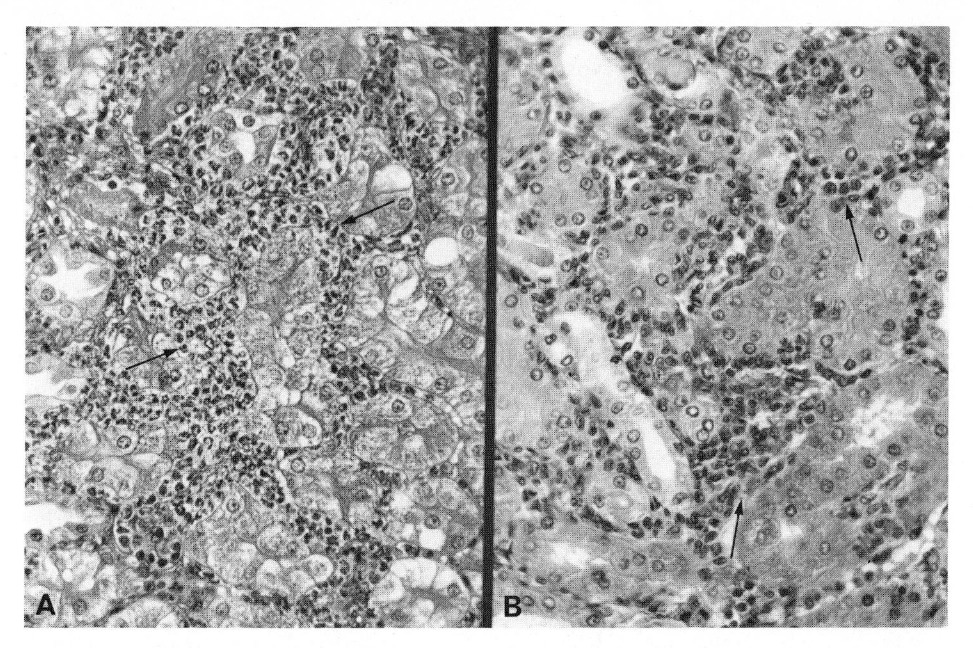

Figure 5. The histologic appearance of anti-TBM nephritis induced in the Brown Norway rat by immunization with bovine renal basement membrane in complete Freund's adjuvant containing pertussis vaccine. In *A*, an acute polymorphonuclear leukocyte infiltration (*arrows*) is observed on day 10 after immunization. By day 13, in *B*, the polymorphonuclear leukocyte infiltration has been largely replaced by a mononuclear infiltration that persists for the duration of the lesion. (Hematoxylin and eosin stain, original magnification × 320.)

only a day or so, and then is replaced with persistent infiltration of mononuclear cells. In the guinea pig model, complement depletion with cobra venom factor appears to protect the recipient from tubulointerstitial nephritis induced by passive transfer of anti-TBM antibody (38). Congenital C4-deficient guinea pigs do develop a lesion, however, suggesting that any participation of complement probably does not involve the classical C142 pathway (39).

ANTI-BASEMENT MEMBRANE ANTIBODY DISEASE IN MAN

Diseases Induced by Anti-GBM Antibodies

Linear immunoglobulin deposits similar to those found in experimental anti-GBM antibody-induced injury were first noted in human renal biopsy specimens in the early 1960s. In 1967, Lerner et al. clearly demonstrated the nephrotoxic potential of these antibodies in man by transferring nephritis to subhuman primates with anti-GBM antibodies isolated from the sera or eluted from the kidneys of patients with linear GBM deposits (40). The most convincing evidence of the nephritogenicity of the antibody came when nephritis was accidentally transferred into a renal transplant placed in a patient who had residual circulating anti-GBM antibody (40). Several examples in which anti-GBM nephritis was transferred to transplanted kidneys have now been reported; however, the nephritis produced was not always severe enough to result in graft failure (27).

Clinical Features. As we gain experience with anti-basement membrane antibody-induced tissue injury in man, it is apparent that a spectrum of clinical presentations can occur (2). Rapidly progressive nephritis and the so-called Goodpasture's syndrome are the most common presentations, with Goodpasture's syndrome seen in roughly two-thirds of the patients with recognized anti-basement membrane antibody disease (27). Goodpasture's syndrome simply denotes the presence of nephritis and pulmonary hemorrhage. Some investigators have used the term Goodpasture's syndrome synonymously with anti-GBM antibody disease; however, this usage excludes other immunologic causes of a similar clinical presentation, such as immune complex-induced injury (2). Since the diagnostic tools are at hand to make an immunopathologic diagnosis, it is wise to do so, eventually replacing the syndrome designation with an immunopathologic classification. In addition to the severe forms of nephritis seen with anti-GBM antibodies, mild and self-remitting nephritic processes are now being recognized. Injury may also be confined to the lung, with the presentation resembling idiopathic pulmonary hemosiderosis (2,41). Anti-TBM antibodies can complicate anti-GBM antibody disease, or occur in association with immune complex-induced renal injury, transplantation, or drug toxicity, or perhaps primarily induce tubulointerstitial nephritis (2).

Persons who have anti-GBM disease, either rapidly progressive glomerulonephritis or Goodpasture's syndrome, often have a preceding flu-like illness (27). Recently, a few patients have presented with arthritis or arthralgia as a prominent early complaint. Males are more commonly affected than females, and the peak incidence of the disease is in the second and third decades of life, although the disease has been identified in persons of all ages, including some under 10 and over 70. In patients with Goodpasture's syndrome, the pulmonary and renal symptoms often begin almost simultaneously, but one set may precede the other by several months. The pulmonary hemorrhage may be mild, with only blood-flecked sputum, or severe, leading to death of hypoxia. Pulmonary hemorrhage may occur episodically during the course of the disease.

The renal histologic alterations in anti-GBM antibody disease, with or without Goodpasture's syndrome, are, most often, those of proliferative, sometimes necrotizing, crescent-forming nephritis with variable amounts of tubulointerstitial alteration that may relate to the amount of accompanying anti-TBM antibody (2) (Fig. 6). Thickening of the GBM is sometimes apparent by light microscopy, particularly as the disease process progresses. In less severely involved patients, or early in the course of involvement, the lesions are typically focal. Electron microscopy reveals diffuse thickening of the GBM with breaks or gaps in its continuity, and with PMNs near or extending into the areas of discontinuation. Electron-dense deposits are generally not observed in humans with this disease, although animals in late stages of experimentally induced anti-GBM nephritis sometimes have such deposits. The related pulmonary pathology is characterized by severe alveolar hemorrhage, with numerous hemosiderin-laden macrophages within alveoli and moderate numbers of PMNs in the pulmonary interstitium (2) (Fig. 6).

Immunopathologic Diagnosis. The diagnosis of anti-GBM nephritis is based primarily on the detection of anti-GBM antibodies in renal or lung tissue and in

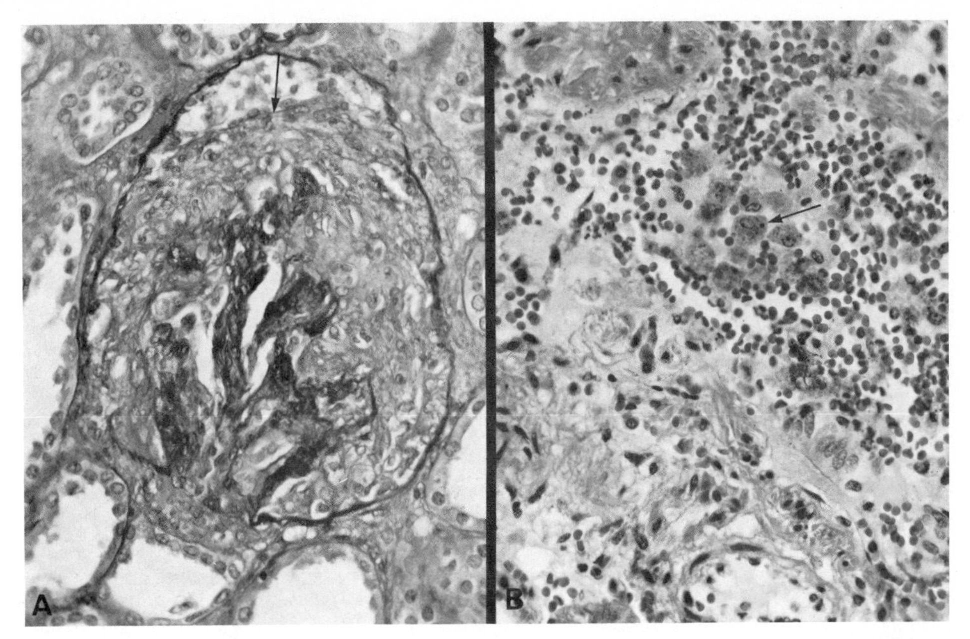

Figure 6. The histologic changes of anti-GBM antibody-induced glomerulonephritis in man are most frequently those of proliferative, crescent-forming glomerulonephritis, as seen in a glomerulus from a patient with elution-confirmed anti-GBM antibody (*A*). In anti-GBM antibody-induced Goodpasture's syndrome, the pulmonary lesion is typified by diffuse alveolar hemorrhage and hemosiderin-laden macrophages *(arrow)* (B). (*A*, Periodic acid Schiff stain; *B*, Hematoxylin and eosin stain, original magnification × 230.)

the circulation (2,27,41). The classical linear deposit of IgG, and much less frequently IgA or IgM, along the GBM is evidence to suggest this diagnosis (Fig. 7). Unfortunately, nonimmunologic linear accentuation of the GBM is being found with increasing frequency in kidneys, such as those obtained at autopsy or after perfusion for transplantation, those from patients with diabetes mellitus, and occasionally those from relatively normal individuals (41). Elution studies from such kidneys show that the deposition noted by immunofluorescence has no specificity for the GBM and represents only entrapment of serum proteins within the basement membrane structure. Indeed, IgG composes roughly 2% of the purest preparation of human GBM isolated. Immunofluorescence studies, then, must be only the first step in making the diagnosis of anti-GBM antibody-induced nephritis. Confirmation of the diagnosis comes by demonstrating the specificity of the presumed anti-GBM antibody eluted from the patient's kidney, when sufficient tissue is available, or by detecting anti-GBM antibody in the patient's serum (2,41).

Early in the course of the disease, the glomerular immunoglobulin deposit is smooth and linear, but later it becomes less regular as the basement membrane becomes damaged and distorted (Fig. 7). Even when the disease process is advanced, however, one can generally appreciate the continuity of the immunofluorescent staining. Anti-TBM antibodies, evidenced as circumferential linear deposits of IgG, involving the TBM of some or most renal tubules are also observed in about 70% of patients (27,42). This observation helps to establish the

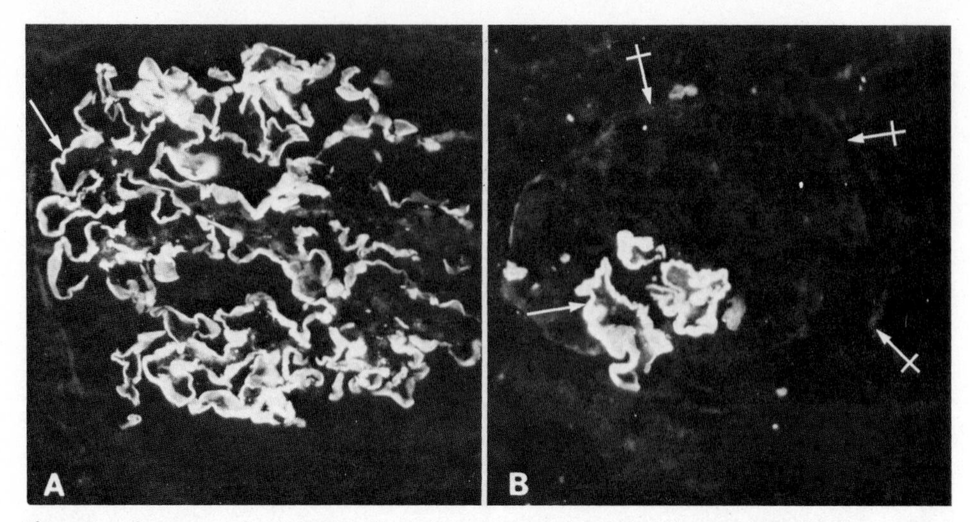

Figure 7. The pattern of anti-GBM antibody fixation in the glomerulus of man is typically linear. In *A*, in the early stage of the disease, when the glomerular architecture is still well preserved, the smooth, continuous nature of the deposits (*arrow*) can be easily observed. Even in later stages of the disease, when crescent formation has compressed and corrugated the GBM, the linear nature of the deposits can generally be appreciated (*B*). The location of Bowman's capsule is outlined by the *hatched arrows*. (Fluorescein-isothiocyanate conjugated antihuman IgG, original magnification × 250.)

diagnosis even when extensive glomerular disruption has occurred. At least two types of anti-TBM reactivity have been recognized in patients with anti-GBM disease (Fig. 8). In one, the antibody reacts with only a few tubules, both in vivo and in vitro, and in the other, the reactivity is diffuse. Histologic changes accompany the TBM deposits and signify their immunopathologic significance (2). The frequency with which anti-TBM antibodies accompany anti-GBM antibodies suggests that the process might more properly be designated anti-basement membrane antibody-induced disease.

The specificity of immunofluorescently detected anti-basement membrane reactivity is confirmed in eluted kidney samples. Elution studies generally involve dissociating antibody from a washed kidney homogenate or glomerular isolates in buffers using acid or alkaline pH, or chaotropic ions (43). Tissue samples as small as those from needle biopsies are sometimes adequate if sensitive enough methods are available to detect any recovered antibody, e.g., radioimmunoassay. The nephritogenic potential of the eluted antibody can be shown by transfer studies using subhuman primates.

Circulating Anti-GBM Antibodies. Detection of circulating anti-GBM antibodies is helpful in establishing the diagnosis, as well as in following the progression of disease. Indirect immunofluorescence has been the standard method of detecting anti-GBM or anti-TBM antibodies in serum (2,44). Sections from normal human kidney are overlaid with the test serum, and any bound immunoglobulin is subsequently detected with a fluorescein-isothiocyanate-labeled antihuman immunoglobulin antibody. The method is limited by the availability of normal human kidney but remains the best technique for detecting anti-TBM reactivity. Gel precipitation methods to detect circulating anti-basement antibodies have been described but are relatively insensitive. Hemagglutination methods have increased sensitivity, but may also have more unexplained positive reactions. Recently, radioimmunoassays have become available for detection of circulating anti-GBM antibodies (2,41,45,46). In the assay developed in our laboratory, the noncollagenous glycoproteins of the GBM remaining after collagenase digestion are used as antigens (2,41,46). The antibody activity is expressed as percent binding of the radiolabeled antigen. The collagenase digest of the GBM contains the nephritogenic GBM antigens, as demonstrated by its ability to absorb antibody activity of serum or eluate previously detected by indirect immunofluorescence.

Results of the radioimmunoassay using collagenase-solubilized GBM correlate excellently with the immunopathologic diagnosis of the patient's renal disease, as determined by immunohistochemical study (47). Seventy-six of 78 patients with anti-GBM antibody-induced Goodpasture's syndrome, and 43 of 52 patients with anti-GBM antibody-induced nephritis alone, had detectable circulating anti-GBM antibodies by this technique. Only 2 of 392 patients with immune complex nephritis were positive. In both of these patients the antibody developed during the course of a membranous glomerulonephritis, as has been previously reported (48). Four of 59 patients with systemic lupus erythematosus had low levels of circulating anti-GBM antibody. In one lupus patient, serial serum samples were available to demonstrate the appearance of the antibody during the course of disease activity. None of 52 patients with glomerular deposits of complement in the absence of immunoglobulin, and none of 36 patients with atypical and presumably nonimmunologic linear accumulations of immunoglobulin, had circulating anti-GBM antibody. Only 1 of 222 patients with

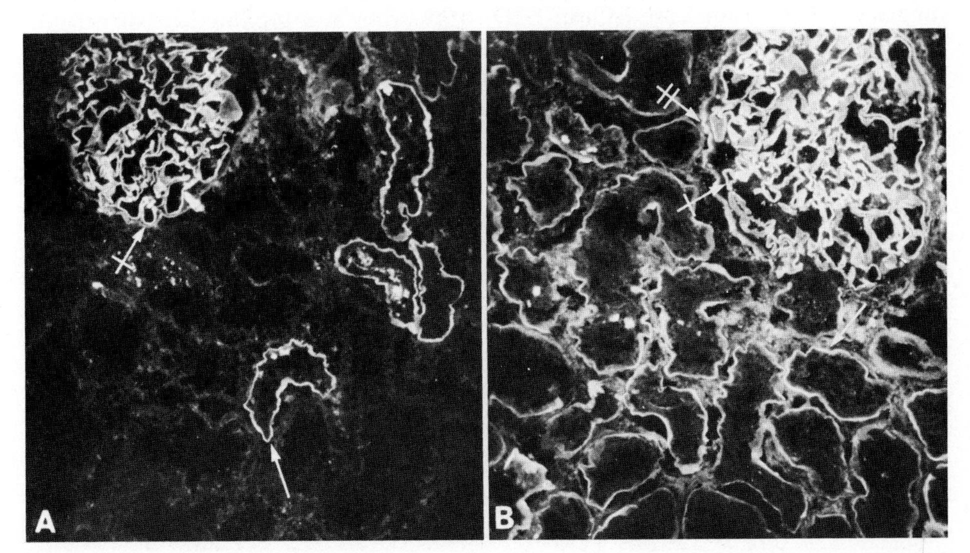

Figure 8. The different patterns of reactivity of anti-TBM antibodies that frequently accompany anti-GBM antibodies are shown by indirect immunofluorescence. Two different sera were used to stain sections from the same normal human kidney. The serum used to stain section *A* reacts only with the TBM of a few scattered tubules (*arrow*) and the GBM (*hatched arrow*). The serum used in *B* reacts with the TBM of virtually all tubules (*arrow*), the GBM (*hatched arrow*), and Bowman's capsule (*double-hatched arrow*). (Fluorescein-isothiocyanate conjugated antihuman IgG, original magnification × 160.)

negative renal immunofluorescence studies had evidence of circulating anti-GBM antibody. In this patient anti-GBM antibody-induced nephritis subsequently developed in a transplant, suggesting the inadequacy of the original immunofluorescent diagnosis.

The anti-GBM antibody response appears to be almost always transient, lasting from a few weeks to months. This observation suggests that the immunologic stimulus is probably also transitory (27). To date, only very loose clinical associations are available to suggest what some of the immunologic stimuli might be. Infectious or noxious environmental stimuli, such as influenza A2 infection or hydrocarbon solvent inhalation, have been observed in association with the development of anti-GBM antibodies (27,49,50). Renal injury, either ischemic or in association with immunologic processes such as immune complex-induced glomerulonephritis, or in association with transplant rejection, has been associated with anti-basement membrane antibody formation (2). The noxious stimuli, infectious, toxic, or immunologic, then, could conceivably act to expose basement membrane in the lung or kidney in a way that is conducive to the formation of an anti-basement membrane response. In the case of Goodpasture's syndrome, noxious stimuli may expose pulmonary antigens that are otherwise inaccessible to react with circulating anti-basement membrane antibodies formed for other reasons. The possible induction of anti-basement membrane antibodies after renal transplantation, or the occasionally observed enhanced disappearance of circulating anti-GBM antibodies following nephrectomy, suggests that the kidney may, in some instances, be the source of the antigenic stimulus.

The possible effects of nephrectomy on the level of circulating anti-GBM antibodies have been a point of interest. Early studies in sheep and man suggested that an increase in anti-GBM antibodies accompanied nephrectomy, presumably through the loss of immunoabsorptive properties of the kidney. More recently, however, it is apparent that nephrectomy does not generally result in a dramatic increase in circulating antibody, presumably because the damaged kidney is no longer exerting much immunoabsorptive capacity (2). Nephrectomy, similarly, does not seem to be essential for the disappearance of circulating anti-basement membrane antibodies; however, observations suggest that in some patients bilateral nephrectomy may enhance the rate of the antibody's disappearance.

Pulmonary Lesions Induced by Anti-Basement Membrane Antibodies. Goodpasture's syndrome, the association of severe and sometimes fatal pulmonary hemorrhage with nephritis, is observed in roughly two-thirds of patients with anti-GBM antibody-induced nephritis (27). Pulmonary hemorrhage is frequently intermittent and may occur at any time during the course of anti-GBM antibody production. There is no absolute relationship between the level of circulating antibodies as detected by radioimmunoassay and the occurrence or severity of pulmonary hemorrhage. It is currently unknown if patients with anti-GBM antibody-induced nephritis alone have antibody fixed to pulmonary basement membranes without overt lung damage. In some instances, the hemorrhage seems to be precipitated by some event, such as fluid overload or pulmonary or systemic infection (51).

Anti-basement membrane antibodies are implicated in the pulmonary lesion of Goodpasture's syndrome in several ways (52). Fixation of antibody can be observed along the alveolar basement membrane by direct immunofluorescence, where it appears in a smooth, linear deposit (Fig. 9). Antibodies reactive with both the alveolar basement membrane and the GBM can be eluted from the lung tissues of such patients, indicating the communal antigenicity of the basement membranes in the two organs (53). Heterologous antilung antibodies produce both pulmonary hemorrhage and glomerulonephritis (23,24), and lung tissue can be used to induce autologous anti-GBM nephritis in sheep. Experimentally produced heterologous anti-GBM antibodies also sometimes have a pneumotoxic effect (22). In fact, anti-GBM antibodies from patients with lung involvement may simply have a more widespread anti-basement membrane reactivity than antibodies from patients with kidney involvement alone (53).

It should be noted that anti-basement membrane antibodies are not the only cause of pulmonary hemorrhage in nephritis of the Goodpasture's syndrome variety. Immune complex deposits, as in systemic lupus erythematosus, vasculitis, or cryoglobulinemia, can also sometimes cause identical clinical presentations, so that immunopathologic classification is imperative (52,54,55,56).

Nephrectomy has been advocated by some investigators as beneficial, or even lifesaving, in patients with severe pulmonary hemorrhage of the Goodpasture's type (57,58,59). A favorable response has not been uniformly noted, however, since some patients continue to have severe pulmonary hemorrhages after ne-

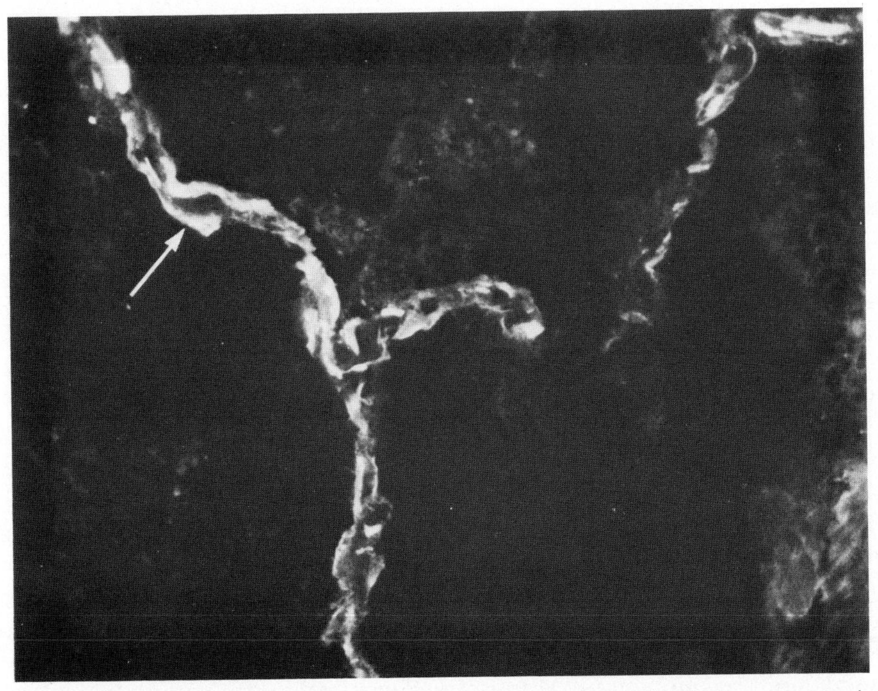

Figure 9. The fixation of anti-basement membrane antibodies to the alveolar basement membrane (*arrow*) of the lung of a patient with elution-confirmed anti-GBM antibody-induced Goodpasture's syndrome is shown. (Fluorescein-isothiocyanate conjugated antihuman IgG, original magnification × 250.)

phrectomy (27,60). Of course, it is difficult to evaluate the unpredictable response to nephrectomy in the often critically ill patient with Goodpasture's syndrome. However, nephrectomy does not generally immediately change the levels of circulating antibody; consequently, any beneficial effect of nephrectomy on pulmonary hemorrhage may relate more to mediator systems of immunologic injury than to the immune response itself. Since spontaneous recovery of renal function does sometimes occur, nephrectomy as a form of management should be considered only as a last resort.

Therapeutic Considerations. Although detailed therapeutic considerations are beyond the scope of this presentation, two areas deserve mention since they pertain to the immunopathogenicity of anti-GBM antibodies. One deals with measures to reduce acutely the levels of circulating anti-GBM antibody through a combination of plasmapheresis and immunosuppressive therapy, and the other deals with the anticipated results of transplantation in patients with anti-basement membrane antibody-induced disease.

It is reasonable to assume that decreasing the circulating anti-GBM antibody would be beneficial in treating anti-basement membrane-induced nephritis and Goodpasture's syndrome. In the past, immunosuppression has been attempted, but without uniform responses (27). Recently, plasmapheresis has been suggested as a means of rapidly removing circulating anti-GBM antibody to augment immunosuppressive therapy (61). In some patients, the combined immunosuppression and plasmapheresis do appear to hasten, if only temporarily, the expected decrease in anti-basement membrane antibody production and may be of benefit. At least three patients with renal failure treated with variations of this management recovered sufficient renal function to discontinue dialysis (51,61,62). Although theoretically this is a rational way of managing patients with anti-basement membrane antibody-induced disease, carefully controlled studies will be necessary to judge its true usefulness. The occurrence of mild and self-remitting forms of the disease in patients who may have responded without intensive therapy complicates the evaluation (63). Evidence already becoming available indicates that once antibody produces severe histologic damage, measures to lower the antibody cannot be expected to result in a recovery of function. As already noted, pulmonary hemorrhage may not directly relate to the level of circulating antibody, and in several instances, intensive plasmapheresis therapy, even with significant diminution in levels of circulating antibody, has not proved sufficient to prevent fatal pulmonary hemorrhaging.

Since renal injury produced by anti-GBM antibodies is often severe, resulting in irreversible renal failure, it is frequently necessary to consider renal transplantation in the patient's long-term management. As noted earlier, the transplanted kidney is subject to the possible recurrence of anti-GBM antibody-induced injury if the recipient's immune response is still active. Transplantation has been generally successful, however, if postponed until the patient's anti-GBM antibody production has ceased (2,27). Once quiescent, the disease process usually does not recur, even with the introduction of a new kidney. However, in a very recent observation, a second anti-GBM response developed in one patient transplanted with a kidney from an identical twin almost two years after the patient's antibody production had ceased.

Initial observations, using the new radioimmunoassay for circulating anti-GBM antibody, suggest that the severity of recurrence may be related to the amount of antibody present at the time of transplantation. Experience is insufficient at this point to determine if a so-called "safe" level of antibody exists, at which a clinically severe recurrence would be avoided. One could shorten the period of maintenance dialysis and its attendant problems in the candidate for transplantation if it were possible to determine the level of antibody that should not produce a severe recurrence. It is also unknown if bilateral nephrectomy is necessary for successful transplantation, although, up to this time, virtually all patients have been nephrectomized, based on the thinking that this hastened the disappearance of antibody. As it becomes evident that nephrectomy is not necessary for cessation of antibody production, pretransplant management may be modified. Any departure from the relatively successful current management, however, will need careful monitoring to avoid deleterious effects.

It is also of interest that when a renal transplant recipient lacks a GBM antigen that is present in the donor and, consequently, in the transplant, the recipient can form antibodies to this "new" antigen. An example is a patient with hereditary nephritis and neurosensory hearing loss (Alport's syndrome) in whom transplantation of a "normal" kidney resulted in the formation of anti-basement membrane antibodies that caused severe nephritis in the graft (64).

Diseases Induced by Anti-TBM Antibodies

Anti-TBM antibodies are present in about 70% of patients with anti-GBM nephritis. As noted earlier, these anti-TBM antibodies can induce tubulointerstitial injury (42). Anti-TBM antibodies also have been infrequently observed in immune complex forms of glomerular injury, in methicillin-induced tubulointerstitial nephritis, in renal transplant recipients, and in "primary" tubulointerstitial nephritis (Fig. 10). When studied in the laboratory, human anti-TBM antibodies have often had the same sort of reactivity noted in the Brown Norway rat model of interstitial nephritis induced with bovine TBM antigen in adjuvant (36). That is, the human antibodies react with the TBM of Brown Norway, but not Lewis, rat kidneys (Fig. 11).

Anti-TBM antibodies developed in a patient with prior severe, acute post-streptococcal glomerulonephritis, 28 weeks after the onset of his apparent immune complex-induced injury (65). The anti-TBM response was probably triggered by the preceding immunologic damage. Anti-TBM antibodies, complicating immune complex glomerulonephritis, have also been observed in children. Anti-TBM antibodies and Fanconi syndrome may also develop after the onset of immune complex-induced injury (66,67). In one such child, with intractable diarrhea, anti-TBM antibodies, which also reacted with intestinal mucosal basement membrane, developed in association with immune complex-induced glomerulonephritis and nephrotic syndrome (68). The immune complexes in this patient appeared to contain a renal tubular antigen that may also have been present in the jejunal mucosa.

Anti-TBM antibodies occasionally develop in patients with methicillin-associated tubulointerstitial nephritis (42,69,70). In this instance, the di-

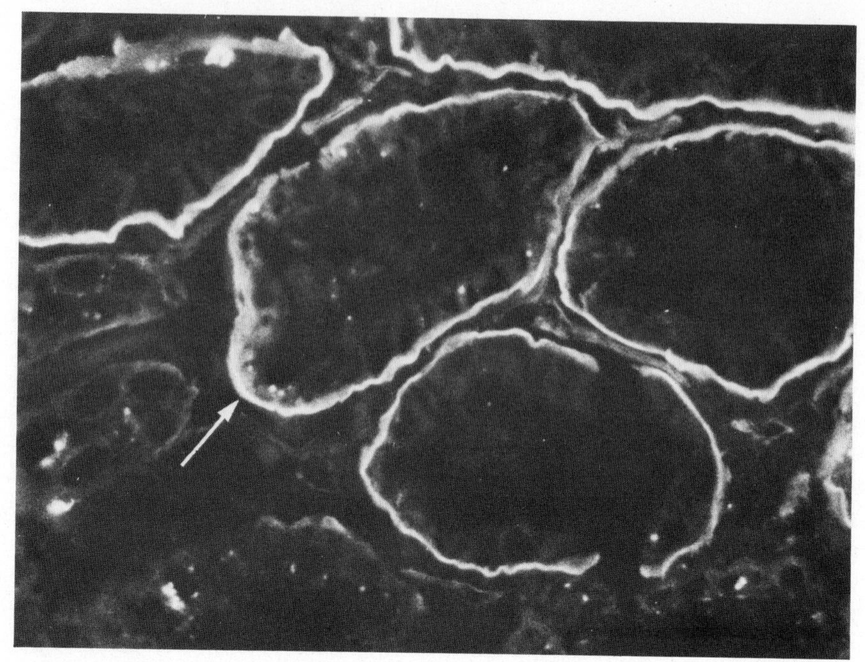

Figure 10. Anti-TBM antibodies eluted from a human renal transplant are shown reacting with the TBM of a normal human kidney (*arrow*). (Fluorescein-isothiocyanate conjugated antihuman IgG, original magnification × 400.)

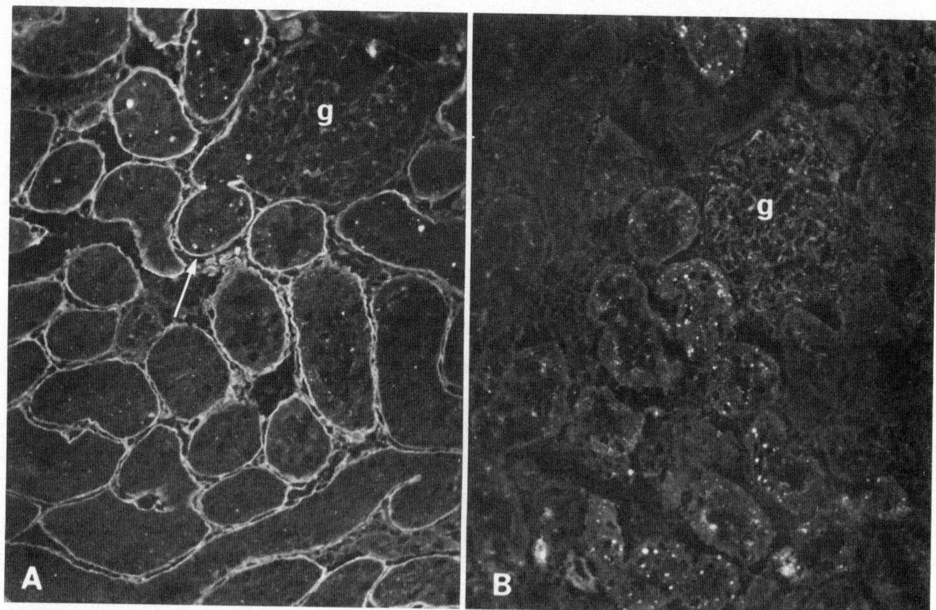

Figure 11. The different reactivities of human anti-TBM antibodies with Brown Norway (*A*) and Lewis (*B*) rat kidney sections are shown by indirect immunofluorescence. The anti-TBM antibody was recovered from the circulation of a patient with combined immune complex-induced glomerulonephritis and anti-TBM antibody-associated tubulointerstitial nephritis. The antigen reactive with the antibody is present in the Brown Norway (*A*) stain, but lacking in the Lewis (*B*) stain. The anti-TBM antibody has no reactivity with the GBM of the glomerulus (g) of either strain. (Fluorescein-isothiocyanate conjugated antihuman IgG, original magnification × 160.)

methoxyphenylpenicilloyl breakdown product of methicillin apparently becomes attached to the TBM, leading to a hapten-carrier conjugate, with antibody produced to the TBM or carrier portion of the conjugate. Since the antibodies are not detectable in all patients with methicillin-associated tubulointerstitial nephritis, presumably the anti-TBM antibodies themselves are not the underlying pathogenic mechanism responsible for methicillin-induced renal injury.

In at least two children anti-TBM antibodies have developed along with tubulointerstitial nephritis, perhaps as a primary process (71,72). Some associated glomerular damage, with minimal or no evidence of an immunologic causation, was also noted in these patients, so that it is difficult to differentiate these patients from those noted earlier who had anti-TBM antibodies associated with immune complex-induced glomerular injury. Another patient has recently been identified who had anti-TBM antibodies and anti-GBM antibodies confined to the IgA class of immunoglobulins (73). Semiquantitative estimates of the amount of antibody present suggested that the anti-TBM antibodies were predominant in this patient, who manifested a clinical presentation of both nephritis and mild pulmonary hemorrhage.

Anti-TBM antibodies have been found in several transplant recipients (42,74,75,76). One patient with anti-TBM antibody after transplantation contained antibodies reactive with his transplant, but not his native kidney, suggesting that he had responded to a TBM antigen that he lacked and was exposed to for the first time through transplantation (77). This observation is similar to that described in the preceding section for the development of anti-basement membrane activation in a patient with Alport's syndrome who received a kidney containing basement membrane antigens absent in his own kidney. These observations in man are reminiscent of those in rats undergoing cross-strain transplantation, which resulted in the formation of anti-TBM antibodies. That is, Brown Norway/Lewis F_1 hybrid "TBM antigen-positive" transplants placed in "TBM antigen-negative" Lewis rats induced anti-TBM antibodies in the recipients (37).

Antigenic differences are not always detected in patients in whom anti-TBM antibodies develop after transplantation; therefore, anti-TBM antibody production may also arise from the rejection process itself. The clinical significance of anti-TBM antibodies in transplant "rejection," and in human renal disease with complicating glomerular injury, is unclear; however, similar antibodies can cause severe tubulointerstitial nephritis in experimental animals, and there is little reason to discount their importance in contributing to human renal injury.

REFERENCES

1. Unanue, E. R., and Dixon, F. J., *Adv. Immunol.* **6**, 1 (1967).
2. Wilson, C. B., and Dixon, F. J., in *The Kidney* (B. M. Brenner and F. C. Rector, Jr., eds.), W. B. Saunders, Philadelphia, 1976, p. 838.
3. Krakower, C. A., and Greenspon, S. A., *Arch. Pathol.* **51**, 629 (1951).
4. Steblay, R. W., *J. Exp. Med.* **116**, 253 (1962).
5. Cochrane, C. G., *Adv. Immunol.* **9**, 97 (1968).
6. Cochrane, C. G., and Janoff, A., in *The Inflammatory Process* (B. W. Zweifach, L. Grant, and R. T. McCluskey, eds.), Academic Press, New York, 1974, p. 85.
7. Unanue, E. R., and Dixon, F. J., *J. Exp. Med.* **121**, 697 (1965).
8. Lerner, R., and Dixon, F. J., *J. Exp. Med.* **124**, 431 (1966).

9. Unanue, E. R., Dixon, F. J., and Feldman, J. D., *J. Exp. Med.* **125**, 163 (1967).
10. Ward, P. A., *Am. J. Pathol.* **77**, 520 (1974).
11. Henson, P. M., in *Progress in Immunology* (D. B. Amos, ed.), Academic Press, New York, 1971, p. 155.
12. Unanue, E. R., and Dixon, F. J., *J. Exp. Med.* **121**, 715 (1965).
13. Shigematsu, H., *Virchows Arch. (Zellpathol.)* **5**, 187 (1970).
14. Gang, N. F., Trachtenberg, E., Allerhand, J., Kalant, N., and Mautner, W., *Lab. Invest.* **23**, 436 (1970).
15. Hawkins, D., and Cochrane, C. G., *Immunology* **14**, 665 (1968).
16. Feldman, J. D., Hammer, D., and Dixon, F. J., *Lab. Invest.* **12**, 748 (1963).
17. Blantz, R. C., and Wilson, C. B., *J. Clin. Invest.* **58**, 899 (1976).
18. Maddox, D. A., Bennett, C. M., Deen, W. M., Glassock, R. J., Knutson, D., Daugherty, T. M., and Brenner, B. M., *J. Clin. Invest.* **55**, 305 (1975).
19. Allison, M., Wilson, C. B., and Gottschalk, C. W., *J. Clin. Invest.* **53**, 1402 (1974).
20. Chang, R. L. S., Deen, W. M., Robertson, C. R., Bennett, C. M., Glassock, R. J., and Brenner, B. M., *J. Clin. Invest.* **57**, 1272 (1976).
21. Bennett, C. M., Glassock, R. J., Chang, R. L. S., Deen, W. M., Robertson, C. R., and Brenner, B. M., *J. Clin. Invest.* **57**, 1287 (1976).
22. Freire-Maia, L., Lenos Fernandes, A. D., Azevedo, A. D., Oliveira, S. B., and Dias da Silva, W., *Agents Actions* **3**, 326 (1973).
23. Hagadorn, J. E., Vazquez, J. J., and Kinney, T. R., *Am. J. Pathol.* **57**, 17 (1969).
24. Willoughby, W. F., and Dixon, F. J., *J. Immunol.* **104**, 28 (1970).
25. Steblay, R. W., *Fed. Proc.* **24**, 693 (1965).
26. Couser, W. G., Stilmant, M., and Lewis, E. J., *Lab. Invest.* **29**, 236 (1973).
27. Wilson, C. B., and Dixon, F. J., *Kidney Int.* **3**, 74 (1973).
28. Lerner, R., and Dixon, F. J., *J. Immunol.* **100**, 1277 (1968).
29. McPhaul, J. J., Jr., and Dixon, F. J., *J. Exp. Med.* **130**, 1395 (1969).
30. Banks, K. L., and Henson, J. B., *Lab. Invest.* **26**, 708 (1972).
31. Steblay, R. W., and Rudofsky, U. H., *J. Immunol.* **107**, 589 (1971).
32. Lehman, D. H., Marquardt, H., Wilson, C. B., and Dixon, F. J., *J. Immunol.* **112**, 241 (1974).
33. Sugisaki, T., Klassen, J., Milgrom, F., Andres, G. A., and McCluskey, R. T., *Lab. Invest.* **28**, 658 (1973).
34. Edgington, T. S., Glassock, R. J., and Dixon, F. J., *Science* **155**, 1432 (1967).
35. Steblay, R. W., and Rudofsky, U., *Science* **180**, 966 (1973).
36. Lehman, D. H., Wilson, C. B., and Dixon, F. J., *Kidney Int.* **5**, 187 (1974).
37. Lehman, D. H., Lee, S., Wilson, C. B., and Dixon, F. J., *Transplantation* **17**, 429 (1974).
38. Rudofsky, U. H., Steblay, R. W., and Pollara, B., *Clin. Immunol. Immunopathol.* **3**, 396 (1975).
39. Rudofsky, U. H., McMaster, P. R. B., Ma, W. S., Steblay, R. W., and Pollara, B., *J. Immunol.* **112**, 1387 (1974).
40. Lerner, R., Glassock, R. J., and Dixon, F. J., *J. Exp. Med.* **126**, 989 (1967).
41. Wilson, C. B., and Dixon, F. J., *Kidney Int.* **5**, 389 (1974).
42. Lehman, D. H., Wilson, C. B., and Dixon, F. J., *Am. J. Med.* **58**, 765 (1975).
43. Woodroffe, A. J., and Wilson, C. B., *J. Immunol.* **118**, 1788 (1977).
44. McPhaul, J. J., Jr., and Dixon, F. J., *J. Immunol.* **103**, 1168 (1969).
45. Mahieu, P., Lambert, P. H., and Miescher, P. A., *J. Clin. Invest.* **54**, 128 (1974).
46. Wilson, C. B., Marquardt, H., and Dixon, F. J., *Kidney Int.* **6**, 114a (1974).
47. Wilson, C. B., and Dixon, F. J., in *Immunological Diseases,* 3d ed. (M. Samter, ed.), Little, Brown, Boston (in press).
48. Klassen, J., Elwood, C., Grossberg, A. L., Milgrom, F., Montes, M., Sepulveda, M., and Andres, G. A., *N. Engl. J. Med.* **290**, 1340 (1974).
49. Wilson, C. B., and Smith, R. C., *Ann. Intern. Med.* **76**, 91 (1972).
50. Beirne, G. J., and Brennan, J. T., *Arch. Environ. Health* **25**, 365 (1972).
51. Johnson, J. P., Whitman, W., Briggs, W. A., and Wilson, C. B., *Am. J. Med.* **65**, 354 (1978).
52. Wilson, C. B., in *Pulmonary Diseases* (A. P. Fishman, ed.), McGraw-Hill/Blakiston, New York (in press).
53. McPhaul, J. J., Jr., and Dixon, F. J., *J. Clin. Invest.* **49**, 308 (1970).
54. Martinez, J. S., and Kohler, P. F., *Ann. Intern. Med.* **75**, 67 (1971).
55. Lewis, E. J., Schur, P. H., Busch, G. J., Galvanek, E., and Merrill, J. P., *Am. J. Med.* **54**, 507 (1973).

56. Beirne, G. J., Kopp, W. L., and Zimmerman, S. W., *Arch. Intern. Med.* **132**, 261 (1973).
57. Maddock, R. K., Stevens, L. E., Reemtsma, K., and Bloomer, H. A., *Ann. Intern. Med.* **67**, 1258 (1967).
58. Nowakowski, A., Grove, R. B., King, L. H., Jr., Antonovych, T. T., Fortner, R. W., Knieser, M. R., Carter, C. B., and Knepshield, J. H., *Ann. Intern. Med.* **75**, 243 (1971).
59. Silverman, M., Hawkins, D., and Ackman, C. F. D., *Can. Med. Assoc. J.* **108**, 336 (1973).
60. Eisinger, A. J., *Am. J. Med.* **55**, 565 (1973).
61. Lockwood, C. M., Boulton-Jones, J. M., Lowenthal, R. M., Simpson, I. J., Peters, D. K., and Wilson, C. B., *Br. Med. J.* **2**, 252 (1975).
62. Lockwood, C. M., Rees, A. J., Pearson, T. A., Evans, D. J., Peters, D. K., and Wilson, C. B., *Lancet* **1**, 711 (1976).
63. Cohen, L. H., Wilson, C. B., and Freeman, R. M., *Arch. Intern. Med.* **136**, 835 (1976).
64. McCoy, R. C., Johnson, H. K., Stone, W. J., and Wilson, C. B., *Lab. Invest.* **34**, 325 (1976) (abstr.).
65. Morel-Maroger, L., Kourilsky, O., Mignon, F., and Richet, G., *Clin. Immunol. Immunopathol.* **2**, 185 (1974).
66. Tung, K. S. K., and Black, W. C., *Lab. Invest.* **32**, 696 (1975).
67. Levy, M., Gagnadoux, M. F., and Habib, R., in *Third Int. Symp. on Pediatr. Nephrol.,* Washington, D.C., 1974, p. 13 (abstr.).
68. Harner, M. H., Nolte, M., Wilson, C. B., Talwalker, Y. B., Musgrave, J. E., Brooks, R. E., and Campbell, R. A., in *Third Int. Symp. on Pediatr. Nephrol.,* Washington, D.C., 1974, p. 8 (abstr.).
69. Border, W. A., Lehman, D. H., Egan, J. D., Sass, H. J., Glode, J. E., and Wilson, C. B., *N. Engl. J. Med.* **291**, 381 (1974).
70. Mayaud, C., Kanfer, A., Kourilsky, O., and Sraer, J. D., *N. Engl. J. Med.* **292**, 1132 (1975).
71. Bergstein, J., and Litman, N., *N. Engl. J. Med.* **292**, 875 (1975).
72. Golbus, S., Channick, M., and Wilson, C. B., in preparation.
73. Border, W. A., Baehler, R. W., Bhathena, D., and Glassock, R. J., *N. Engl. J. Med.* (submitted).
74. Klassen, J., Kano, K., Milgrom, F., Menno, A. B., Anthone, S., Anthone, R., Sepulveda, M., Elwood, C. M., and Andres, G. A., *Int. Arch. Allergy Appl. Immunol.* **45**, 675 (1973).
75. Andres, G. A., and McCluskey, R. T., *Kidney Int.* **7**, 271 (1975).
76. Berger, J., Noël, H., and Yianeva, H., *Sixth Int. Cong. on Nephrol.,* Florence, Italy, June 8–12, 1975, p. 134 (symposia abstr.).
77. Wilson, C. B., Lehman, D. H., McCoy, R. C., Gunnels, J. C., Jr., and Stickel, D. L., *Transplantation* **18**, 447 (1974).

Chapter Eleven

Human Immune Complex Diseases

CLIVE L. HALL, ROBERT B. COLVIN,
AND ROBERT T. McCLUSKEY

Departments of Pathology, Massachusetts General Hospital and Harvard Medical School, Boston, Massachusetts

In this chapter we will evaluate evidence indicating that many, and perhaps most, forms of vasculitis and glomerulonephritis in man are mediated by immune (antigen-antibody) complexes. On the basis of experimental studies such as those described in Chapter 3, as well as certain clinical studies to be described here, it is believed that such lesions are usually initiated by complexes formed within the circulation. These complexes are usually modified considerably following deposition in tissue, particularly through combination of additional antibody, antigen, complement components, or rheumatoid factors. Immune complexes may also be initially formed within tissues, and this may be an important mechanism responsible for immune complex formation in the thyroid, renal interstitium, dermal-epidermal junction, and synovium—these forms of immune complex-mediated injury will not be extensively discussed.

DETECTION OF IMMUNE COMPLEXES IN TISSUE

No histologic criteria permit identification of immune complex-mediated glomerular or vascular injury, and recognition depends largely on evidence that complexes are present at the sites of tissue damage. In glomeruli the evidence generally consists of the demonstration by immunofluorescence or im-

The authors are grateful for the support of USPHS Grant AM 18729 and for the excellent secretarial assistance of Mary Lahey, Nadja McGahn and Judy Jensen.

munoperoxidase techniques of granular or irregular deposits of immunoglobulins and complement components. Usually, electron microscopy reveals corresponding dense deposits. (The other major immunologically mediated glomerular disease, due to anti-glomerular basement membrane antibodies, is characterized by completely continuous, so-called linear, accumulation of IgG along the glomerular basement membrane (GBM); electron-dense deposits are generally not found.) From experimental studies and from observations on human glomerular lesions known to be mediated by immune complexes (especially lupus nephritis), it is clear that complexes may accumulate in various portions of the glomerulus, notably in the mesangium and along either side of, or within, the glomerular basement membrane. Although the finding of granular or irregular immunoglobulin-containing deposits provides presumptive evidence for immune complexes, especially if the deposits are present in patterns closely resembling established models, the possibility that certain deposits represent nonimmunologically trapped plasma proteins should be considered. If various plasma proteins (albumin, certain immunoglobulin classes) are not demonstrable in the deposits, nonspecific trapping can be considered unlikely. Nevertheless, to provide rigorous proof that immunoglobulin-containing deposits are immune complexes, it must be shown that they contain specific antibodies and corresponding antigens.

The specificity of the antibodies can best be examined by analysis of immunoglobulins eluted from renal tissue or isolated glomeruli. Woodroffe and Wilson have recently reported on the most effective elution techniques (1). Substantial amounts of tissue are generally required; thus, percutaneous renal biopsy specimens are usually not suitable. Detection of specific antibody activity in eluates is possible only if the corresponding antigen is available for testing. Since in most instances there is no clue as to the identity of the antigen, the only approach is to test a panel of viral or autologous antigens (which are at present the leading candidates for the antigens involved in "idiopathic" immune complex-mediated glomerulonephritis). Moreover, it is not enough to demonstrate antibody activity; it must be shown that a given antibody is more concentrated in the eluate than in the serum. This has been accomplished most convincingly in lupus nephritis, in which high concentrations of anti-DNA antibodies have been demonstrated (2).

In unusual instances, specific antibody activity has been demonstrated by immunofluorescence in tissue sections, through the use of anti-idiotype antibodies (3) or aggregated gamma globulin (to detect rheumatoid factor activity) (3). These methods do not have wide applicability and cannot be used to measure the concentration of specific antibodies in deposits.

The demonstration of a specific antigen within glomerular deposits also provides evidence for the presence of immune complexes. This approach has the advantage of being feasible with small biopsy specimens. However, there are serious problems with such studies, which we believe are not widely enough understood. For one thing, it is difficult to be certain that a given antiserum is truly monospecific; a common practice is to measure specificity by immunoelectrophoresis, but this technique is less sensitive than immunofluorescence. Furthermore, unless there is some clue as to the antigen, the chances of identifying it, through the use of a battery of antisera, are small indeed. Even if the appropriate antiserum is used, antigens present in immune complexes may not be detected because the determinants are saturated with antibodies. This obstacle can sometimes be surmounted by partial elution of the antibodies, which may uncover reactive antigenic sites without dislodging the antigen. When positive staining is obtained, at least three conditions should be met before it is concluded that a specific antigen has indeed been demonstrated within immune complexes: (1) the staining for antigen should be in the same location as the deposits of immunoglobulin and complement; (2) the antigen should not be demonstrable in unrelated conditions characterized by deposits of immunoglobulins and complement; and (3) staining should be abolished by absorption of the antisera with a purified preparation of antigen.

Even when an antigen has been convincingly demonstrated within glomerular deposits, the possibility remains that it is material that has become trapped in immune complexes of other specificities. This has been clearly shown to occur in an experimental model (4). Rats with autologous immune complex disease (Heymann nephritis) were injected intravenously with proteins that can be traced by electron microscopy (peroxidase, catalase, ferritin), and the tracer proteins were found to become concentrated within the subepithelial deposits. Obviously, this may provide a mechanism for intensification of the glomerular injury, if specific antibody combines with the secondarily trapped antigen. There is reason to suspect that HBs Ag may sometimes be secondarily trapped in immune deposits (see below).

Demonstration of complexes in the circulation also provides evidence for an immune complex pathogenesis; however, unless it can be shown that complexes are of the same specificity as those deposited in glomeruli, this cannot be considered conclusive evidence, especially since it is now apparent that complexes without any pathogenetic significance are found in a variety of diseases, and even in apparently healthy individuals. In the majority of human glomerular diseases in which an immune complex pathogenesis is thought likely, there is no clue concerning the identity of the postulated antigen, and in these instances one must regard the mechanism as unproved. If, however, there is an established experimental model of immune complex glomerulonephritis that very closely resembles the human disease, especially in terms of immunofluorescence and electron-microscopic findings, an immune complex pathogenesis can be considered highly probable. On this basis, it seems quite likely that membranous glomerulonephritis and poststreptococcal glomerulonephritis are mediated by immune complexes.

The significance of small, irregular deposits in glomeruli is generally obscure. Irregular, and usually faint, staining for IgM and C3 in mesangial regions is seen fairly often in the absence of other evidence of glomerular disease. It is possible that such findings do sometimes represent immune complexes that have failed to produce detectable glomerular damage. However, this conclusion should be viewed with caution, since it has been shown experimentally that certain proteins, especially in aggregated form, can localize in mesangial regions (5). Partially sclerotic glomeruli, as in end-stage kidneys or focal glomerular sclerosis, often contain some immunoglobulin, especially IgM and C3, but it is not certain that these represent immune deposits.

It is even more difficult to evaluate the significance of immunoglobulins or complement components in blood vessel walls. C3 (usually alone but sometimes with IgM) is commonly found in renal arterioles that appear normal histologically or show only hyaline thickening. Immunoglobulins and complement components are often found in damaged vessels in malignant hypertension or scleroderma, but the significance of these findings is unknown (6). In necrotic arteries, as in the lesions of polyarteritis nodosa, nonspecific trapping of plasma proteins or irrelevant circulating exogenous antigens would be expected to occur regularly. Even in this circumstance, however, staining for different plasma proteins is variable. Obviously, elution of immunoglobulins from vessel walls is generally not feasible. Identification of antigenic material by immunofluorescence may be attempted, if there is reason to suspect a particular antigen. As discussed later, hepatitis B antigens have been reported to be within vessel walls in some cases of polyarteritis nodosa.

When immune complexes are convincingly demonstrated at a site of tissue damage, it is reasonable to assume that they are responsible for the initiation of the injury. However, it is also possible that other immunologic mechanisms (cell-mediated, IgE-mediated) or nonimmunologic mechanisms sometimes participate.

It should also be recognized that the absence of deposits of immunoglobulins and complement does not necessarily exclude an immune complex pathogenesis. In some rabbits with acute serum sickness, immunoglobulins are not demonstrable in glomeruli, even in the face of severe glomerular lesions, presumably because the complexes are rapidly degraded (7). Furthermore, in the late stages of acute serum sickness, deposits may stain for C3 but not for Ig or antigen (8); this has also been described in the Arthus reaction (9).

DETECTION OF IMMUNE COMPLEXES IN THE CIRCULATION

Until recently, circulating immune complexes were demonstrated principally by physicochemical methods, such as analytical ultracentrifugation, sucrose gradient centrifugation, and column chromatography, which detect immune complexes by their large molecular size. Lately, various biologic systems, often using the principle of radioimmunoassay (RIA), have been developed (Table 1). These are considerably more sensitive and permit the processing of larger numbers of specimens. The biologic assays may be divided into three main groups: (1) those in which purified proteins such as C1q, monoclonal (mRF), or polyclonal (pRF) rheumatoid factor bind to the Fc portion of IgG or IgM in immune complexes; (2) those in which living cells interact with immune complexes, including binding of complexes by complement receptors on lymphoblastoid cells (Raji cells), phagocytosis of complexes by macrophages, and aggregation of human platelets; and (3) anticomplementary assays in which complexes consume complement and render it functionally unavailable.

Most assays are calibrated by measuring the activity of artificial soluble "complexes" of heat-aggregated human IgG (AHG). Comparison of sensitivities is usually based on the micrograms per milliliter of AHG detectable. However, the sensitivity to different sizes and types of complexes varies (all methods are more sensitive to larger complexes, and as yet no single technique detects all types of

Table 1. Some Recently Developed Assays for Immune Complexes

Assay	Property of Complex Required	Potential Interfering Substances[a]	Approximate Sensitivity[b] (AHG μg/ml)
Raji cell (43)	C3b, d bound	Antibodies reactive with Raji cells	10
C1q polyethylene glycol (PEG)(28)	Binds free C1q; insoluble in 2.5% PEG	Polyanions	10
C1q-solid phase (30,33)	Binds free C1q; Ig present	Polyanions	4
C1q-deviation (29)	Binds free C1q	Polyanions	4
Monoclonal rheumatoid factor (RF) (30,31)	IgG Fc reactive with RF	RF	0.5–15
Polyclonal RF (37)	IgG Fc reactive with RF	RF	1–10
Platelet aggregation (46)	IgG Fc reactive with platelets	Platelet antibodies; RF	4
Macrophage uptake (44)	IgG Fc reactive with macrophages	RF; ?others	20–30

[a] All tests will detect Ig artifactually aggregated by improper storage. The Raji test seems rather insensitive to this phenomenon, perhaps because active complement components must also be present in the serum. The C1q-PEG test may be less sensitive to polyanions because only macromolecular complexes are detected.

[b] The sensitivity is highly dependent on the nature of the complexes and is given as a very rough approximation in equivalent concentrations of heat-aggregated IgG (AHG).

circulating complexes). Further improvement of the sensitivities of the assays may not be of substantial benefit, since small amounts of circulating complexes are apparently sometimes present in normal persons.

Physicochemical Techniques

Three physiochemical methods—ultracentrifugation, gel filtration, and cryoprecipitation—have been of value in detecting and characterizing circulating soluble immune complexes.

Ultracentrifugation. Complexes can be obtained from the test specimen in a relatively unaltered state, and the ultracentrifugation technique can provide information about the size of the complexes. For example, complexes of human serum albumin and rabbit antialbumin formed in extreme antigen excess are of a small size, sedimenting at 9S (10). In slight to moderate antigen excess, the complexes are larger, sedimenting between 9S and 11S. At equivalence or in antibody excess, complexes that remain soluble have sedimentation coefficients of more than 30S. The ultracentrifugal technique is not particularly sensitive and is not readily adaptable for the analysis of large numbers of samples. Its principal use now is to validate biologic assays and to determine the size of complexes.

Gel Column Chromatography. C3 bound to immune complexes ("macromolecular C3") can be separated by size from native plasma C3 by gel filtration (11,12). The C3 can be determined by microhemagglutination inhibition, able to detect 0.2 μg of C3 per ml (11). Macromolecular C3 in the void peak is believed to represent C3 bound to complexes. This approach, while allowing large quantities of serum to be processed, does not yield purified complexes.

Cryoprecipitation. Cold-precipitable proteins (cryoglobulins) have been observed in the serum in a variety of diseases (13,14). Cryoglobulins may represent immune complexes or altered immunoglobulin with the biologic properties of immune complexes (15). On the basis of immunochemical analysis, cryoglobulins have been classified into three categories (16). Type I cryoglobulins are composed of single monoclonal immunoglobulins. Types II and III are mixed cryoglobulins, that is, they contain more than one immunoglobulin class. In type II there is a monoclonal component (usually IgM), possessing antibody activity against the other component, which is polyclonal IgG. In type III cryoglobulin, all the immunoglobulin components are polyclonal. The majority of type III cryoglobulins contain IgM and IgG, and in most instances the IgM component exhibits antibody activity against IgG. Thus, type II and most type III cryoglobulins can be considered to be in part IgG-anti-IgG immune complexes. However, in some cases it has been shown that the complexes also contain an exogenous antigen (HBs Ag) (17) or an endogenous antigen (DNA) (18), against which the IgG component and, to a lesser extent, the IgM component exhibit antibody activity. Probably most, if not all, IgG-anti-IgG cryoglobulins will eventually be shown to contain exogenous or endogenous antigens. Cryoglobulins sometimes contain antigens and specific antibodies at concentrations many times greater than those in the circulation (19). Cryoprecipitates therefore provide an excellent source of material in which to search for antigens involved in immune complex disease. Complement components, especially C3, are commonly found in the precipitates. The physicochemical basis of cryoprecipitation is not known. The common presence of IgM RF suggests that RF may be one factor that favors cryoprecipitation.

C1q Techniques

The C1q molecule is a subunit of the first component of complement, which binds with a receptor on the Fc portion of IgG_1, IgG_2, IgG_3, and IgM (20). The binding is greatly enhanced by aggregation of the immunoglobulins, either by heating or during the formation of immune complexes (21). Under suitable conditions, soluble complexes can be precipitated by C1q (22), and the reaction of C1q with AHG or immune complexes can be demonstrated by gel diffusion (23).

The C1q Gel Diffusion Test. As developed by Agnello and others, this test has been used to detect circulating immune complexes in patients with systemic lupus erythematosus (SLE) and rheumatoid arthritis (23), dermatitis herpetiformis (24), leprosy (25), and arteritis (26). However, gel diffusion detects complexes only at concentrations greater than 100 μg of AHG per ml, and is essentially a qualitative test (27).

^{125}I-C1q Radioimmunoassays. In recent years radioimmunoassays employing ^{125}I-labeled C1q have been developed for the quantitative measurement of immune complexes (28,29,30,31). In the ^{125}IC1q binding assay (28,32), ^{125}I-C1q is added to the test serum and becomes incorporated in complexes able to bind C1q. Polyethylene glycol (PEG) is added (2.5%), which precipitates C1q bound in macromolecules and allows free C1q to remain in solution. To prevent the incorporation of ^{125}I-C1q into the C1qrs complex (which is precipitable by PEG), the test serum is initially heat-inactivated (28). This decreases the sensitivity of the test, probably by causing the formation of IgG aggregates, or destroying labile complexes; however, this difficulty can be overcome by using edetic acid (EDTA), which blocks the reaction of ^{125}I-C1q with C1rs, but not with complexes, and increases the sensitivity of the test to 10 μg/ml of AHG (32).

Other C1q-dependent radioimmunoassays use the competitive inhibition of the binding of ^{125}I-C1q to a substrate by C1q-reactive immune complexes in the test serum. ^{125}I-C1q is added to the test serum, and the distribution of ^{125}I-C1q between the soluble phase and the C1q-reactive substrate is measured. In the "C1q deviation test" (29), the substrate consists of sheep erythrocytes coated with antisheep erythrocyte IgG. The uptake of ^{125}I-C1q by the red cells with and without the test serum is determined. This test has a maximum sensitivity of 5 μg/ml for AHG in heat-inactivated normal human serum. In the "solid phase C1q deviation test" (30), IgG bound to agarose beads is used as the C1q-reactive substrate. The binding of ^{125}I-C1q to the IgG linked to the sepharose is sufficiently specific and stable to eliminate significant interference from monomeric IgG in the test serum, and heat inactivation is not required. The test has a maximum sensitivity of 4 μg/ml of AHG. Other successful assays employ C1q bound to polystyrene plastic tubes as the "solid phase" and measure IgG in the test serum which binds to the immobilized C1q with ^{125}I-anti-IgG (33).

The radioimmunoassays using ^{125}I-C1q detect only those complexes with available C1q binding sites. Immune complexes that activate complement only via the alternative pathway and those that do not activate complement at all are not detected. In addition, C1q can bind to a variety of polyanionic molecules, including single- and double-stranded DNA, and single- and double-stranded polyribonucleotides (23,28), endotoxin lipopolysaccharides (34), meningococcal group A polysaccharides (35), and certain poorly defined low-molecular-weight substances in the sera of some patients with SLE (3). The C1q-PEG test may be relatively insensitive to these polyanions, because this assay depends upon the formation of macromolecular complexes with C1q, which precipitate in PEG. All ^{125}I-C1q assays detect predominantly larger-sized complexes; the sensitivity increases threefold as the complexes increase in size from 19S to 45S (30,32). Iodinated C1q can form aggregates, which may increase the background and decrease the sensitivity of the assays (27). Despite these limitations, assays using ^{125}I-C1q have been refined into quantitative and sensitive methods for detecting IgG- and IgM-containing immune complexes.

Rheumatoid Factors

Both monoclonal (mRF) and polyclonal (pRF) rheumatoid factors are IgM antibodies that react with IgG in immune complexes (or in aggregates), but not with monomeric IgG or other immunoglobulins. mRF is more efficient than pRF (36) and detects small complexes, which escape precipitation by most pRFs or C1q reagents (27). mRF is present in the serum of certain patients with lymphoproliferative disorders, mixed cryoglobulinemia, rheumatoid arthritis, and Waldenström's macroglobulinemia (30). RF can be used to precipitate IgG complexes either in gels or in solution (36). In recent years, RF radioimmunoassays have been developed.

In the mRF radioimmunoassay of Gabriel and Agnello (30), complexes in the test serum compete with IgG linked to agarose beads for the binding of ^{125}I-mRF. Immune complexes in the test specimen are detected by inhibition of uptake of ^{125}I-mRF by the IgG-beads. The assay has a maximum sensitivity for AHG of 0.5 μg/ml and detects immune complexes as small as 8S, as well as larger complexes. In another solid-phase radioimmunoassay (31), mRF is in the solid phase (microcrystalline cellulose). The inhibition of binding of ^{125}I-AHG caused by the presence of immune complexes in the test specimen is measured. Although the affinity for monomeric 7S IgG of the mRF employed is less than 1/50 of that for AHG, it is necessary to adjust each serum to a uniform IgG concentration to obtain consistent results. The assay has a maximum sensitivity for AHG of 25 μg/ml and detects preferentially larger immune complexes ($>$ 19S). The mRF assay yields a higher incidence of positive results in patients with rheumatoid arthritis than the other assays. The reasons are unclear, but may be due either to the detection of complexes of small size, which are not detected by the Raji cell or C1q assays, or to the fact that mRF possesses some selectivity for immune complexes in patients with rheumatoid arthritis (27).

Analogous assays employ pRF obtained from the serum of patients with active rheumatoid arthritis (37). The pRF assay has a maximum sensitivity of 1 μg/ml for immune complexes formed at equivalence, and decreases to 5 to 10 μg/ml for immune complexes formed in five- to tenfold antigen or antibody excess. The pRF assay cannot be employed to detect complexes in sera which contain rheumatoid factors (e.g., sera from many patients with rheumatoid arthritis and some patients with SLE), as the serum RF competes with the pRF of the assay.

The Raji Cell Test

Raji cells, derived from a patient with Burkitt's lymphoma (38), are human lymphoblastoid cells with some B cell characteristics, maintained in continuous suspension culture (39). Raji cells lack surface Ig and have low avidity receptors for Fc and high avidity receptors for C3, C3b, C3d (39,40,41), and other complement components (42). The cells detect complexes largely, if not entirely, by binding complement components contained in the complexes. In the radioimmunoassay method, Raji cells are first incubated with the test specimen and then with ^{125}I-labeled rabbit antihuman IgG antibody. The radioactivity bound to the cells is measured and compared with that obtained with known amounts of AHG that were incubated with fresh human serum. The concentration of immune complexes is determined as equivalents of AHG in micrograms per milliliter (43). Complexes bound to Raji cells can also be detected by immunofluorescence, using antisera directed against IgG or antigen (when this is known); however, this method is not as readily quantitated.

The Raji cell radioimmunoassay method has certain advantages. It is a quantitative and highly reproducible technique, which detects complexes that have bound complement either by the classical or the alternative pathways. As with other techniques, its sensitivity varies with the size of the immune complexes, being 6 μg/ml with large immune complexes (> 35S), 25 μg/ml with intermediate-size immune complexes (19S to 34S), and 50 μg/ml with small immune complexes (11S to 19S) (43). In addition, Raji cells may be used to identify antigens in immune complexes under certain conditions; one approach is by immunofluorescence. Thus, bovine serum albumin, human serum albumin, and mouse thyroglobulin have been demonstrated on the surface of the Raji cells following incubation with the serum of animals with experimental immune complex disease or with immune complexes prepared in vitro (41). Similarly, HBs Ag has been identified bound to the surface of Raji cells following incubation in the serum of patients with HBs Ag-positive chronic active hepatitis (43). Another approach involves the addition of excess complement, which by competing for the Raji cell complement receptors, may release some of the immune complexes into the supernatant (39), from which they can be harvested.

The Raji cell technique also has several disadvantages. It probably detects only immune complexes that bind complement. The cells have to be maintained in continuous tissue culture (although they grow easily and rapidly as suspension cultures). Certain sera, particularly those from patients with SLE or patients who have received multiple blood transfusions or kidney transplants, may contain antilymphocyte or antihistocompatibility antibodies, which can combine with the Raji cells and be detected by the probe antibody, producing a false-positive result. However, antilymphocyte antibodies that react with Raji cells have not been identified in the sera of patients with SLE (43).

Macrophage Radiobioassay

In the macrophage radiobioassay, ^{125}I-AHG and immune complexes compete for receptor sites on guinea pig peritoneal macrophages (44,45). The macrophages are treated with human gamma globulin to block the Fc receptors and are incubated with heat-inactivated test serum that contains ^{125}I-AHG. The uptake by the macrophages is compared with that using ^{125}I-AHG alone. The test has a maximum sensitivity of 20 to 30 μg/ml of AHG. Several factors influence the inhibitory effect of serum on the phagocytosis of ^{125}I-AHG by macrophages (44), including the serum levels of IgG and complement, and the concentration of some electrolytes, particularly calcium. Moreover, the sera of approximately one-third of patients with seropositive rheumatoid arthritis and of some patients with SLE having rheumatoid factor produce enhanced uptake of ^{125}I-AHG uptake, causing difficulties in interpretation (44).

Platelet Aggregation Assay

The platelet aggregation assay (Pl.A.) (46) uses the alteration in the adhesive properties of human platelets that occurs when immune complexes interact with the Fc receptors on the platelet surface. Viable platelets are required, as the surface alteration that results in aggregation is dependent upon the metabolic activity of the platelets. The complexes are measured as the highest serum dilution with a positive aggregation sedimentation pattern, and compared with the titer of solutions of known concentrations of immune complexes. The Pl.A. assay detects IgG-containing immune complexes, whether or not they fix complement, but does not detect complexes formed with IgM. The assay can detect as little as 4 μg of AHG per ml in serum and is most sensitive to relatively large complexes ($> 19S$).

There are several disadvantages to the Pl.A. assay. Viable platelets are required, and they must be used on the day they are obtained. Various platelet preparations show different reactivity, and approximately 10 to 15% of preparations fail to react at all. Platelet aggregation reactions caused by immune complexes are competitively inhibited by some rheumatoid factors, C1q, and to a lesser degree by monomeric IgG. Platelet aggregation can be induced by antiplatelet antibodies in the absence of immune complexes, producing false-positive results. Despite these difficulties, the platelet assay appears to have been used successfully to detect immune complexes in patients with viral infections (47,48), mycoplasmal pneumonia (49), rheumatoid arthritis (50), and SLE (51).

Anticomplementary Assay

The anticomplementary assay (52) is based on the principle that immune complexes bind added C1, in an amount proportional to their concentration, so that the C1 is consumed and unavailable to mediate lysis of antibody-coated red blood cells. The assay detects complement-fixing complexes in antibody excess, or in mild antigen excess. As in other assays based on inhibition, rather than activity, there may be a wide variety of interfering substances. The assay does not detect either small immune complexes, such as those formed in moderate or marked antigen excess, or immune complexes that activate complement by the alternative pathway, since this system is probably not operative at the low temperature at which the test is conducted.

Summary of Methods Used to Detect Immune Complexes in the Circulation

At present there is no one single sensitive assay suitable for the detection of all types of circulating immune complexes. This is due in large part to the varied nature and properties of immune complexes, which may contain antibodies of the IgG, IgM, or other immunoglobulin classes. Some complexes bind complement through the classical pathways, others through the alternative pathway, and still other complexes do not fix complement at all. The size of immune complexes varies considerably from less than 11S to more than 40S. Each of the methods described above will detect only certain kinds of immune complexes, depending upon their size, their ability to fix complement, and other as yet unknown properties. Moreover, virtually all the assays will detect aggregated immunoglobulin, so that positive results cannot be considered to provide conclusive evidence for the presence of immune complexes.

Because no one test is capable of identifying all types of complexes, the ideal study would make use of several different techniques. However, because of the complexities involved in performing these tests, most studies have been based on the use of one or two methods. It is not yet known how useful any of the recently developed methods will be in providing evidence for or against an immune complex pathogenesis in various diseases, in identifying the responsible antigens, or in monitoring the activity of diseases in which circulating immune complexes are of importance. A number of interesting results have been obtained to date. It has been shown that high levels of complexes are often demonstrable in certain diseases in which on other grounds immune complexes are thought to be important, notably SLE, hepatitis B infections, and certain forms of vasculitis and glomerulonephritis. On the other hand, it is apparent that immune complexes cannot always be found by currently available methods in the serum of patients with typical immunofluorescence features of immune complex-mediated glomerular disease, including membranous glomerulonephritis (53). Furthermore, in some cases where circulating complexes are found, their composition differs from that of the glomerular deposits—for example, circulating C1q binding complexes in some patients with membranoproliferative glomerulonephritis have been shown to contain IgG and C3, but the deposits contained IgM and IgA (in addition to IgG and C3) (54). It is also clear that immune complexes are being detected with increasing frequency in diseases in which no other evidence for a pathogenic role of these materials is available, and even in some apparently normal individuals.

There are several possible explanations for the frequent lack of correlation between the presence or amounts of circulating complexes and other evidence of immune complex-mediated tissue damage. First, available methods may fail to detect damaging complexes, either because they are below the threshold of detection or because the complexes are of a composition that does not react with the reagents used. Furthermore, in certain conditions, complexes may be of importance and yet not detected because they appear only intermittently in the circulation. This has been shown to be true in SLE (3). In addition, it is known from experimental studies that certain kinds of complexes may be formed in abundance in the circulation and yet produce no tissue damage. As discussed in Chapter 3, large complexes formed after injection of antigen into rabbits with very high levels of circulating antibodies are efficiently removed by the reticuloendothelial system, and glomerular or vascular lesions are not produced. In addition, very small complexes formed in marked antigen excess generally fail to produce tissue damage. Indeed, on the basis of studies following the fate and distribution of intravenously injected preformed complexes, it seems probable that with most kinds of complexes only a small fraction becomes trapped in glomeruli or blood vessels (55), and the precise physical properties that cause certain kinds of complexes to localize in these tissues have yet to be defined.

Furthermore, different kinds of complexes tend to accumulate in different portions of the glomerulus, and this is an important factor in determining the type of glomerular injury that develops. In particular, accumulation of complexes in mesangial regions often occurs without clinical or histologic evidence of glomerular damage. Aside from differences in intrinsic properties of the complexes themselves, host factors may be important in determining localization of complexes. It has been shown that release of vasoactive amines may be crucial in the vascular or glomerular localization of complexes (see Chapter 3). Thus, in one individual a particular type of immune complex might accumulate within certain tissues under the influence of pharmacologic mediators and yet fail to do so in another individual in whom such mediators are not active.

Finally, although it is generally assumed that immune complex-mediated glomerular and vascular diseases are initiated by complexes formed in the circulation, this may not be true in all cases. In particular, it has been shown in experiments in rats that certain aggregated proteins may localize in mesangial regions; if antibodies are administered subsequently, complexes form within the glomeruli and produce injury (5). Furthermore, it has been suggested that the complexes seen in Heymann nephritis are formed locally, although the evidence on this point is not entirely convincing (56). In view of these considerations, it seems likely that no combination of methods for detection of circulating complexes will provide complete information required to monitor immune complex-mediated glomerular diseases.

CAUSATIVE FACTORS IN IMMUNE COMPLEX-MEDIATED GLOMERULONEPHRITIS AND ARTERITIS

There are a number of facets to the causation of immune complex-mediated glomerular or vascular disease. The basic requirements for the development of circulating complexes are of course the entrance of an antigen (or antigens) into the circulation and the elicitation of an antibody response. Immune complexes will be formed only if the antigen persists in or reenters the circulation when antibodies are present. For reasons mentioned above and discussed elsewhere in this volume, the type of complexes formed is of crucial importance; this depends in large part on the ratio of antigen to antibody in the circulation, as determined by the amount of antigen in the circulation and the intensity of the antibody response. Since the antibody response to many antigens is under genetic control (57), heredity may play a role in the development of certain immune complex-mediated diseases. The kinds of antibodies produced are also important; high-affinity antibodies may lead to the formation of complexes that are rapidly and efficiently removed by the cells of the reticuloendothelial system. The composition of the complex may be considerably modified by the addition of complement components, which may be present in variable amounts in different individuals. Miller and Nussenzweig have shown that C3 may solubilize complexes in vitro (58). It is conceivable that the consumption of C3 in vivo (or suppression of C3 synthesis) could result in decreased solubility of circulating complexes, a change that might obviously influence their distribution. The addition of rheumatoid factor to complexes will obviously modify them considerably. As noted earlier, the release of pharmacologically active substances may determine where certain complexes localize. The length of time during which complexes are present in the circulation is of great importance in determining the type of tissue damage that ensues—if present for only a short interval (as in experimental acute serum sickness), rapidly reversible proliferative glomerulonephritis and necrotizing arteritis may be seen. If complexes are formed for prolonged periods, several forms of chronic and largely irreversible glomerular lesions may develop.

Several antigens have been used to induce immune complex glomerulonephritis experimentally, and it is apparent that the nature of the glomerular injury is frequently independent of the particular antigen used. Thus, either bovine serum albumin or bovine gamma globulin can be used to produce identical lesions. Conversely, the same antigen may be used to produce quite different lesions, depending on the amount injected, the duration of administration, and the intensity of the antibody response. Nevertheless, it may well be that certain antigens possess peculiar properties that are important in the pathogenesis of some immune complex diseases, either by influencing their localization or by modifying the damaging properties of the complexes. For example, it has been suggested that the affinity of DNA for collagen may influence the localization of complexes in SLE (59). Moreover, certain agents appear to be highly effective in producing immune complex glomerulonephritis in man—the incidence of glomerulonephritis following certain types of group A streptococcal infection far exceeds that following comparable infections produced by other organisms. Although the explanation for this is unknown, it is possible that innate properties of an unidentified streptococcal antigen are responsible.

Finally, even if it were possible to explain how complexes are formed and why they localize in glomeruli or blood vessels, the question remains as to how they produce tissue damage. This subject is reviewed in Chapter 3, but it is worth emphasizing how remarkably little has been learned about the mediation of glomerular injury by immune complexes—in the most easily studied model, acute serum sickness, neither the complement system nor leukocytes appear to be required. Furthermore, in a model of chronic immune complex disease, Heymann nephritis, there is no evidence that leukocytes participate, and yet it is clear that immune deposits alter the filtration properties of the glomerulus (4), by mechanisms that remain to be determined.

In view of the above considerations, it should be apparent that identification of the antigen contained in the complex is only one step in understanding immune complex-mediated diseases. It is also important to learn how the antigen gains access to the circulation, why in some instances antigens are persistently or intermittently released into the circulation, what determines the intensity of the antibody response, what factors influence the deposition of complexes in certain sites, and how they mediate the tissue damage. By any of these measures, progress in unraveling human immune complex-mediated disease has been very slow. Nevertheless, there is reason to believe, or at least to hope, that identification of one link might permit the interruption of the chain of events leading to immune complex-mediated tissue injury. For example, if the offending antigen could be identified, it might be possible to induce tolerance or even cause dissolution of immune deposits through administration of excess antigen (60). Obviously, such maneuvers are fraught with difficulty and might make matters worse rather than better. Another possibility is that a critical pathogenetic mechanism might be identified and inhibited.

In the following sections we will discuss the evidence that certain antigens are involved in immune complex-mediated glomerular diseases. Inspection of Table 2 indicates that a variety of antigens have been implicated. However, the percentage of cases accounted for is quite small, since certain antigens have been identified in only a few cases. Moreover, since documentation cannot be considered conclusive in some cases, certain antigens may have to be eliminated from the list. In some cases, the identification of the antigen may provide insight into how the antibody response was initiated. For example, if treponemal antigens are found in glomerular deposits, this provides evidence that a syphilitic infection initiated the process. In other situations, however, even though the antigen is identified, the factors initiating the antibody remain unknown; this is true in lupus nephritis, in which, although DNA has been identified as the major antigen in the deposits, the cause of the anti-DNA response remains unknown. In still other cases, the initiating factor may be identified and the antigen remains unidentified, as in gold- or penicillamine-induced nephropathy.

It is not possible to review all of the evidence concerning the role of immune complexes in glomerular and vascular disease; however, the major diseases will be reviewed.

Table 2. Human Glomerular Diseases Known or Presumed to Be Mediated by Immune Complexes

Disease Category	Antigens Identified in Glomeruli	Disease Category	Antigens Identified in Glomeruli
I. Glomerulonephritis (GN) of known cause		II. GN associated with diseases of unknown causes	
A. Due to bacterial infections		A. Systemic lupus erythematosus	DNA, IgG
Acute post infectious GN		B. Schönlein-Henoch purpura	None
Streptococcal	Streptococcal?	C. "Essential" mixed cryoglobulinemia	IgG
Pneumococcal	Pneumococcal?	III. Glomerulopathy associated with malignancies	
Bacterial endocarditis or shunt infections	Bacterial Ag in some cases	A. Carcinoma GI tract	Carcinombryonic Ag (1 case)
Syphilitic nephropathy	Treponemal antigens	B. Other tumors	Tumor-associated Ag?
B. Glomerulonephritis with parasitic infection	Parasitic Ag?	C. Carcinoma of lung	Tumor-associated Ag or antibody (1 case)
Malaria	Malaria Ag	IV. Primary glomerular disease of unknown cause	
Schistosomiasis	Schistosomal Ag?	A. Membranous GN	None (except for a few cases with thyroglobulin or brush border Ag)
C. Viral infections		B. Membranoproliferative GN with subendothelial deposits (type I)	None
Hepatitis B (various forms of GN) and arteritis (see text)	HBs Ag	C. IgA nephropathy (Berger's)	None
D. Drug-induced (membranous GN)		D. Some cases classified as focal, chronic, or crescenteric	None
Gold	None		
Penicillamine	None		
Mercury	None		
Heroin	None		

RENAL DISEASES

Acute Poststreptococcal Glomerulonephritis (APSGN)

Considerable evidence suggests that acute poststreptococcal glomerulonephritis (APSGN) is caused by the deposition in glomeruli of immune complexes, probably containing streptococcal antigens (61,62). The renal lesions develop after a latent period, generally between 7 and 21 days following certain types of group A hemolytic streptococcal infections. During this period, antibodies to a variety of streptococcal products (streptolysin O, streptokinase, hyaluronidase) are formed. The serum complement levels are usually considerably depressed at the onset of the glomerulonephritis, but return to normal within several weeks. Renal biopsy reveals a diffuse lesion involving all glomeruli, with proliferation of mesangial cells and infiltration of polymorphonuclear and mononuclear leukocytes. Granular deposits of C3 and IgG are usually found, predominantly along the GBM and less prominently in mesangial areas (63–67). In some biopsy specimens, especially those obtained relatively late, C3 deposits are seen without Ig (65). Components of the alternative pathway, particularly properdin, are generally present (68). Electron-dense deposits are usually seen, chiefly along the epithelial side of the GBM (forming the characteristic "humps"), and less often between proliferating mesangial cells and under the endothelium along the GBM (63,69,70). The similarities of the histologic, immunofluorescence, and electron-microscopic findings to those in acute serum sickness in rabbits provides impressive evidence for a short-lived immune complex mechanism.

It seems highly probable that a streptococcal antigen is present in the immune complexes that appear to mediate poststreptococcal glomerulonephritis; nevertheless, the evidence concerning this point is controversial. Although several groups have described streptococcal antigens within glomeruli using fluoresceinated antisera prepared against streptococci or streptococcal products (65,70,71), others have been unable to demonstrate such material (63,64). There are two major reasons for favoring the positive results. First, if streptococcal antigens are present in the deposits, it seems likely that they become quickly saturated with antibodies, which would render them difficult to detect after the very earliest stages of the disease; biopsy specimens are ordinarily obtained only after several days or even weeks of clinically apparent disease. Second, the antisera used in the negative studies may not have contained antibodies against the relevant antigen. On the other hand, antigens within complexes may be detected by immunofluorescence, even without partial elution of antibodies, especially if the antisera used contains antibodies against determinants that have not reacted with host antibodies. Furthermore, the antisera used in one negative study were prepared in the same fashion as for those used to obtain positive results (64).

The most serious objection to the claim that streptococcal antigens have been identified in glomeruli in APSGN is that the published photomicrographs are not entirely convincing, and certainly do not resemble the deposits of immunoglobulins and C3 usually seen. In some pictures, the material appears to be in mesangial regions, where immunoglobulin deposits are usually scanty or absent; in others, the staining could be within leukocytes, which are notoriously prone to produce nonspecific staining. Furthermore, among those who have reported positive results, different conclusions have been reached as to which streptococcal antigen has been demonstrated. Treser et al. claim to have found constituents of the cell membrane (71), whereas Zabriskie's findings point toward cell wall material (62).

Using another approach, Treser et al. claim to have stained streptococcal antigen in glomeruli with fluoresceinated IgG fractions from the sera of patients who had recovered from APSGN (71). Evidence that the reactive material was of streptococcal origin was obtained by showing that absorption of the sera with nephritogenic strains prevented staining. These results await confirmation. Since poststreptococcal glomerulonephritis is (fortunately) rarely fatal, it has not been possible to obtain sufficient renal tissue to perform elution studies, which might allow detection and measurement of antistreptococcal antibodies in the glomerular deposits.

In view of the uncertainty about the presence of streptococcal products in the deposits in APSGN, it is worth considering the possibility that an autologous antigen is involved, possibly rendered immunogenic through release or alteration. In support of this, evidence has been presented that circulating complexes composed of altered IgG and anti-IgG are present in some patients with APSGN (15). It remains to be shown, however, that these complexes are of pathogenetic significance, and if so, whether they are of primary or only secondary significance.

Zabriskie (62) has suggested a different primary pathogenetic mechanism for APSGN, based on experimental observations of Kantor, who showed that M protein forms complexes with fibrinogen, and that these complexes have the property of accumulating in glomeruli (72,73). It was postulated that M protein-fibrinogen complexes localize in mesangial regions of glomeruli during the streptococcal infection. Later, when anti-M antibodies are produced, they combine locally with the M protein and somehow stimulate the proliferation of mesangial cells. In this scheme, epimembranous deposits might be a late and relatively unimportant phenomenon. In support of this interpretation, mesangial deposits of streptococcal products, possibly of cell wall origin, have been described in APSGN, as noted above. Furthermore, diffuse glomerular deposits of fibrinogen (or its derivatives) are often found, apparently within and between proliferating cells; however, similar observations are sometimes made in other forms of proliferative glomerulonephritis (64).

Grupe has observed cryoglobulins in a substantial proportion of a group of patients with APSGN (74), providing evidence for circulating immune complexes. The precipitates contained IgG and C3. As noted above, mixed IgM-IgG cryoglobulins have been found in some patients with APSGN. Antistreptococcal antibodies could not be demonstrated in the cryoprecipitates (15). Ooi et al. (54) have provided further evidence for the presence of circulating complexes in patients with APSGN, through the use of a C1q binding assay and sucrose density gradient analysis. Positive results were obtained in 15 of 20 cases. The sedimentation coefficients of the complexes ranged between 16S and 19S. The composition of the complexes was studied in three cases; IgM and C3 were present in all, and IgG and C4 in two cases. IgA was not found. The complexes were not studied for streptococcal antigens or specific antibodies.

Since only a minority of individuals infected with nephritogenic streptococci develop glomerulonephritis, it seems probable that host factors are of great importance. There are, however, no relevant data, and it is not known to what extent susceptibility may be genetically determined.

Assuming that some form of immune complexes initiates the glomerular damage, what can be said of the secondary pathogenetic mechanism? The presence of neutrophils and complement components in glomeruli suggests that these factors may be involved. However, as mentioned earlier, in the experimental model that most closely resembles the human disease, namely, acute "one-shot" serum sickness in the rabbit, neither the complement system nor leukocytes appear to be necessary for the development of glomerular lesions. It should be noted, however, that neutrophil accumulation is often more conspicuous in the human disease. In those cases characterized by conspicuous crescent formation, it is likely that fibrin deposition in Bowman's space is an important pathogenetic factor (75). Furthermore, the presence of fibrin (or other fibrinogen derivatives) within or between proliferating mesangial cells, and the evidence that increased fibrin formation occurs in APSGN (76), suggest that the coagulation system may play a role even in cases of ordinary severity, without crescents.

Thus, although available evidence indicates that poststreptococcal glomerulonephritis is an acute immune complex disease, there is uncertainty concerning the nature of the antigen and ignorance of factors determining individual host susceptibility and of secondary pathogenetic mechanisms. Unfortunately, there appears to be no entirely satisfactory experimental model of streptococcal-induced glomerulonephritis in which these questions could be more easily explored. In any case, if the glomerular disease is in fact due to immune complexes, it can be assumed that the complexes possess certain distinctive properties that render them extremely efficient in producing glomerular disease, since in many other situations, including other types of acute bacterial infection, where complexes are presumably formed in the circulation, glomerular disease (at least clinically evident) is rarely seen.

The great majority of patients with APSGN survive the acute disease and go on to complete recovery, and the deposits disappear within several weeks. In a few patients, however, the glomerular disease appears to remain active for many months, as manifested by persistence of diffuse proliferation and neutrophil infiltration, and the continued presence of IgG- and C3-containing deposits. It is not possible to document a streptococcal cause with certainty in individual cases, so that such patients may, in fact, be suffering from unrelated diseases of unknown cause. Assuming that some such cases do represent persistently active poststreptococcal disease, it would be difficult to conceive of how a streptococcal product could continue to serve as the antigen, and this consideration again suggests the possibility that an autologous antigen is involved. In addition, in a small percentage of patients slowly progressive glomerulosclerosis has been observed years after an attack of apparently well-documented APSGN (77). The pathogenetic mechanisms in these cases have not been elucidated; there is no evidence that continued deposition of immune complexes is responsible, since granular deposits of immunoglobulin and complement are not found in the glomeruli.

Syphilitic Glomerulonephritis

It has been recognized for many years that renal disease, often manifested by the nephrotic syndrome, may develop in association with either congenital syphilis (78,79,80) or the secondary stage of acquired syphilis (81). The condition often resolves spontaneously (82). Until recently the cause of the renal lesions was obscure and was attributed variously to direct invasion of the kidneys by spirochetes, or a hypersensitivity reaction to the spirochetes or to therapeutic agents (heavy metals or penicillin). Recent evidence indicates that the lesions are mediated by immune complexes containing treponemal antigens (83,84).

Histologic studies of renal biopsy specimens have shown variable degrees of swelling and proliferation of the mesangial cells (82,85,86,87). Cellular proliferation is apparently most severe in patients with gross hematuria or impaired renal function and is accompanied by infiltration of polymorphonuclear leukocytes. In some cases, especially in congenital syphilis, glomerular capillary wall thickening is the only histologic abnormality. Electron microscopy reveals numerous electron-dense deposits, mainly in a subepithelial distribution, although some are also present in subendothelial, intramembranous, and mesangial positions (82–87).

By immunofluorescence, granular deposits of IgG are observed in the mesangium and along the GBM (83–86). Complement components may be present in a similar distribution but sometimes are absent. Several attempts to detect glomerular bound treponemal antigens by immunofluorescence were unsuccessful (85,86,88,89). However, using a rabbit antitreponemal antiserum and a fluoresceinated sheep antirabbit antiserum, Tourville et al. (84) detected treponemal antigens in the glomeruli in a distribution similar to that of the IgG deposits. In addition, Gamble and Rearden (83) found that elution of renal tissue with citric acid yielded specific antibodies that reacted with living *Treponema pallidum.* Thus, both treponemal antigen and specific antitreponemal antibody have been detected in the kidneys, and the distribution of the treponemal antigen in the glomeruli paralleled that of the granular deposits of IgG. Apparently, circulating complexes have not yet been identified.

The causative role of the *Treponema* organisms is also indicated by the rapid clinical response to penicillin, which is accompanied by disappearance of the glomerular immune deposits, usually within 6 to 12 weeks (82,87). However, as noted above, it has been observed that the renal disease may resolve spontaneously in untreated patients (82).

Quartan Malarial Nephropathy

The association between the nephrotic syndrome in tropical countries and quartan malaria was reported by Giglioli in 1932 (90) and was supported by subsequent observations (91–93). Further evidence for the relationship came from the results of the malaria eradication program in British Guiana, which led to the virtual disappearance of the nephrotic syndrome in children and young adults (94). However, once initiated, quartan malarial nephropathy is frequently progressive and does not respond to antimalarial therapy and poorly, if at all, to immunosuppressive therapy (96,97). The most characteristic renal morphologic changes consist of increased mesangial matrix and thickening of the glomerular capillary walls, with duplication of the basement membrane, as seen in silver stains. The process initially involves only a few glomeruli segmentally, but progresses ultimately to diffuse glomerulosclerosis, without conspicuous cellular proliferation or neutrophil infiltration (95,97,98). In the majority of cases, granular deposits containing either IgG or IgM, or both, are found along the glomerular basement membrane and to a lesser extent in the mesangium; in about half of the cases, granular deposits of C3 are observed in a similar distribution (95,99). Electron-microscopic studies have revealed dense deposits in various locations within glomeruli (95,97,98).

Plasmodium malariae antigens have been reported to be demonstrable by direct immunofluorescence along the glomerular capillary walls and in the mesangium of 20 to 35% of patients with malarial nephropathy (95,97,99,100). Although the specificity of the staining was not proved conclusively by absorption of the antiserum with *P. malariae* antigen, the antiserum did not stain normal kidneys or the kidneys of patients with *Plasmodium falciparum.* Moreover, other controls, including the use of fluoresceinated antisera to *P. falciparum*, antistreptolysin O, and rubella virus, were uniformly negative (95,97,99,100). Anti-*P. malariae* antibody has been eluted from the kidney of a patient with malarial nephropathy; on immunodiffusion, the eluate gave a line of precipitation with both the serum and the splenic extracts of a patient with *P. malariae,* but not of a patient with *P. falciparum* (95). Thus, both *P. malariae* antigen and specific anti-*P. malariae* antibody have been demonstrated in the kidneys in malarial nephropathy. It has been shown that ^{125}I-labeled anti-*P. malariae* antibody disappears more rapidly from the circulation of patients with malarial nephropathy than labeled anti-*P. falciparum* antibody or normal IgG, and that shortly after the injection of the labeled anti-*P. malariae* antibody much of it is in a form precipitable by 7.5% PEG (101). Several features of *P. malariae* infections might predispose to prolonged formation of circulating immune complexes, including the prolonged release of antigen and the relatively ineffective nature of the immune response to *P. malariae* infections, which is due at least in part to the fact that predominantly low-affinity antibodies are formed (102).

Infective Endocarditis

Glomerulonephritis has long been recognized as a serious complication of infective endocarditis; in the pre-antibiotic era perhaps as many as 10 to 15% of patients died of renal disease (103). Antibiotic treatment was noted to decrease the incidence of glomerulonephritis considerably, and the incidence of renal failure fell to less than 3% (104). Initially the glomerular lesions were thought to be caused by emboli from the vegetations—hence the term focal embolic glomerulonephritis (a diffuse form of glomerulonephritis was also recognized). More recently it was suggested that immune complexes formed in the circulation are responsible for the renal disease. Patients with infective endocarditis or other forms of persistent sepsis are likely candidates for the development of immune complex-mediated glomerular and vascular disease: whole organisms and presumably their constituents are repeatedly shed into the circulation and stimulate antibody production. A variety of antibody-antigen combinations would be expected, in varied amounts and with various sizes and biologic activities.

Evidence supporting the importance of immune complexes in the glomerulonephritis associated with infective endocarditis has been obtained in the past several years and can be summarized as follows. By immunofluorescence, coarse, broad granular deposits of C3 and usually of IgG and IgM have been found (105–110), both in mesangial regions and along the GBM. However, in some cases, particularly those without clinical signs of renal disease and with sclerotic lesions, only C3 is seen (109). Moreover, a few patients have been described with proliferative glomerulonephritis without immune deposits. Electron microscopy has shown subendothelial and mesangial deposits in most cases studied (107,110,111); in some cases, only mesangial (106) or subepithelial deposits, resembling the "humps" of poststreptococcal glomerulonephritis, (110,112) were found.

Efforts to demonstrate antigen in deposits were unsuccessful in two cases (107), but in one, a rabbit antiserum prepared against the α-hemolytic streptococcus isolated from the patient's blood reacted with material in glomeruli (113). In another case, eluates from renal tissue contained antibodies to the organism (enterococcus), but contamination with serum, which had a high antienterococcus titer, was not excluded (105). Thus, while complexes containing constituents of the organism most likely cause the glomerular injury, further evidence is needed.

Several studies have demonstrated that patients with infective endocarditis frequently develop rheumatoid factor, as well as depression of circulating complement components. One important early study (114) showed that about half of the patients have rheumatoid factor and immunoconglutinin (antibodies for activated complement components). Furthermore, many patients, particularly those with nephritis, were found to have low complement levels (CH50). Other investigators have confirmed the low complement levels and found that C3 is usually decreased (110,106,111,107,113). More complete studies have shown depression of classical pathway components (C4 and occasionally C1q), but normal levels of components of the alternative pathway (C3 proactivator and properdin) (107,111). However, low C3, C3 proactivator with normal C4, and C1q have been found in a patient with endocarditis and pulmonary abscesses (115), suggesting alternative pathway activation.

Evidence for circulating complexes in patients with infective endocarditis has been obtained by several techniques. Cryoprecipitates were detected in 19 of 20 patients with endocarditis, in amounts ranging from 10 to 430 μg/ml (116). The cryoprecipitates contained IgG (19 of 19), IgM (18 of 19), IgA (10 of 19), C3 (4 of 19), and fibrinogen-related antigens (2 of 19). The only antibody regularly detected was rheumatoid factor (12 of 15); this was specifically concentrated in the precipitates, and none was found in the serum of these patients. Antibody to the organism was specifically concentrated in only one of four cryoprecipitates; in two it was undetectable. Complexes were detected by the Raji cell assay in 29 of 30 endocarditis patients (117). The amounts of Raji cell-reactive complexes were higher in patients with extracardiac signs (arthritis, glomerulonephritis, splenomegaly), with disease for more than four weeks and with low CH50 values. Although 75% of the patients in this study were addicts, none was HBs Ag-positive. The presence and concentration of circulating complexes generally correlated with positive blood cultures, but in two instances complexes persisted longer. These studies suggest that immune complex assays may prove to have a role in monitoring therapy in endocarditis.

Shunt Nephritis

In patients with chronically infected cerebrospinal fluid shunts that drain into the venous circulation, glomerular lesions sometimes develop that appear to be mediated by immune complexes. In 19 of 22 reported cases, the organism was *Staphylococcus albus;* in the others the organisms were *Staphylococcus aureus* and *Listeria monocytogenes* (118–126). All patients had proteinuria, and most were nephrotic (14 of 17). This contrasts with endocarditis patients, who are rarely nephrotic (111). Hematuria was found in all but one nephritis patient and in about half was macroscopic. Low C3 levels were reported in 8 of 11 patients analyzed. More detailed studies in five patients revealed consistently low levels of classical pathway components (C1q, C4, C2) and inconstant depression of alternative pathway components (C3 proactivator and properdin); C5 was normal (120,122). Depressed complement levels have been observed to persist for several weeks after onset of therapy. Other features are anemia, splenomegaly, azotemia, fever, and arthralgias.

The renal lesion in patients with infected shunts is typically a diffuse mesangial, proliferative glomerulonephritis, usually with neutrophil accumulation. Crescents are occasionally seen. Electron-microscopic studies have shown duplication of the GBM, as well as subendothelial and mesangial deposits (119–121,125). By immunofluorescence, granular deposits of C3 (10 of 10), IgG (8 of 10), IgA (3 of 5), and C1q (2 of 2) have been observed along the GBM and in mesangial regions (118,120–122,125,126). Overall, the findings closely resemble those of membranoproliferative glomerulonephritis, type I (120).

The effect of shunt removal has generally been to reduce the proteinuria, hematuria, and azotemia. The evolution of the lesion has been studied in a few patients. One patient who remained infected showed progressive mesangial proliferation and glomerular loss over a 23-month period (121). Biopsies were done on three patients after shunt removal. In specimens obtained at three and seven months there was persistence of proliferative changes and of deposits; the biopsy obtained at 22 months showed resolution. These findings indicate that the glomerular injury and deposits may be very slow to resolve, despite the removal of the apparent source of antigens.

Attempts have been made to demonstrate bacterial antigens in the glomerular deposits and in circulating complexes in patients with shunt nephritis. Kaufman and McIntosh reported staining of material in glomeruli in one case with an anti-*S. albus* antiserum (126). Absorption with bacteria abolished the staining. Cryoglobulins occur commonly and have been found to contain IgG (4 of 4), C3 (4 of 4), C4 (3 of 3), and rheumatoid factor (2 of 2) (120). Antibacterial antibodies were detected in the cryoprecipitate in a case with *Listeria* infection

(120), but not in a patient with *S. albus* infection (126). Bacterial antigens have been detected only indirectly: antibodies to teichoic acid (a cell wall constituent of *S. albus*) and to *Listeria* were found in rabbits immunized with cryoprecipitates from two patients infected with *S. albus* and *L. monocytogenes,* respectively.

Other Forms of Chronic Infection

Glomerulonephritis presumably due to immune complexes is seen in some patients with other types of chronic bacterial infections, and sometimes causes renal failure. Of seven patients who had renal failure and visceral abscesses (caused by *S. aureus, Escherichia coli, Pseudomonas aeruginosa,* and *P. mirabilis*) without endocarditis, four had diffuse or focal mesangial proliferation and three had abundant crescents (115). Granular glomerular deposits of C3 were found in all cases, sometimes without Ig. In the three patients studied, no abnormality of complement components was detected (C1, C4, C3, C5, and C3 proactivator). The guinea pig macrophage-IgG uptake inhibition test was positive with the serum of the patients tested. Bacterial antigens were detected with an antibody to capsular polysaccharide in the glomeruli of three patients who died of *Klebsiella* pneumonia (127). Although focal proliferative glomerulonephritis was present in each of these three patients, none had clinical evidence of renal disease. This latter study suggests that subclinical immune complex disease may occur rather frequently in bacterial infections.

IMMUNE COMPLEXES IN HEPATITIS

In recent years evidence has been obtained that immune complexes containing hepatitis B antigens are important pathogenic agents in various forms of disease, in particular in the prodromal syndrome of acute hepatitis, in certain forms of vasculitis and glomerulonephritis, and in mixed cryoglobulinemia. The evidence for each of these associations will be discussed after consideration of the nature of the complexes themselves.

The immune complexes occurring in the serum of some patients with hepatitis have been well characterized, because some of the antigens can be seen by electron microscopy (128,129,130,19). Ultrastructural analysis of particles obtained by ultracentrifugation of serum reveals 20 nm diameter spheres and rods (129) believed to be surface coat proteins (HBs Ag), which are proteins of 3.7 to 416 $\times$ 10^6 daltons (131). Larger, 40-nm "Dane" particles with a dense core, believed to be the intact virus (130), or bare 27-nm core particles, are also present in some cases (129,132). Clumps of spheres and rods are found in some sera; these are believed to represent immune complexes. It seems probable that other complexes are formed with smaller antigenic fragments that are not detected by electron microscopy.

Further information about the complexes has come from immunochemical analysis of cryoprecipitates. Wands et al. (19) found that cryoprecipitates from patients with acute hepatitis often contained IgG, IgM, and HBs Ag; in those patients with arthritis, complement components (C3, C4, C5) were also present.

Both antigen (HBs Ag) and antibody (anti-HBs Ag) are concentrated in the cryoprecipitates (19,133). In fact, as noted earlier, in some instances HBs Ag or anti-HBs is detectable only in the cryoprecipitate (17). Almost certainly in most cases the cryoprecipitates represent only a portion of the complexes in the circulation. Of interest, even at 37°C, at which temperature cryoprecipitates do not form in serum, C3 activation can occur (19).

Two studies have used sensitive techniques to detect circulating complexes in various forms of liver disease (28,43). In acute HBs Ag-positive hepatitis, 30 and 63% of patients had detectable complexes by the C1q-PEG (28) or Raji cell (43) assays, respectively. Patients with HBs Ag-negative acute hepatitis also were commonly positive (40%) (43). In contrast, asymptomatic carriers of HBs Ag had complexes detected much less frequently (0 to 13%).

There is uncertainty about the role of antibody and complexes in the liver damage in acute or chronic hepatitis. Prince and Trepo and co-workers (128,134) have noted that there is little correlation between liver damage and HBs Ag-containing complexes and suggest that liver cells are injured by other immunologic means (135).

Alpert et al. (136) drew attention to the possibility that immune complexes are responsible for the prodromal syndrome that resembles serum sickness, characterized by transient arthritis and urticaria, which precedes by a week or more the icteric phase of acute viral hepatitis in some patients. Among 18 patients with hepatitis, nine who had arthritis or urticaria had very low CH50, C4, and C3 levels; the other nine patients, without arthritis or rash, had normal complement values. In a later study it was shown that although immune complexes (cryoglobulins) were present in all six patients with acute hepatitis, only in those three patients with arthritis or urticaria was there evidence of complement-fixing complexes (19). There are only a few pathologic studies of the affected joints in patients with hepatitis, and so far no direct evidence has been reported for the presence of immune complexes in synovial tissue. In one study, no inflammatory infiltrate was seen in two synovial biopsies, and the most prominent change was endothelial damage (137). Some evidence, although not conclusive, was obtained by electron microscopy and immunofluorescence that the virus was present in the endothelial and synovial cells.

Glomerular disease is rare in acute hepatitis, despite the high frequency of circulating complexes. Histologically, only minimal mesangial abnormalities are seen (138,139); by electron microscopy, amorphous granular material can be found in mesangial and subendothelial locations (140,138); and by immunofluorescence, IgG, IgM, and C3 deposits have been noted in several patients. HBs Ag deposition was not detected in two patients (141).

In recent years, increasing evidence has been obtained for a pathogenic role of HBs Ag in some cases of necrotizing arteritis. There are now over 50 patients reported with "polyarteritis" and HBs Ag (134,142–148). Overall, in about 40 to 50% of cases of polyarteritis nodosa or necrotizing arteritis reported in recent years, patients have HBs Ag in their serum (134). In most patients the arteritis has been transient, and unless there was irreversible damage to the brain or other organs, recovery ensued (134,144,145). In this respect, the arteritis differs from most cases of idiopathic polyarteritis nodosa. No correlation has been noted between the arteritis and the presence or severity of liver disease. Serum complement levels have been normal. The pathologic features have not received detailed analysis, but judging from published reports, small arterial branches are usually involved and grossly apparent aneurysms typical of polyarteritis nodosa are rare. The term "generalized necrotizing vasculitis" has been suggested for this pattern (144).

Although the conclusion that HB virus infection may cause arteritis in man seems inescapable, the mechanisms are not known. It is generally assumed that circulating complexes containing HBs Ag are responsible. In support of this is the finding of an association between immune complexes and arteritis, e.g., clumps of HBs are present in the serum during active vasculitis (134,144). However, it is also possible that lesions depend upon replication of the virus in the vessels or on other types of immunologic mechanisms, possibly involving cell-mediated reactions. In a few patients HBs Ag has apparently been found in arterial walls (147,148), usually with Ig and C3. This important finding should be confirmed.

In some patients with chronic infection or the chronic carrier state, HBs Ag may be involved in the pathogenesis of glomerulonephritis (141,149–151). The evidence consists principally of the demonstration in glomeruli by immunofluorescence or the immunoperoxidase (150) technique of HBs Ag in association with deposits of immunoglobulins and complement components. On pathologic grounds, the glomerular lesions have classified in most cases as membranous glomerulonephritis, or membranoproliferative glomerulonephritis (type I), or rarely as focal glomerulosclerosis or acute glomerulonephritis. In many of the patients there was no evidence of chronic hepatitis.

Most of the reports have dealt with relatively few patients and do not provide evidence that HBs Ag is involved in an appreciable percentage of cases of chronic glomerulonephritis. However, in a report from Poland (152), HBs Ag was detected in glomerular deposits in 18 of 52 children with various forms of glomerular disease, including 12 of 15 with membranoproliferative glomerulonephritis, in each of 2 patients with membranous glomerulonephritis, and 2 of 13 patients with "endocapillary proliferation." In contrast, HBs Ag was not found in any of 20 patients without deposits (minimal change disease). If one assumes that the results are technically valid, one must conclude either that HBs Ag is in fact a major antigen involved in glomerulonephritis, at least in Poland, or that this antigen often becomes secondarily trapped in glomerular immune complex deposits of other specificities. In support of the latter possibility is the fact that plasma or blood transfusions are used in Poland for treatment of the nephrotic syndrome. Resolution of this problem may come from further elution studies, which might show whether or not antibodies to HBs Ag are present in the glomerular deposits in higher concentrations than in serum (151).

Levo et al. (17) have recently reported evidence that hepatitis B virus is involved in the pathogenesis "essential" mixed cryoglobulinemia. As noted earlier, mixed cryoglobulins most often contain IgM and IgG; the IgM component possesses antibody activity against IgG. Patients with essential mixed cryoglobulinemia (that is, unassociated with classifiable disease, such as systemic lupus erythematosus or lymphoproliferative disease) often develop purpura, arthralgia, weakness, and diffuse proliferative glomerulonephritis (153). Immunofluorescence has revealed granular deposits of IgM and IgG in glomeruli, and rheumatoid factor activity has been demonstrated in glomerular deposits (154). These findings support a pathogenic role of IgM anti IgG complexes. However, it had been suspected that IgG component consisted of antibodies directed against unidentified antigens in the complex. The findings of Levo et al. (17) indicate that in most cases HBs Ag is that antigen. Thus 14 of 19 cryoprecipitates from patients with mixed cryoglobulinemia were positive either for HBs Ag or its antibodies. Electron microscopy of the cryoprecipitates showed the 20-nm and 27-nm spheres and tubules, as well as Dane particles.

SYSTEMIC LUPUS ERYTHEMATOSUS (SLE)

It has been thoroughly documented that the renal lesions of SLE are mediated by immune complexes, especially DNA-containing complexes. There is also abundant, if not entirely conclusive, evidence that the same mechanism is responsible for other important manifestations of SLE—arteritis, endocarditis, arthritis, and skin and cerebral involvement. This discussion is largely restricted to the pathogenetic role of immune complexes in SLE, and we will not review the substantial literature on etiologic factors or on the immunologic defects found in patients with SLE.

SLE is characterized by the production of numerous autoantibodies, including antibodies reactive to nuclear and cytoplasmic constituents, platelets, clotting factors, erythrocytes, lymphocyte surface components, and altered IgG (rheumatoid factor) (3). The antinuclear antibodies have received particularly intensive study. Several nuclear substances are antigens, notably native (double-stranded) deoxyribonucleic acid (DS-DNA) (155,156), denatured (single-stranded) DNA (SS-DNA) (157,158), nucleoproteins (159,160), a periodate-sensitive carbohydrate protein (Sm) (161), RNA protein-extractable nuclear antigen (ENA) (162), and double-stranded RNA (DS-RNA) (163,164). It is apparent that patients with SLE are as distinctive in the diversity of autoantibodies produced as in their specificities. It is chiefly anti-DS-DNA that distinguishes SLE from other conditions in which autoantibodies are produced. Even anti-DS-DNA antibodies are apparently not pathognomic for SLE, since they are said to be present in 2 to 3% of patients with rheumatoid arthritis, chronic active hepatitis, or "chronic glomerulonephritis" (3); however, some of these results are apparently attributable to contamination of SS-DNA in the reagents used for assay (165). Some of the autoantibodies are directed against cell surface components and are thus able to damage certain target cells—platelets, red cells, or lymphocytes. However, most of the autoantibodies are directed against antigens normally intracellular, and in such cases antigen-antibody interaction can generally occur only if the antigens are released from the cells. Some antigens, formerly considered to be exclusively intracellular, notably DS-DNA and SS-DNA, have been detected free in the circulation. Release of nuclear material may occur during normal cell turnover, but can be increased by cell damage. In this respect, hemodialysis has been shown to increase circulating DNA levels (166). Other causes of cell damage, such as sunlight, toxins, and infection, also may cause release of DNA antigens.

Depression of serum complement levels usually occurs during exacerbations of the disease, providing indirect evidence for immune complexes (167–170). Depressed levels of all components of the classical pathway (C1, C1q, C4, C2, C3) have been demonstrated (168). In some patients the alternative pathway appears to be activated also, as indicated by low serum levels of properdin and C3 proactivator (171). Metabolic studies, which have been performed in a few patients using radiolabeled complement components, indicate that the low levels are due largely to increased catabolism rather than decreased synthesis (172). Presumably this is due to consumption by immune complexes, and there is indirect evidence to support this mechanism. Complement degradation fragments appear in the serum during active disease (173). Moreover, the ability of certain complexes to bind complement has been demonstrated by C1q binding assays (174) for immune complexes (28,43), and by the presence of C1q in cryoprecipitates (168). Local consumption of complement in SLE patients with active cerebral disease is suggested by decreased levels of C4 in the cerebrospinal fluid (CSF) (175,176). Indirect evidence for the presence of DNA-containing complexes in the CSF has been obtained in a few patients (177,178).

Evidence for circulating DNA-containing complexes in SLE has been obtained in several studies. The serum levels of antigens (DS-DNA, SS-DNA) have been noted to increase during exacerbation and alternate with detectable levels of their corresponding antibodies (179,180). More direct evidence for DNA-anti-DNA complexes was obtained by measuring serum DNA binding capacity before and after incubation in DNase, which would be expected to degrade DNA antigens bound to antibodies and increase the number of available combining sites (177,181,182). Using this approach, evidence for DNA-anti-DNA complexes has been found only in patients with SLE and almost exclusively in those with "active" nephritis or central nervous system disease. Moreover, DNA-containing complexes were present in a high percentage of patients with "active" lupus nephritis and disappeared with subsidence of signs of active renal involvement (182).

The use of recently developed assays has revealed evidence for high levels of circulating immune complexes in many patients with SLE; in fact, most assays are first tested on SLE sera and are not considered satisfactory unless positive in a high percentage of cases. Only a few recent reports can be reviewed here. In general, there is a good correlation between clinical activity and evidence of circulating immune complexes, based on the following tests: (1) C1q binding assay (28,30,32,183); (2) Raji cell test (43); (3) the bovine conglutinin test (184); (4) the monoclonal rheumatoid factor assays (30,183); (5) the macrophage inhibition assay (145); or (6) the presence of cryoglobulins (168). It is likely that not all antibodies in SLE are pathogenetically significant. Analysis in one series suggested that small IgG complexes (1 to 1.5 $\times$ 10^6 daltons) may be preferentially associated with renal disease and that larger complexes (2.5 to 5 $\times$ 10^6 daltons) may be found without evidence of renal involvement (183). Some antibodies do not correlate with renal disease, e.g., anti-DS-RNA (37), and anti-RNA even shows a negative correlation (185).

Direct evidence as to the nature of at least a subpopulation of the complexes in SLE has been obtained by analysis of serum cryoprecipitates, which have been shown to contain IgG, IgM, C1q, and C3 (18,168,174,186,187). Certain antibodies have been shown to be selectively concentrated in the cryoprecipitates, namely anti-IgG (RF) (18,168,174,186), antilymphocyte antibody (186), anti-DS-DNA, anti-SS-DNA, antiribonucleoprotein, and to a lesser degree anti-DS-RNA. The mean enrichment of anti-DS-DNA was over 100-fold that in the serum, and in the two cryoprecipitates analyzed, 65 to 80% of the IgG (but not the IgM) was removed by absorption with red cells coated with DS-DNA and SS-DNA. DNA has also been demonstrated in cryoprecipitates (18).

The most direct evidence for the role of immune complexes in lupus nephritis has come from the demonstration that complexes, especially DNA-containing complexes, are present in abundant amounts in glomeruli. A variety of forms of glomerular injury are observed, and to a considerable extent the nature of the damage correlates with the site of immune complex accumulation within glomeruli. Four basic patterns of glomerular damage can be recognized (Table 3), although there is some overlap among these patterns. In most cases the glomerular injury does not shift from one pattern to another in the course of the disease (188). (1) Patients with minimal morphologic changes (principally equivocal or slight increase in mesangial cells and matrix) usually have deposits of IgG and C3 confined to mesangial regions. In most cases there is no clinical evidence of renal disease (189,190). A few patients have been found to have linear IgG staining (163) along the GBM; in most cases this probably does not result from anti-GBM antibodies (191), although such antibodies have been found in at least one case (192). Electron-dense deposits are largely restricted to the mesangium. (2) Mild (or focal) lupus nephritis is characterized histologically by segmental lesions in some of the glomeruli, typically with irregular mesangial proliferation, necrosis, neutrophil accumulation, and segmental GBM thickening. Usually, diffuse Ig and C3 deposits are found both in mesangial regions and segmentally along the GBM. Electron-dense deposits are found in the mesangium and also on both sides of the GBM. These patients often have proteinuria or hematuria (188). (3) The severe (diffuse) proliferative form of lupus nephritis shows similar histologic abnormalities, but is considerably more widespread. Subendothelial deposits are usually large and numerous. The patients may have severe proteinuria, hematuria, and/or renal failure usually accompanied by profound hypocomplementemia and evidence of circulating immune complexes. (4) In the membranous form the histologic picture resembles idiopathic membranous glomerulonephritis, with diffuse capillary wall thickening and usually only slight, irregular mesangial hypercellularity. Electron microscopy shows numerous subepithelial deposits, and usually some mesangial deposits. Immunofluorescence shows granular deposits of Ig and C3 along the GBM. The patients usually have moderate to severe proteinuria and tend to have a prolonged stable course. A fifth pattern of lupus nephritis has also been described, in which the predominant change is glomerular sclerosis (193). In addition, tubulointerstitial immune complex deposition and associated injury may be seen (see below).

The immunoglobulins present in the glomerular deposits in lupus nephritis include IgG and often IgM and IgA. Both classical and alternative pathway complement components are found, including C1q, C4, C2, C3, properdin, and rarely C3 proactivator (171,194–196).

DNA (163) and nucleotides (194,197) have been demonstrated in the glomeruli in some patients with SLE. Koffler et al. (2) showed that glomerular

Table 3. Incidence of Different Morphologic Patterns of Lupus Nephritis and Life Expectancy

	Approximate Incidence (%)	Approximate Survival at 5 Years (%)
Minimal lupus nephritis	30–40	80–90
Mild (focal) proliferative lupus nephritis	10–20	80
Severe (diffuse) proliferative lupus nephritis	40–50	30–40
Membranous lupus nephritis	10–15	60–80

deposits in a patient with severe lupus nephritis stained with fluoresceinated human anti-DNA, particularly after 2 M NaCl treatment. Free DNA abolished the staining. One of five other renal specimens had detectable DNA deposition, but none had appreciable SM antigen or nucleoprotein (2). Andres et al. (197) showed that antibodies to thymine and cytosine, which react with these components in SS-DNA, bound to the glomeruli of eight of nine patients with active lupus nephritis, in a distribution similar to that of Ig and C3. No DNA antigens were detected in the glomeruli of four patients with minimal or "burned-out" glomerular disease. Only one patient of 53 with idiopathic membranous glomerulonephritis showed staining for DNA. Antibodies to thymidine were also found to react (particularly after acid treatment) with glomerular deposits in eight of ten patients with lupus nephritis (194); it was noted that the staining correlated with the presence of C1q, which is known to bind SS-DNA under physiologic conditions (30). Elution studies have identified antinuclear antibodies in almost all cases; crucial evidence for the presence of complexes has been provided by the demonstration that these antibodies are found in higher concentrations in eluates than in the serum (when adjusted for equal IgG concentrations) (2).

Other studies further identified the antibodies concentrated in the glomeruli of patients with lupus nephritis (194). Antibody activity (per milligram of IgG) was increased in the glomerular eluates as compared with serum, when tested against DS-DNA (six of nine), SS-DNA (eight of nine), and RNA protein (four of nine); in one case there was no anti-DNA in the eluate. No anti-DS-RNA was found in any patient, further indicating that this system has little if any role in lupus nephritis. Deposition of a different type of antibody, namely anti-IgG rheumatoid factor (RF), has also been shown in one case—by reaction of the glomerular deposits with an anti-idiotypic antibody to a monoclonal IgM (174).

Although presumably most of the DNA in the glomerular deposits is endogenous, this has not been directly shown, and efforts have been made to determine whether some of the nucleic acid is of viral origin (198,199). Using immunofluorescence, RNA viral antigens have been detected in glomeruli in lupus (198). In one study it was found that an antiserum to a mammalian C-type virus stained all lupus-affected kidneys but not several other kidneys (199). Proof of antibody specificity is absolutely essential to the proper interpretation of these potentially important findings. Efforts to relate the tubuloreticular structures found by electron microscopy in glomerular endothelial cells in most patients with SLE cells to paramyxoviruses (200) were short lived (201), and these structures are now generally considered to be manifestations of cell injury, possibly related to viral infection. In any case, the structures are not specific for SLE (202).

Deposition of Ig and complement components frequently occurs in sites other than the glomeruli in SLE, in particular along renal tubular basement membranes and in the renal interstitium (203–205). Deposits are also found outside the kidney. In the skin, deposits are seen along the dermal-epidermal junction (196,206–208). Deposits have also been described in the spleen, lungs (204), and choroid plexus (209,210). These deposits often appear to be of pathogenetic significance; the extra glomerular deposits in the kidney are usually accompanied by tubulointerstitial damage, which has been observed even in the absence of glomerular disease (211). In the skin, deposits can be present in clinically normal skin (207), although microscopic evidence of inflammation is often seen.

The mechanism of deposition of the complexes in various tissues in SLE has not been established. In analogy to experimental models, complexes formed in the circulation probably initiate the glomerular, vascular, and possibly the tubulointerstitial deposits. However, local complex formation may also occur, due to the strong avidity of SS-DNA for basement membranes (59). By this means, free antigen could preferentially accumulate along the GBM, and antibody and complement components could subsequently bind locally. The factors accounting for the various patterns of intraglomerular deposition are also unknown. However, experimental studies suggest that very large complexes localize principally in mesangial regions and small complexes along the outside of the GBM. It seems most likely that in situ formation accounts for the accumulation of complexes along the dermal-epidermal junction, as a consequence of release of intracellular antigens from injured epidermal cells. This hypothesis might account for the preferential accumulation of deposits in sites exposed to the sun. The ensuing inflammation might serve as a perpetuating mechanism, by causing further release of DNA from cells.

Although many of the lesions of SLE can be attributed to autoantibodies or their immune complexes, little is known either of causative agents or of the basis of the abnormal immune responses. Until further progress is made in these areas, treatment will continue to be symptomatic, as by suppression of the immune response and the inflammatory process with drugs or, as suggested by recent studies, by removal of the circulating complexes by plasmapheresis (212,183).

MALIGNANCIES

Although there is increasing evidence that patients with a variety of malignancies have circulating immune complexes (47,213–217), few have signs of immune complex-mediated tissue damage (218). However, at least 27 patients with malignancies have been reported to have immune deposits in the kidney (219). Only in five cases was evidence obtained that antigens or antibodies related to the tumor were present in the glomeruli. All these cases were classified pathologically as membranous glomerulonephritis. Fluoresceinated eluates of renal tissue and serum in one case stained the patient's own squamous carcinoma (220);

however, no specific glomerular concentration was demonstrated, so that might have been due to serum contamination. In another patient, with carcinoma of the colon, serum obtained after resection of the tumor stained glomerular deposits in a renal biopsy performed prior to surgery; a specimen obtained four months later did not react (221). Another patient with colonic carcinoma had deposits of carcinoembryonic antigen in glomeruli (222), which was not found in the case cited above (221). Glomerular eluates from a patient with melanoma reacted by indirect immunofluorescence with a monkey antimelanoma serum; however, the controls reported in the abstract did not include other diseased kidneys (223). Finally, Feulgen positive material was found in glomeruli in a patient with oat-cell carcinoma and antinuclear antibodies; the source was suggested to be the necrotic tumor (224). In three patients with renal cell carcinoma, serum cryoprecipitates and glomerular eluates contained antibody reactive with normal brush border antigens (225).

Many patients with malignancies (especially with Hodgkin's disease) have been found to have glomerular disease resembling minimal change disease (219) without evidence of immune complex deposition. Further studies are needed to determine the significance and pathogenetic mechanisms involved in these cases.

IMMUNE COMPLEX-MEDIATED DISEASES INITIATED BY THERAPEUTIC AGENTS

There has been considerable speculation (and some evidence) that certain therapeutic agents can initiate immune complex-mediated lesions in man. For the most part, before a drug can elicit an immune response a stable conjugate must be formed between a host protein and the drug, or one of its breakdown products. If such immunogenic conjugates are formed within the circulation and persist there until antibodies are formed, complexes will be produced, which might be expected to bring about glomerulonephritis or necrotizing arteritis. Indeed, it is widely believed that reaction to certain drugs, especially in the penicillin group, is responsible for such lesions. There appears to be little solid support for this view, however; for the most part, the evidence consists of isolated case reports of arteritis occurring in the course of therapy, and no findings are recorded that strongly support a causative role of the therapy (61). It is, of course, well established that a variety of drugs, including the penicillin group, can induce hypersensitivity reactions, including a serum sickness-like syndrome—and although vasculitis occurs in this syndrome, the vessels involved are venules and evidence of necrotizing arteritis, glomerulonephritis, or other visceral lesions is lacking (226). It is possible that drug-induced serum sickness-like syndromes are in fact mediated by immune complexes, but this has not been thoroughly documented. Insofar as they affect the kidneys, well-documented reactions to penicillin and certain other drugs are characterized by tubulointerstitial nephritis, rather than arteritis or glomerulonephritis (227). The mechanisms responsible for these lesions have not been entirely elucidated, in large part because no experimental model is available.

There is, nevertheless, good reason to believe that several therapeutic agents, namely gold (228), penicillamine (229), probably mercury, and possibly certain other agents can occasionally induce immune complex-mediated glomerular disease, manifested clinically by the nephrotic syndrome and pathologically by a picture that resembles membranous glomerulonephritis. The evidence that the renal lesions seen in patients receiving penicillamine or gold are due to the treatment rather than the underlying disease is compelling. Similar lesions are not seen in untreated patients with the diseases that may be treated with these agents (rheumatoid arthritis, Wilson's disease). Furthermore, in some cases, evidence of renal disease has been discovered soon after treatment was started, and in most cases has disappeared after cessation of therapy (although sometimes only after many months). In addition, immune complex-mediated lesions have been produced experimentally by injection of gold or mercury (230).

The evidence that the glomerular lesions associated with gold or penicillamine therapy are produced by immune complexes consists entirely of their very striking resemblance to certain well-documented immune complex-mediated lesions—notably the membranous form of lupus nephritis in man and the model of Heymann nephritis (see below). The mechanisms leading to immune complex formation have not been clarified. One possibility is that the agents form immunogenic conjugates with host constituents and that these conjugates serve as the antigens in the complexes. There is no direct evidence supporting this view, and in the case of gold-induced nephropathy there is rather compelling evidence against it. Gold has not been demonstrated by spectroscopic analytical examination within glomerular deposits, although by this technique gold was readily demonstrable within tubular cells (228). Attempts have been made to provide evidence for penicillamine within glomerular deposits by incubating renal sections in high concentrations of penicillamine, with the expectation that penicillamine-containing complexes would dissociate and cause disappearance of the deposits; this did not succeed (231).

Another conceivable mechanism is that an autologous constituent serves as the antigen, possibly rendered immunogenic by structural alteration or release from damaged sites in which it is normally sequestered. There is no direct evidence for this mechanism in man. However, Roman-Franco et al. have provided some evidence in an experimental model (230). Rabbits were repeatedly injected with mercuric chloride. At first, the animals were found to produce anti-basement membrane antibodies, which caused typical linear accumulation of IgG along the GBM. Later, granular Ig-containing deposits were found along glomerular and other basement membranes. Mercury was not detectable in the deposits. The authors suggested that the immune complexes were formed by autoantibodies and basement membrane antigens.

Another possible causative agent of immune complex-mediated glomerular disease is heroin. There appears to be a higher than expected incidence of the nephrotic syndrome in heroin addicts. A variety of glomerular lesions have been described, usually resembling either focal glomerulosclerosis or membranoproliferative glomerulonephritis. In some cases the immunoflourescence findings in renal specimens suggest immune complex deposition—in the form of focal granular deposits of IgM, C3, and C1q along the GBM (232). Furthermore, some patients have depressed serum complement levels and C1q precipitins, providing evidence of circulating complexes (232). It is possible that heroin, or a contaminant, serves as a hapten in the putative antigen, or that infections, which are common in addicts, lead to complex formation. No direct information about the responsible antigen(s) is available.

AUTOLOGOUS IMMUNE COMPLEX-MEDIATED GLOMERULAR DISEASE

It has been thoroughly documented in experimental models that autologous substances can serve as antigens in immune complex-mediated glomerular disease. The most extensively studied model is Heymann nephritis (autologous immune complex disease). Heymann et al. (233) reported in 1959 that when rats are injected with preparations of homologous renal tissue in Freund's adjuvant, there develops a chronic glomerular disease, manifested by severe proteinuria and characterized histologically by mild glomerular changes, principally capillary wall thickening. Later studies showed finely granular deposits of IgG along the GBM, with corresponding deposits of electron-dense material along the epithelial side of the GBM. As noted earlier, the findings are strikingly similar to those of membranous glomerulonephritis in man. Studies by Grupe and Kaplan (234,235) and by Edgington et al. (236) have shown that the responsible antigen is normally present in the brush border region of proximal convoluted tubules. Thus, rats with the glomerular disease have circulating autoantibodies that react with brush border regions (235). Furthermore, immunoglobulin eluted from cortical tissue of diseased kidneys reacts with brush border-associated antigens, but not with normal glomeruli. In addition, the glomerular deposits have been shown by immunofluorescence to contain brush border-associated antigen (236). Finally, the glomerular disease can be induced by injections of very small amounts of material (3 to 6 μg of protein N) purified from renal tubules (236). It has generally been assumed that the complexes are formed within the circulation. Obviously this mechanism would require entrance of the renal tubular antigen into the circulation—at least intermittently. Recently, it has been suggested that the complexes are formed in glomeruli (56). This is supported by the observation that epimembranous deposits form in kidneys perfused with rabbit antiserum prepared against renal tubular antigen. However, because heterologous antisera were employed, it is not certain that the reacting antigens are the same as those involved in Heymann nephritis. In fact, as noted above, sera or renal eluates from rats with Heymann nephritis do not appear to have antibody activity against normal glomerular constituents.

The only other experimentally induced model of autologous immune complex-mediated glomerular disease is that described by Weigel and Nakamura (237), who reported that rabbits immunized with thyroglobulin sometimes develop glomerular lesions due to thyroglobulin-containing immune complexes. Autologous antigens, in particular DNA, may also participate in the spontaneously occurring immune complex-mediated glomerular lesions in NZB/W mice (although some of the DNA may be of viral origin) (238). Autologous antigens also appear to be involved in experimentally induced tubulointerstitial immune complex renal disease in rabbits. The antigen is believed to be derived from the cytoplasm of proximal tubular cells, and the complexes appear to be formed locally (239).

Autoantibodies and autologous antigens appear to be involved in certain human immune complex-mediated glomerular diseases. The most important example is lupus nephritis, in which, as discussed above, DNA-containing complexes are of paramount importance (we are assuming that most of the DNA in the complexes is of host rather than viral origin). Rheumatoid factor, presumably combined with IgG, has been shown to be present in the glomerular deposits in cases of mixed cryoglobulinemia and lupus nephritis, and IgM-anti-IgG complexes may also participate as secondary pathogenetic agents in APSGN, as discussed earlier.

In addition, the same two antigens that have been used experimentally to induce autologous immune complex glomerular disease—renal tubular antigen and thyroglobulin—may be involved in human glomerular disease in rare instances.

Naruse et al. (240) reported that a brush border-associated antigen was demonstrable by immunofluorescence within glomerular deposits in four of nine patients in Japan with membranous glomerulonephritis. In these studies they employed antisera from rabbits immunized with human tubular antigen preparations. Others, however, have failed to obtain similar results, even though fairly large numbers of patients with membranous glomerulonephritis were studied (241). One possible explanation for these discordant results is that in Japan, but not in Britain or America, certain etiologic agents act to induce the formation of autoantibodies against renal tubular antigens, and account for some cases of membranous glomerulonephritis. A more likely explanation is that the antisera used in the various laboratories have different specificities. In this respect, Miyakawa et al. (242) have reported that only one of three antisera raised against different preparations of renal tubular antigens reacted with glomerular deposits, although all three stained the luminal portion of proximal tubules. The "nephritogenic tubular antigen" was studied further and found to be present in pronase-digested extracts of all organs tested, including kidney, intestine, liver, spleen, stomach, heart, and lung. The antigen was also identified in the serum, even in anephric patients. In view of these properties, it seems unlikely that the material is comparable to that responsible for Heymann nephritis. At the present time, the claim that renal tubular antigens are involved in human membranous glomerulonephritis cannot be considered substantiated.

Renal tubular antigenic material has also been described in glomerular deposits in seven patients with sickle cell anemia in whom diffuse proliferative glomerular disease was present (243). Moreover, in some of the patients, cryoprecipitable complexes were obtained from the circulation and were found to contain renal tubular antigens (244). Similar findings were reported in a 6-year-old patient with immune complex-mediated glomerular lesions and tubulointerstitial nephritis, manifested by the nephrotic syndrome and Fanconi's syndrome (245).

Fairly convincing evidence has been presented that thyroglobulin can be demonstrated in the deposits of immune complex-mediated glomerular disease. To date, however, only two such cases have been reported in detail (246,247). In one case the clinical findings suggested that the glomerular disease was exacerbated by radioiodine treatment for thyrotoxicosis, presumably due to release of thyroglobulin into the circulation (246).

Primary Glomerular Disease of Unknown Cause

The diseases in this category (Table 2) are classified on the basis of histologic, immunofluorescence, and electron-microscopic findings. A majority of these diseases are assumed to be mediated by immune complexes because of their resemblance to experimental models or to documented forms of immune complex-mediated disease in man, especially with respect to the immunofluorescence and electron-microscopic findings. By definition, neither causative agents nor responsible antigens have been identified.

Idiopathic Membranous Glomerulonephritis

As noted earlier, it seems almost certain that membranous glomerulonephritis results from immune complexes because of the very close resemblance of the glomerular abnormalities to those of Heymann nephritis and to the membranous form of lupus nephritis. Furthermore, as has been discussed, in a few cases classified on pathologic grounds as membranous glomerulonephritis, specific antigens may have been identified. To date, it has not been demonstrated that circulating complexes are found in patients with membranous glomerulonephritis. Possible explanations for this have been discussed.

Membranoproliferative Glomerulonephritis (MPGN) and Dense Deposit Disease (DDD)

It now appears that the condition generally referred to as membranoproliferative (or mesangiocapillary) glomerulonephritis includes two pathologic entities, which can be designated membranoproliferative glomerulonephritis with subendothelial deposits (MPGN) type I and dense deposit disease (MPGN type II) (248). The immunofluorescence findings in MPGN type I are consistent with an immune complex pathogenesis. In most cases broad, irregular deposits of immunoglobulins and complement components are found along the GBM, and electron microscopy shows corresponding subendothelial deposits. Further support for an immune complex mechanism is provided by the observation that in some patients with infected shunts, morphologically indistinguishable lesions develop (120). In addition, Ooi et al. have detected complexes in the serum of some patients with MPGN type I by C1q binding and sucrose density gradient ultracentrifugation (54). The nature of the postulated antigen(s) is unknown.

The pathogenesis of dense deposit disease (MPGN type II) is obscure. In this condition, broad, extensive intramembranous electron-dense deposits are found by electron microscopy in glomerular and tubular basement membranes, which are unlike the deposits seen in any experimental model of immune complex glomerulonephritis. Moreover, immunoglobulins are not usually found in the deposits, and IgG in particular is almost never observed. Nevertheless, in some cases of dense deposit disease, epimembranous deposits (humps) are found, suggesting the participation of immune complexes. In addition, evidence for the presence of circulating complexes has been obtained in a few cases (54).

Considerable efforts have been directed at elucidating the derangements of the complement system that are seen in patients with MPGN types I and II (248). Briefly, it appears that in most patients with MPGN type I, the serum complement profile is indicative of classical pathway activation, whereas in patients with MPGN type II, the findings are more often suggestive of alternative pathway activation. The immunofluorescence findings in glomeruli tend to support these conclusions, in that in MPGN type I, immunoglobulins, C1q, and C4 are generally found in addition to C3, whereas in type II, C3 is found often without associated immunoglobulins (especially IgG) or early complement components. It has been suggested that the lesions of dense deposit disease may result from an agent (or agents) that activates the complement system via the alternative pathway. Unfortunately, there is no entirely satisfactory experimental model of glomerular injury induced by alternative pathway activation; in fact, as noted earlier, little enough is known about how any components of the complement system produce glomerular damage. It is possible that some unidentified material accumulates for unknown reasons in glomerular and tubular basement membranes in dense deposit disease and that the role of the complement system is secondary.

IgA/IgG Nephropathy (Berger's Disease)

Berger's disease is characterized in most instances by recurrent hematuria; renal function is usually normal. The bouts of hematuria often occur in association with upper respiratory tract infections, which are presumed to be viral in origin (249). Histologically, there is usually little to be seen except for slight, irregular increase in mesangial cells. Immunofluorescence reveals features that are consistent with an immune complex pathogenesis, namely, conspicuous mesangial deposits of immunoglobulins, especially IgA, and complement. Once again, the nature of the postulated antigen(s) is unknown. The frequent association of attacks of hematuria with upper respiratory tract infections suggests a viral etiology. It is not known how frequently circulating complexes are present in Berger's nephropathy.

Focal Glomerulonephritis, Rapidly Progressive Glomerulonephritis, and Unclassifiable Glomerular Diseases

In some cases classified as rapidly progressive glomerulonephritis (crescenteric glomerulonephritis), focal glomerulonephritis, and in some cases of unclassifiable or end-stage glomerular disease, irregular granular deposits of immunoglobulins and complement components are found in glomeruli, suggesting the presence of immune complexes. Further documentation is obviously required in each of these categories.

CONCLUDING REMARKS

Following a rapid expansion in the 1960s of knowledge concerning basic pathogenetic mechanisms and classification of human glomerular diseases, progress has slowed considerably. In particular, responsible antigens and causative factors have been identified in only a small minority of cases assumed to be mediated by immune complexes. A series of recent findings suggests that HBs Ag is involved in a variety of immune complex-mediated lesions, including several forms of glomerulonephritis and arteritis, but further observations are required to assess its overall importance. The search for other viral antigens or autologous antigens has been largely unsuccessful, although these remain the leading candidates at present. Furthermore, very little has been learned about how immune complexes actually mediate glomerular injury. Experimental studies point to the importance of factors that influence the intensity and quality of the antibody response, which may be at least in part genetically determined; there is as yet almost no information concerning these factors in human renal disease. The role of the recently described C3 receptors in glomeruli in the accumulation and fate of complexes in glomeruli is currently under investigation (250,251). Interest is now focused on methods that permit the detection of small amounts of immune complexes in the circulation; however, it is not yet clear how much useful information these methods will provide in the study of immune complex-mediated lesions in man. At present, these assays seem to detect complexes in many diseases in which complexes are not known to cause tissue injury. Further characterization of the material in the complexes is of central importance and may yield clues to causative factors and broaden our concepts of the pathogenetic effects of immune complexes.

REFERENCES

1. Woodroffe, A. J., and Wilson, C. B., *J. Immunol.* **118**, 1178 (1977).
2. Koffler, D., Schur, P. H., and Kunkel, H. G., *J. Exp. Med.* **126**, 607 (1967).
3. Agnello, V., Koffler, D., and Kunkel, H. G., *Kidney Int.* **3**, 90 (1973).
4. Schneeberger, E. E., Leber, P. D., Karnovsky, M. J., and McCluskey, R. T., *J. Exp. Med.* **139**, 1283 (1974).
5. Maurer, M., Sutherland, D. E. R., Howard, R. J., Fish, A. J., Najarian, J. S., and Michael, A. F., *J. Exp. Med.* **137**, 553 (1973).
6. Burkholder, P. M., *Atlas of Human Pathology*, Harper and Row, New York, 1973, p. 317.
7. McCluskey, R. T., and Vassalli, P., *Inflammation, Immunity and Hypersensitivity*, Hoeber Med. Div., Harper and Row, New York, 1971.
8. Fish, A. J., Michael, A. F., Vernier, R. L., and Good, R. A., *Am. J. Pathol.* **49**, 997 (1966).
9. Cream, J. J., Bryceson, A. D., and Ryder, G., *Br. J. Dermatol.* **84**, 106 (1971).
10. Steensgaard, J., and Hill, R. J., *Anal. Biochem.* **34**, 485 (1970).
11. Williams, B. D., Clarkson, A. R., Groves, R. J., and Lessof, M. M., *J. Immunol. Methods* **7**, 219 (1975).

12. Amlot, P. L., Slaney, J. M., and Williams, B. D., *Lancet* **1**, 449 (1976).
13. Wintrobe, M. M., and Buell, M. V., *Bull. Johns Hopkins Hosp.* **52**, 156 (1933).
14. Lerner, A. B., and Watson, C. J., *Am. J. Med. Sci.* **214**, 410 (1947).
15. McIntosh, R. W., Kaufman, D. B., Kulvinskas, C., and Grossman, B. J., *J. Lab. Clin. Med.* **75**, 566 (1970).
16. Brouet, J. C., Clauvel, J. P., Danon, F., Klein, M., and Seligmann, M., *Am. J. Med.* **57**, 775 (1974).
17. Levo, Y., Gorevic, P. D., Kassab, H. J., Zucker-Franklin, D., and Franklin, E. C., *N. Eng. J. Med.* **229**, 1501 (1977).
18. Winfield, J. B., Koffler, D., and Kunkel, H. G., *J. Clin. Invest.* **56**, 563 (1975).
19. Wands, J. R., Mann, E., Alpert, E., and Isselbacher, K. J., *J. Clin. Invest.* **55**, 930 (1975).
20. Müller-Eberhard, H. J., and Calcott, M. A., *Immunochemistry* **3**, 500 (1966).
21. Augener, W., Grey, H. M., Cooper, N. R., and Müller-Eberhard, H. J., *Immunochemistry* **8**, 1011 (1971).
22. Müller-Eberhard, H. J., and Kunkel, H. G., *Proc. Soc. Exp. Biol. Med.* **106**, 291 (1961).
23. Agnello, V., Koffler, D., Eisenberg, J. W., Winchester, R. J., and Kunkel, H. G., *J. Exp. Med.* **134**, 2285 (1971).
24. Mowbray, J. F., Hoffbrand, A. V., Holborow, E. J., Seah, P. P., and Fry, L., *Lancet* **1**, 400 (1973).
25. Rojas-Espinosa, O., Mendez-Navarrate, I., and Estrada-Parra, S., *Clin. Exp. Immunol.* **12**, 215 (1972).
26. Gocke, D., Hsu, J. K., Morgan, C., Bombarderi, S., Lockshin, M., and Christian, C. L., *J. Exp. Med.* **134**, 3305 (1971).
27. Agnello, V., in *Manual of Clinical Immunology* (N. R. Rose and H. Freedman, eds.), American Society for Microbiology, Washington, D.C., 1976, p. 699
28. Nydeggar, U. E., Lambert, P. H., Gerberg, H., and Miescher, P. A., *J. Clin, Invest.* **54**, 297 (1974).
29. Sobel, A. T., Bokisch, V. A., and Müller-Eberhard, H. J., *J. Exp. Med.* **142**, 139 (1975).
30. Gabriel, A., and Agnello, V., *J. Clin. Invest.* **59**, 990 (1977).
31. Luthra, H. S., McDuffie, F. C., Hunder, G. G., and Samayoa, E. A., *J. Clin. Invest.* **56**, 458 (1975).
32. Zubler, R. H., Lange, G., Lambert, P. H., and Miescher, P. A., *J. Immunol.* **116**, 232 (1976).
33. Hay, F. C., Nineham, L., and Roit, I. M., *Clin. Exp. Immunol.* **24**, 396 (1976).
34. Müller-Eberhard, H. J., Bokisch, V. A., and Budzko, D. B., in *Sixth International Symposium on Immunopathology* (P. A. Miescher, ed.), Grune and Stratton, New York, 1971.
35. Loos, M., Bitter-Suermann, D., and Dierich, M., *J. Immunol.* **112**, 935 (1974).
36. Winchester, R. J., Kunkel, H. G., and Agnello, V., *J. Exp. Med.* **134**, 2865 (1971).
37. Cowdery, J. S., Treadwell, P. E., and Fritz, R. B., *J. Immunol.* **114**, 5 (1975).
38. Pulvertaft, R. J. V., *J. Clin. Pathol.* **18**, 261 (1965).
39. Theofilopoulos, A. N., Dixon, F. J., and Bokisch, V. A., *J. Exp. Med.* **140**, 877 (1974).
40. Theofilopoulos, A. N., Bokisch, V. A., and Dixon, F. J., *J. Exp. Med.* **139**, 696 (1974).
41. Theofilopoulos, A. N., Wilson, C. B., Bokisch, V. A., and Dixon, F. J., *J. Exp. Med.* **140**, 1230 (1974).
42. Gupta, R. C., McDuffie, F. C., Tappeiner, G., and Jordan, R. E., *Immunology* **34**, 751 (1978).
43. Theofilopoulos, A. N., Wilson, C. B., and Dixon, F. J., *J. Clin. Invest.* **57**, 169 (1976).
44. Onyewotu, I. I., Johnson, P. B., Johnson, G. D., and Holborow, E. J., *Clin. Exp. Immunol.* **19**, 267 (1975).
45. Stühlinger, W. D., Verroust, P. J., and Morel-Maroger, L., *Immunology* **30**, 43 (1976).
46. Penttinen, K., *Ann. Rheum. Dis.* **36**, 55 (1977).
47. Myalla, G., Vaheri, A., and Penttinen, K., *Clin. Exp. Immunol.* **8**, 399 (1971).
48. Penttinen, K., *Am. J. Dis. Child.* **123**, 418 (1972).
49. Biberfeld, G., and Norberg, R., *J. Immunol.* **112**, 413 (1974).
50. Norberg, R., *Scand. J. Immunol.* **3**, 229 (1974).
51. Wager, O., Penttinen, K., Rasanen, J. A., and Myalla, G., *Clin. Exp. Immunol.* **15**, 393 (1973).
52. Johnson, A. H., Mowbray, J. F., and Porter, K. A., *Lancet* **1**, 762 (1975).
53. Rossen, R. D., Reisberg, M. A., Singer, D. B., Schloeder, F. X., Suki, W. N., Hill, L. L., and Eknoyan, G., *Kidney Int.* **10**, 256 (1976).
54. Ooi, Y. M., Vallota, E. H., and West, C. D., *Kidney Int.* **11**, 275 (1977).

55. Mannik, M., and Arend, W. P., *J. Exp. Med.* **134**, 19s (1971).
56. Van Damme, B., Flevren, G. J., Bakker, W. W., Hoedemaeker, P. J., and Vernier, R. L., *Kidney Int.* **10**, 551 (1976).
57. Benacerraf, B., and Katz, D. M., *Adv. Cancer Res.* **21**, 121 (1975).
58. Miller, G. W., and Nussenzweig, V., *Proc. Natl. Acad. Sci.* **72**, 418 (1975).
59. Izu, S., Lambert, P.-H., and Miescher, P. A., *J. Exp. Med.* **144**, 428 (1976).
60. Valdes, A. J., Senterfit, L. B., Pollack, A. S., and Germuth, F. G., *Johns Hopkins Med. J.* **124**, 9 (1969).
61. McCluskey, R. T., and Leber, P. D., in *Controversy in Internal Medicine* II (F. J., Ingelfinger, R. H. Ebert, M. Finland, and A. S. Relman, eds.), W. B. Saunders, Philadelphia, 1974.
62. Zabriskie, J. B., in *The Immune System and Infectious Diseases,* Fourth Int. Convoc. Immunol. (E. Neter and F. Milgrom, eds.), Karger, Basel, 1975.
63. Feldman, J. D., Mardiney, M. R., and Shuler, S. E., *Lab. Invest.* **15**, 283 (1966).
64. McCluskey, R. T., Vassalli, P., Gallo, G., and Baldwin, D. S., *N. Eng. J. Med.* **274**, 695 (1966).
65. Michael, A. F., Drummond, K. N., Good, R. A., and Vernier, R. L., *J. Clin. Invest.* **45**, 237 (1966).
66. Fish, A. J., Herdman, R. C., Michael, A. F., Pickering, R. J., and Good, R. A., *Am. J. Med.* **48**, 28 (1970).
67. Morel-Maroger, L., Leatham, A., and Richet, G., *Am. J. Med.* **53**, 170 (1972).
68. Michael, A. F., and McLean, R. H., *Adv. Nephrol.* **4**, 49 (1974).
69. Movat, H. Z., Steiner, J. W., and Huhn, D., *Lab. Invest.* **11**, 117 (1962).
70. Andres, G. A., Accini, L., Hsu, K. C., Zabriskie, J. B., and Seegal, B. C., *J. Exp. Med.* **123**, 339 (1966).
71. Treser, G., Semar, M., McVicas, M., Franklin, M., Ty, A., Sagel, I., and Lange, K., *Science* **163**, 676 (1969).
72. Kantor, F. S., *J. Exp. Med.* **121**, 849 (1965).
73. Kantor, F. S., *J. Exp. Med.* **121**, 861 (1965).
74. Grupe, W. E., *Pediatrics* **42**, 474 (1964).
75. Vassalli, P., and McCluskey, R. T., *Am. J. Pathol.* **45**, 653 (1964).
76. Alkjaersig, N. K., Fletcher, A. P., Lewis, M. L., Cole, B. R., Ingelfinger, J. R., and Robson, A. M., *Kidney Int.* **10**, 319 (1976).
77. Baldwin, D. S., Gluck, M. C., Schacht, R. G., and Gallo, G., *Ann. Intern. Med.* **80**, 342 (1974).
78. Yampolsky, J., and Mullins, D. P., *Am. J. Dis. Child.* **69**, 163 (1945).
79. Taitz, L. S., Isaacson, C., and Stein, H., *Br. Med. J.* **2**, 152 (1961).
80. Pollner, P., *J.A.M.A.* **198**, 173 (1966).
81. Hermann, G., and Marr, W. L., *Am. J. Syph. Neurol.* **14**, 1 (1935).
82. Falls, W. F., Jr., Ford, K. L., Ashworth, C. T., and Carter, N. W., *Ann. Intern. Med.* **63**, 1047 (1965).
83. Gamble, C. N., and Rearden, J. B., *N. Eng. J. Med.* **292**, 449 (1975).
84. Tourville, D. R., Byrd, L. H., Kim, D. U., Zajd, D., Lee, I., Reichman, L. B., and Baskin, S., *Am. J. Pathol.* **82**, 479 (1976).
85. Braunstein, G. D., Lewis, E. F., Galvanek, E. G., Hamilton, A., and Bell, W. R., *Am. J. Med.* **48**, 643 (1970).
86. Bhorade, M. S., Carag, H. B., Lee, H. J., Potter, E. V., and Dunea, A. B., *J.A.M.A.* **216**, 1159 (1971).
87. Yuceoglu, A. M., Sages, I., Treser, G., Wasserman, E., and Lange, K., *J.A.M.A.* **229**, 1085 (1974).
88. Hill, L. L., Singer, D. B., Falletta, J., and Stasney, R., *Pediatrics* **49**, 260 (1972).
89. Kaplan, B. S., Wigglesworth, F. W., Marks, M. I., and Drummond, K. N., *J. Pediatr.* **81**, 1154 (1972).
90. Giglioli, G., *Trans. R. Soc. Trop. Med.* **26**, 177 (1932).
91. Carothers, J. C., *East Afr. Med. J.* **10**, 335 (1934).
92. Gilles, H. B., and Hendrickse, R. G., *Br. Med. J.* **2**, 27 (1963).
93. Kibukamusoke, J. W., Hutt, M. S. R., and Wilks, N. E., *Q. J. Med.* **36**, 393 (1967).
94. Giglioli, G., *Ann. Trop. Med. Parasitol.* **56**, 225 (1962).
95. Allison, A. C., Houba, V., Hendrickse, R. G., DePetris, S., Edgington, G. M., and Adenayi, A., *Lancet* **1**, 1232 (1969).
96. Adenayi, A., Hendrickse, R. G., and Houba, V., *Lancet* **1**, 644 (1970).

97. Hendrickse, R. G., Adenayi, A., Edington, G. M., Glasgow, E. F., White, R. H. R., and Houba, V., *Lancet* **1**, 1143 (1972).
98. White, R. H. R., *Nephron* **11**, 147 (1973).
99. Ward, P. A., and Kibukamusoke, J. W., *Lancet* **1**, 283 (1969).
100. Houba, V., Allison, A. C., Adenayi, A., and Houba, J. E., *Clin. Exp. Immunol.* **8**, 761 (1971).
101. Houba, V., Lambert, P. H., Voller, A., and Soyanow, M. A. O., *Clin. Immunol. Immunopathol.* **6**, 12 (1976).
102. Steward, M. W., and Voller, A., *Br. J. Exp. Pathol.* **54**, 198 (1973).
103. Bell, E. T., *Am. J. Pathol.* **8**, 639 (1932).
104. Spain, D. M., and King, D. W., *Ann. Intern. Med.* **36**, 1086 (1952).
105. Levy, R. L., and Hong, R., *Am. J. Med.* **54**, 645 (1973).
106. Dathan, J. R., and Heyworth, M. F., *Br. Med. J.* **1**, 376 (1975).
107. Boulton-Jones, J. M., Sissons, J. G., Evans, D. J., and Peters, D. K., *Br. Med. J.* **2**, 11 (1974).
108. Kesslin, M. H., Messner, R. P., and Williams, R. C., Jr., *Arch. Intern. Med.* **132**, 578 (1973).
109. Morel-Maroger, L., Sraer, J. D., Herreman, G., and Godeau, P., *Arch. Pathol.* **94**, 205 (1972).
110. Gutman, R. A., Striker, G. E., Gilliland, B. C., and Cutler, R. E., *Medicine* **51**, 1 (1972).
111. Rifle, G., Justrabo, R., Genin, J. M., and Faivre-Guillaumie, J., *Kidney Int.* **10**, 188 (1976).
112. Tu, W. H., Shearn, M. A., and Lee, J. C., *Ann. Intern. Med.* **71**, 355 (1969).
113. Perez, G. O., Rothfield, N., and Williams, R. C., *Arch. Intern. Med.* **136**, 334 (1976).
114. Williams, R. C., Jr., and Kunkel, H. G., *J. Clin. Invest.* **41**, 666 (1962).
115. Beaufils, M., Morel-Maroger, L., Sraer, J.-D., Kanfer, A., Kourilsky, O., and Richet, G., *N. Engl. J. Med.* **295**, 185 (1976).
116. Hurwitz, D., Quismorio, F. P., and Friow, G. J., *Clin. Exp. Immunol.* **19**, 131 (1975).
117. Bayer, A. S., Theofilopoulos, A. N., Eisenberg, R., Dixon, F. J., and Guze, L. B., *N. Eng. J. Med.* **295**, 1500 (1976).
118. Black, J. A., Challacombe, D. N., and Ockenden, B. G., *Lancet* **2**, 921 (1965).
119. Moncrieff, M. W., Glasgow, E. F., Arthur, L. J. H., and Hargreaves, H. M., *Arch. Dis. Child.* **48**, 69 (1973).
120. Strife, C. T., McDonald, B. M., Riley, E. J., McAdams, A. J., and West, C. D., *J. Pediatr.* **88**, 403 (1976).
121. Rames, L., Wise, B., Goodman, J. R., and Piel, C. F., *J.A.M.A.* **212**, 167 (1970).
122. Stickler, G. B., Shin, M. H., Burke, E. C., Holley, K. E., Miller, R. H., and Segar, W. E., *N. Engl. J. Med.* **279**, 1077 (1968).
123. McKenzie, S. A., and Hayden, S. K., *Pediatrics* **54**, 806 (1974).
124. Stauffer, U. G., *Dev. Med. Child Neurol.* **12**, 161 (1970).
125. Wegmann, W., and Leumaun, E. P., *Virchows Arch. Pathol. Anat.* **359**, 185 (1973).
126. Kaufman, D. B., and McIntosh, R. M., *Am. J. Med.* **50**, 262 (1971).
127. Forrest, J. W., Jr., John, F., Mills, L. R., Buxton, T. B., Moore, W. L., Jr., Hudson, J. B., and Ozawa, T., *Clin. Nephrol.* **7**, 76 (1977).
128. Prince, A. M., and Trepo, C. G., *Lancet* **1**, 1309 (1971).
129. Almeida, J. D., and Waterson, A. P., *Lancet* **2**, 983 (1969).
130. Dane, D. S., Cameron, C. H., and Briggs, M., *Lancet* **1**, 695 (1970).
131. Chairez, R., Hollinger, F. B., Brunschwig, J. P., and Dressman, G. R., *J. Virol.* **15**, 182 (1974).
132. Farivar, M., Wands, J. R., Benson, G. D., Dienstag, J. L., and Isselbacher, K. J., *Gastroenterology* **71**, 490 (1976).
133. McIntosh, R. M., Koss, M. N., and Gocke, K. J., *Q. J. Med.* **45**, 23 (1976).
134. Trepo, C. G., Zuckerman, A. J., Bird, R. C., and Prince, A. M., *J. Clin. Pathol.* **27**, 86 (1974).
135. Sabesin, S. M., and Levinson, M. J., *Adv. Intern. Med.* **22**, 421 (1977).
136. Alpert, E., Isselbacher, K. J., and Schur, P. H., *N. Engl. J. Med.* **285**, 185 (1971).
137. Schumacher, H. R., and Gall, E. P., *Am. J. Med.* **57**, 655 (1974).
138. Eknoyan, O., Gyorkey, E., Dichoso, C., Martinez-Maldonaldo, M., Suki, W. N., and Gyorkey, P., *Kidney Int.* **1**, 413 (1972).
139. Conrad, M. E., Schwartz, F. D., and Young, A. A., *Am. J. Med.* **37**, 789 (1964).
140. Sakaguchi, H., Dachs, S., Grishman, E., Fiorenzo, P., Salomon, M., and Churg, J., *Lab. Invest.* **14**, 533 (1965).
141. Combes, B., Stastny, P., Shorey, J., Eigengrodt, E. H., Barrera, A., Hall, A. R., and Carter, N. W., *Lancet* **2**, 234 (1971).
142. Baker, A., Sidel, J., and Kaplan, M., *Gastroenterology* **60**, 183 (1971).

143. Heathcote, E. J. L., Dudley, F. L., and Sherlock, S., *Gut* **13**, 319 (1972).
144. Sergent, J. S., Lockshin, M. D., Christian, C. L., and Gocke, D. J., *Medicine* **55**, 1 (1976).
145. Duffy, J., Lidsky, M. D., Sharp, J. T., Davis, J. S., Person, D. A., Hollinger, F. B., and Min, K.-W., *Medicine* **55**, 19 (1976).
146. Fye, K. H., Becker, M. J., Theophilopoulos, A. N., Moutsopoulos, H., Feldman, J.-H., and Talal, N., *Am. J. Med.* **62**, 783 (1977).
147. Gocke, D. J., Hsu, K., Morgan, C., Bombardieri, S., Lockshin, M., and Christian, C. L., *J. Exp. Med.* **134**, 330s (1971).
148. Gerber, M. A., Brodin, A., Steinberg, D., Vernace, S., Yang, E. M., and Paronetto, F., *N. Engl. J. Med.* **286**, 14 (1972).
149. Nowoslawski, A., Krawczynski, K., Brzosko, W. J., and Madalinski, K., *Am. J. Pathol.* **68**, 31 (1972).
150. Knieser, M. R., Jenis, E. H., Lowenthal, D. H., Bancroft, W. H., Burns, W., and Shalboub, R., *Arch. Pathol.* **97**, 193 (1974).
151. Ozawa, T., Levisohn, P., Orsini, E., and McIntosh, R. M., *Arch. Pathol. Lab. Med.* **100**, 484 (1976).
152. Brzosko, W. J., Krawczynski, J., Nazarewicz, T., Morzycka, M., and Nowolawski, A., *Lancet* **2**, 477 (1974).
153. Meltzer, M., Franklin, E. C., Elias, K., McCluskey, R. T., and Cooper, N., *Am. J. Med.* **40**, 837 (1966).
154. Asamer, H., Weiser, G., and Michlmayr, G., *Schweiz. Med. Wochenschr.* **105**, 1057 (1975).
155. Holman, H. R., and Kunkel, H. G., *Science* **126**, 162 (1957).
156. Seligmann, M., and Milgrom, F., *C. R. Acad. Sci.* **245**, 1472 (1957).
157. Diecher, H. R., Holman, H. R., and Kunkel, H. G., *J. Exp. Med.* **109**, 97 (1959).
158. Stollar, D., and Levine, L. *J. Immunol.* **87**, 477 (1961).
159. Holman, H. R., and Deicher, H. R., *J. Clin. Invest.* **38**, 2059 (1959).
160. Tan, E. M., *J. Lab. Clin. Med.* **70**, 800 (1967).
161. Tan, E. M., and Kunkel, H. G., *J. Immunol.* **96**, 464 (1966).
162. Holman, H. R., *Ann. N. Y. Acad. Sci.* **124**, 800 (1965).
163. Koffler, D., Agnello, V., Carr, R. I., and Kunkel, H. G., *Am. J. Pathol.* **56**, 305 (1969).
164. Schur, P. H., and Monroe, N., *Proc. Natl. Acad. Sci.* **63**, 1108 (1969).
165. Steinman, C. R., Grishman, E., Spiera, H., and Deesomochok, U., *Am. J. Med.* **62**, 319 (1977).
166. Steinman, C. R., and Ackad, A., *Am. J. Med.* **62**, 693 (1977).
167. Schur, P. H., and Sandson, J., *N. Engl. J. Med.* **278**, 533 (1968).
168. Hanauer, L. B., and Christian, C. L., *J. Clin. Invest.* **46**, 400 (1967).
169. Kohler, P. F., and Ten Bensel, R., *Clin. Exp. Immunol.* **4**, 191 (1969).
170. Ruddy, S., Hunsicker, L. G., Schur, P. H., and Austen, K. F., *J. Clin. Invest.* **51**, 82a (1972).
171. Westberg, N. G., Naff, G. B., Boyer, J. T., and Michael, A. F., *J. Clin. Invest.* **50**, 642 (1971).
172. Carpenter, C. B., Ruddy, S., Shehadeh, I. H., Müller-Eberhard, H. J., Merrill, J. P., and Austen, K. F., *J. Clin. Invest.* **48**, 1495 (1969).
173. Perrin, L. H., Lambert, P. H., and Miescher, P. A., *J. Clin. Invest.* **56**, 165 (1975).
174. Agnello, V., Koffler, D., Elsenberg, J. W., Winchester, R. J., and Kunkel, H. G., *J. Exp. Med.* **134**, 228s (1971).
175. Hadler, N. M., Gerwin, R. D., Rank, M. M., Whitaker, J. N., Baker, M., and Decker, J. L., *Arthritis Rheum.* **16**, 507 (1973).
176. Petz, L. D., Sharp, G. C., Cooper, N. R., and Irvin, W. S., *Medicine* **50**, 259 (1971).
177. Carr, R. I., Harbeck, R. J., Hoffman, A. A., Pirofsky, B., and Bardana, E. J., *J. Rheumatol.* **2**, 184 (1975).
178. Keeffe, E. B., Bardana, E. J., Jr., Harbeck, R. J., Pirofsky, B., and Carr, R. I., *Ann. Intern. Med.* **80**, 58 (1974).
179. Tan, E. M., Schur, P. H., Carr, R. I., and Kunkel, H. G., *J. Clin. Invest.* **45**, 1732 (1966).
180. Koffler, D., Agnello, V., and Kunkel, H. G., *J. Clin. Invest.* **52**, 198 (1973).
181. Harbeck, R. J., Bardana, E. J., Kohler, P. F., and Carr, R. I., *J. Clin. Invest.* **52**, 789 (1973).
182. Bardana, E. J., Jr., Harbeck, R. J., Hoffman, A. A., Pirofsky, B., and Carr, R. I., *Am. J. Med.* **59**, 515 (1975).
183. Levinsky, R. J., Cameron, J. S., and Soothill, J. F., *Lancet* **1**, 564 (1977).
184. Eisenberg, R. A., Theofilopoulos, A. N., and Dixon, F. J., *J. Immunol.* **118**, 1428 (1977).
185. Reichlin, M., and Mattioli, M., *N. Engl. J. Med.* **286**, 908 (1972).

186. Winfield, J. B., Winchester, R. J., Wernef, P., and Kunkel, H. G., *Clin. Exp. Immunol.* **19**, 399 (1975).
187. Stastny, P., and Ziff, M., *N. Eng. J. Med.* **280**, 1376 (1969).
188. Morel-Maroger, L., Mery, J. P., Droz, D., Godin, M., Verroust, P., Kourilsky, O., and Richet, G., *Adv. Nephrol.* **6**, 79 (1976).
189. Cavallo, T., Cameron, W. R., and Lapenas, D., *Am. J. Pathol.* **87**, 1 (1977).
190. Cruchaud, A., Chenais, F., Fournie, G. J., Humair, L., Lambert, P. H., Mulli, J. C., and Chatelanat, F., *Eur. J. Clin. Invest.* **5**, 297 (1975).
191. Gallo, G. R., *Am. J. Pathol.* **61**, 377 (1970).
192. Wilson, C. B., and Dixon, F. J., in *The Kidney* (B. A. Brenner and F. C. Rector, eds.), W. B. Saunders, Philadelphia, 1976, p. 838
193. Baldwin, D. S., and Gallo, G. R., *Clin. Rheum. Dis.* **1**, 639 (1975).
194. Koffler, D., Agnello, V., and Kunkel, H. G., *Am. J. Pathol.* **74**, 109 (1974).
195. Verroust, P. J., Wilson, C. B., Cooper, N. R., Edgington, T. S., and Dixon, E. J., *J. Clin. Invest.* **53**, 77 (1974).
196. Rothfield, N., Ross, H. A., Minta, J. D., and Lepow, I. H., *N. Engl. J. Med.* **287**, 681 (1972).
197. Andres, G. A., Accinni, L., Beiser, S. M., Christian, C. L., Cinotti, G. A., Erlanger, B. F., Hsu, K. C., and Seegal, B. C., *J. Clin. Invest.* **49**, 2106 (1970).
198. Mellors, R. C., and Mellors, J. W., *Proc. Natl. Acad. Sci.* **73**, 233 (1976).
199. Panem, S., Ordenez, N. G., Kirstein, W. H., Katz, A. I., and Spargo, B. H., *N. Engl. J. Med.* **295**, 470 (1976).
200. Gyorkey, F., *N. Engl. J. Med.* **280**, 333 (1969).
201. Pincus, T., Blacklow, N. R., Grimley, P. M., and Bellanti, J. A., *Lancet* **2**, 1058 (1970).
202. Bariety, J., Ricker, D., Appay, M. D., Gossette, J., and Callard, P., *J. Clin. Pathol.* **26**, 24 (1973).
203. Klassen, J., Andres, G. A., Brennan, J. C., and McCluskey, R. T., *Clin. Immunol. Immunopathol.* **1**, 69 (1972).
204. Brentjens, J. R., Sepulveda, M., Baliah, T., Bentzel, C., Erlanger, B. V., Elwood, C., Montes, M., Hsu, K. C., and Andres, G. A., *Kidney Int.* **7**, 342 (1975).
205. Lehman, D. J., Wilson, C. B., and Dixon, F. J., *Am. J. Med.* **58**, 765 (1975).
206. Tan, E. M., and Kunkel, H. G., *Arthritis Rheum.* **9**, 37 (1966).
207. Gilliam, J. N., Cheatum, D. E., Hurd, E. R., Stastny, P., and Ziff, M., *J. Clin. Invest.* **53**, 1434 (1974).
208. Jordan, R. E., Schroeter, A. L., and Winkelmann, R. K., *Br. J. Dermatol.* **92**, 263 (1975).
209. Atkins, C. F., Kondon, J. J., Quismorio, F. P., and Friou, G. J., *Ann. Intern. Med.* **76**, 65 (1972).
210. McIntosh, R. M., and Koss, M. M., *Ann. Intern. Med.* **81**, 111 (1974).
211. Case Records of the Massachusetts General Hospital, Case 2–1976, *N. Engl. J. Med.* **294**, 100 (1976).
212. Jones, J. V., Cumming, R. H., Bucknall, R. C., and Asplin, C. M., *Lancet* **1**, 709 (1976).
213. Rossen, R. D., Reisberg, M. A., Hersh, E. M., and Gutterman, J. U., *Clin. Res.* **24**, 462A (1976).
214. Heimer, R., and Klein, G., *Int. J. Cancer* **18**, 310 (1976).
215. Day, N. K., Winfield, J. B., Gee, T., Winchester, R., Teshima, H., and Kunkel, H. G., *Clin. Exp. Immunol.* **26**, 189 (1976).
216. Samayoa, E. A., McDuffie, F. C., Nelson, A. M., Go, V. L., Luthra, H. S., and Brumfield, H. W., *Int. J. Cancer* **19**, 12 (1977).
217. Long, J. C., Hall, C. L., Brown, C. A., Stamatos, C., Weitzman, S. A., and Laver, K., *N. Engl. J. Med.* **297**, 295 (1977).
218. Pascal, R. R., Iannoccone, P. M., Rollwagen, F. M., Harding, T. A., and Bennett, S. J., *Cancer Res.* **36**, 43 (1976).
219. Egan, J. W., and Lewis, E. J., *Kidney Int.* **11**, 297 (1977).
220. Lewis, M. G., Loughridge, L. W., and Phillips, T. M., *Lancet* **2**, 134 (1971).
221. Couser, W. G., Wagonfeld, J. B., Spargo, B. H., and Lewis, E. J., *Am. J. Med.* **57**, 962 (1974).
222. Costanza, M. E., Pinn, V., Schwartz, R. S., and Nathanson, L., *N. Engl. J. Med.* **289**, 520 (1973).
223. Weksler, M. E., Carey, T., Day, N., Susin, M., Sherman, R., and Becker, C., *Kidney Int.* **6**, 112A (1974).
224. Higgins, M. R., Randall, R. E., and Still, W. J. S., *Br. Med. J.* **3**, 450 (1974).
225. Ozawa, T., Pluss, R., Lacher, J., Boedecker, E., Guggenheim, S., Hammond, W., and McIntosh, R., *Q. J. Med.* **44**, 523 (1975).

226. Soter, N. A., Mihm, M. C., Gigli, I., Dvorak, H. F., and Austen, K. F., *J. Invest. Dermatol.* **66**, 344 (1976).
227. McCluskey, R. T., and Colvin, R. B., *Ann. Rev. Med.* **29**, 191 (1978).
228. Watanabe, I., Whittier, F. C., Moore, J., and Cuppage, F. E., *Arch. Pathol. Lab. Med.* **100**, 632 (1976).
229. Bacon, P. A., Tribe, C. R., Mackenzie, J. C., Verrier-Jones, J., Cummings, R. H., and Amer, B. *Q. J. Med. Neuro Ser.* **45**, 661 (1976).
230. Roman-Franco, A. A., Turiello, M., Albini, B., Ossi, E., Milgrom, F., and Andres, G. A., *Clin. Immunol. Immunopathol.* **9**, 464 (1978).
231. Lachmann, P., *Postgrad. Med. J.* **44**, Suppl. 23 (1968).
232. Kilcoyne, M. M., Daly, J. J., Gocke, D. J., Thompson, G., Meltzer, J. T., Hsu, K. D., and Tannenbaum, M., *Lancet* **1**, 17 (1972).
233. Heymann, W., Hackel, D. B., Harwood, S., Wilson, S. G. F., and Hunter, J. L. P., *Proc. Soc. Exp. Biol. Med.* **100**, 660 (1959).
234. Grupe, W. E., and Kaplan, M. H., *Fed. Proc.* **26**, 573 (1967).
235. Grupe, W. E., and Kaplan, M. H., *J. Lab. Clin. Med.* **74**, 400 (1969).
236. Edgington, T. S., Glassock, R. J., and Dixon, F. J., *J. Exp. Med.* **127**, 555 (1968).
237. Weigle, W. O., and Nakamura, R. M., *Clin. Exp. Immunol.* **4**, 645 (1969).
238. Yoshiki, T., Mellors, R. C., Strand, M., and August, J. T., *J. Exp. Med.* **140**, 1011 (1974).
239. Klassen, J., McCluskey, R. T., and Milgrom, F., *Am. J. Pathol.* **63**, 333 (1971).
240. Naruse, T., Kitamura, K., Miyakawa, Y., and Shibata, S., *J. Immunol.* **110**, 1163 (1973).
241. Whitworth, J. A., Leibowitz, S., Kennedy, M. D., Cameron, J. S., Evans, D. J., Glassock, R. J., and Schoenfeld, L. S., *Clin. Nephrol.* **5**, 159 (1975).
242. Miyakawa, Y., Kitamura, K., Shibata, S., and Naruse, T., *J. Immunol.* **117**, 1203 (1976).
243. Pardo, V., Strauss, J., Kramer, H., Ozawa, T., McIntosh, R. M., *Am. J. Med.* **59**, 650 (1975).
244. Strauss, J., Koss, M., Griswold, W., and McIntosh, R. M., *Ann. Intern. Med.* **81**, 114 (1974).
245. Shwayder, M., Ozawa, T., Boedecker, B. A., Guggenheim, S., and McIntosh, R. M., *Ann. Intern. Med.* **84**, 433 (1976).
246. Ploth, D. W., Fitz, A., Schnetzler, D., Seidenfeld, J., and Wilson, C. B., *Clin. Immunol. Immunopathol.* **9**, 327 (1978).
247. O'Regan, S., Fong, J. S. C., Kaplan, B. S., Chad Revian, J. P., Lapointe, N., and Drummond, K. N., *Clin. Immunol. Immunopathol.* **6**, 341 (1976).
248. West, C. D., *Kidney Int.* **9**, 1 (1976).
249. Berber, J., Yanera, H., Nabarra, B., and Barbanel, C., *Kidney Int.* **7**, 232 (1975).
250. Gelfand, M. D., Frank, M. M., and Green, I., *J. Exp. Med.* **142**, 1029 (1975).
251. Pettersson, E. E., Bhan, A. K., Schneeberger, E, E., Collins, A. B., Colvin, R. B., and McCluskey, R. T., *Kidney Int.* **13**, 245 (1978).

Chapter Twelve

Immunopathology of Rheumatoid Arthritis

NATHAN J. ZVAIFLER AND PHILIP D. GREENBERG

Department of Medicine, University of California, San Diego

It might seem odd, at first, that a book on mechanisms of immunopathology should include a chapter on rheumatoid arthritis. On reflection, however, the reason becomes clear, for perhaps no other human disease displays so many facets of the immune response. Let us cite just a few examples. Loss of tolerance to tissue constituents and proteins is represented by the multiple autoantibodies found in the synovial fluid and circulation. Immune complexes are primarily responsible for inflammation of the articular tissues (synovitis) and the widespread vasculitis occasionally seen in "systemic rheumatoid disease." Lymphocytes fill the congested synovial membrane and directly, or by the factors they elaborate, are responsible for much of the injury to cartilage and other joint tissues. Unique granulation tissues, like the subcutaneous nodule or the pannus that destroys bone and cartilage, are the pathologic hallmarks of rheumatoid arthritis. And, finally, although rheumatoid arthritis still has no known etiology, the importance of immunologic mechanisms in its pathogenesis is persuasively demonstrated by the therapeutic efficacy of immunosuppressive drugs and the dramatic response to lymphocyte depletion by thoracic duct drainage.

THE IMMUNOLOGIC STATUS OF PATIENTS WITH RHEUMATOID ARTHRITIS

As noted in earlier chapters, the lymphocyte occupies a central position in the immune system. It is not surprising, therefore, that lymphocyte numbers and functions would be analyzed in great detail in a disease such as rheumatoid arthritis (RA), which is purported to be immunologically mediated. Several reports have cited normal percentages of T cells in the blood of patients with RA (1,2). Williams et al., using anti-T cell antisera (3), and Zeiders et al., using E rosette formation (4), found normal percentages of T cells, although both noted a tendency for the proportion of T cells to decrease below normal with the development of severe disease activity or vasculitis. Utsinger and Bluestein (5) demonstrated an overall decrease in the absolute number of lymphocytes, as well as a preferential decrease in T cells, associated with increases in disease activity (Table 1). Fröland et al. (6) found an increased percentage of E rosette-forming cells in RA patients, although the normal percentage in their laboratory was considerably lower than in others.

Most investigators have used anti-immunoglobulin antisera to assess the percentage of B cells in peripheral blood. RA patients are generally equivalent to normal controls for these values (1–6), but an increased (7) or decreased (8) percentage of B cells in peripheral blood has been reported. In addition, several studies have noted increased numbers of "null" cells, i.e., cells not identifiable by conventional T and B markers, in patients with RA (2–4).

Since data from peripheral blood analysis have been of only limited usefulness, some investigators have attempted to classify lymphocytes present in synovial effusions. Again the results are conflicting. The percentage of T cells was increased in some studies (6,9). Winchester et al. (10) demonstrated a normal percentage of T cells in RA effusions, but the synovial fluid absolute lymphocytosis resulted in an increase in the total number of T cells as compared to peripheral blood. Large numbers of "null" cells were observed in joints with marked diminution of synovial fluid complement. The percentage of B cells has been variably reported to be increased when measured by EAC rosettes and surface immunoglobulins (8); normal, measured by surface immunoglobulins (9); and decreased, using aggregated IgG receptors and surface immunoglobulins (10).

Thus, when grouped together, the data on T and B lymphocytes in RA are somewhat confusing (11). In general, the percentage of B cells in the blood is normal, whereas that in synovial fluid is quite variable. The percentage of T cells in blood, although often normal, may be decreased, especially in the presence of

Table 1. Lymphocyte Counts in Rheumatoid Arthritis (RA) and Sjögren's Syndrome

	No.[1]	Total[2]	T[3]	B[4]
a. Normal	25	2700±180	1701± 62	694±86
b. Seropositive RA	50	1806±120	1101± 68	452±40
c. Seronegative RA	20	2401±182	1478±101	561±42
d. Sjögren's syndrome	11	2021±139	1197± 89	513±35
a vs. b		$p < .001$	$< .001$	$< .02$
b vs. c		$p < .01$	$< .01$	$< .05$
a vs. c		$p < .05$	$< .02$	$< .05$
a vs. d		$p < .01$	$< .01$	$< .02$

[1]Number of subjects studied—most with more than 2 determinations.
[2]Cells per mm^3 ± SE.
[3]T cells determined as E rosette-forming cells.
[4]B cells determined as immunoglobulin-bearing cells using a polyvalent antiserum.

very active arthritis or in patients with extra-articular manifestations. T cells in synovial fluid are probably increased, if not in percentage, then in absolute numbers.

There are many reasons for the variability in results. Few studies define the criteria used for inclusion of patients, the level of disease activity, or the presence of systemic (extra-articular) rheumatoid disease. Most data are presented only as percentages, and the absolute number of lymphocytes is omitted. The methods used for identifying T and B cells differ among laboratories, as does the normal range for the same detection system. In addition, biologic fluids from RA patients contain substances that introduce important artifacts. For instance, Mellbye et al. (8) showed that the number of normal B lymphocytes identified by EAC rosettes could be sharply reduced by incubating them with rheumatoid synovial fluid, thus increasing the number of "null" cells. Several investigators have demonstrated that RA sera contain warm- and cold-reactive antilymphocyte antibodies which can coat lymphocyte surfaces, potentially increasing the number of B cells identified by anti-immunoglobulin antisera (12,13). It seems likely that progress in this area must await new techniques, similar to those being developed for mouse lymphoid cells, which categorize subpopulations within the T and B cell classes.

In vivo cellular immunity has been evaluated in rheumatoid patients by using skin test reactions to a panel of common antigens (i.e., PPD, streptokinase-streptodornase, mumps virus, and *Candida albicans*), and immunization with compounds such as dinitrochlorobenzene (DNCB) or keyhole limpet hemocyanin (KLH). Although not unanimous, most studies of responses to memory antigens suggest an impairment of delayed hypersensitivity (14–16). Some of the conflict derives from different methods of scoring, such as the time when maximal responses are recorded, or measurement of edema as well as induration. In general, however, the rheumatoid population when compared to matched controls demonstrates a diminution in the total number of indurative responses at 48 hours to a panel of antigens. Waxman et al. (14), using sedimentation rate and rheumatoid factor titers to assess disease activity, suggested that the diminished skin test responsiveness is correlated best with disease duration rather than disease activity. The reason for this disturbance in immune function is uncertain. It has been observed that prolonged stimulation by a single antigen (i.e., in this instance the putative pathogen of RA) can lead to poor responses to other antigens due to antigenic competition (17).

Sensitization of RA patients with new antigens results in normal or somewhat decreased cellular immune responses. Waxman et al. (14) showed that the response to immunization with DNCB was suppressed in RA patients with long-standing disease and correlated with skin test reactivity to a panel of common antigens. Another group, using patients with noninflammatory joint diseases as controls, confirmed this reduction in DNCB responsiveness (16). Others, however, have demonstrated normal reactivity to brucella antigen (18), as well as to DNCB (19). Perhaps, as suggested by Epstein and Jessar, if subtle deficiencies in RA lymphocyte function exist, they will only be identified by titration of the DNCB dose or use of less potent antigens (20).

In vitro function of rheumatoid T cells has been evaluated by mitogen- and antigen-induced blastogenesis and mediator production. The majority of data suggest that the response of RA lymphocytes to phytohemagglutinin (PHA) is identical to, or only slightly less than, that of control lymphocytes (21–23). The problems inherent in these kinds of investigations are illustrated in the studies of Lockshin and his associates. Initially, they noted normal PHA responses in many RA patients, even in the presence of diminished cutaneous delayed hypersensitivity (14). Subsequently, they found that rheumatoid subjects had a diminished PHA responsiveness when compared to healthy subjects, although the responses of the rheumatoid patients were not significantly different from those of comparably ill patients (24). Lymphocytes from some patients with RA have a high spontaneous uptake of ^{3}H-thymidine, and respond poorly to PHA, possibly due to prior commitment to antigen (25). Stimulation with suboptimal doses of PHA sometimes accentuates the abnormal responses. RA lymphocytes transform normally when stimulated by Concanavalin A and pokeweed mitogens (24,26). Preliminary results of in vitro antigenic stimulation of lymphocytes suggest diminished responsiveness (21,27), consistent with in vivo antigen reactivity.

Identification of antigens unique to RA would obviously be important. A number of investigators have studied cellular immunity to IgG because of the well-recognized association of serum antibodies to IgG (rheumatoid factors) in the majority of patients with RA. The results have been contradictory. Three groups of investigators failed to demonstrate transformation of rheumatoid lymphocytes challenged with pooled human IgG, autologous native IgG, or aggregated IgG (28–30). Kinsella, on the other hand, observed lymphocyte transformation to aggregated IgG in 8 of 12 rheumatoid subjects (31). In contrast, results with leukocyte migration inhibition assays have consistently demonstrated a delayed hypersensitivity type of response to IgG in all its forms—autologous, aggregated, or in immune complexes (32–35). The group working with autologous IgG also obtained positive results in some family members of patients with RA, suggesting that the immune response to IgG may be under genetic control (36). Additional evidence for an association of RA with specific immune response genes comes from studies of mixed leukocyte cultures.

The MLC (mixed leukocyte culture) test was developed as an in vitro model for the recognition phase of the homograft reaction. The test is generally constructed to measure the DNA synthetic response of one set of lymphocytes responding to foreign transplantation antigens on a second set of stimulating lymphocytes, pretreated with mitomycin or irradiation to block their own thymidine incorporation. Genetic studies suggest that the lymphocyte surface antigens responsible for stimulation in MLC are coded for by genes in the major histocompatibility complex (MHC), which also code for HLA antigens (37).

RA lymphocytes usually respond and stimulate appropriately in an MLC reaction with normal lymphocytes (38). An early report noting decreased responsiveness was ascribed to an antibody in some RA patients' serum (12,39). Subsequently, it has been confirmed that deficient responses are generally found when both sets of cells are derived from rheumatoid patients (40).

A number of human diseases are correlated with an increased frequency of antigens coded for by the MHC; the most notable rheumatic disease being ankylosing spondylitis with HLA antigen B-27. Studies of inbred mouse strains revealed that immune response genes (dominant genes controlling response to foreign antigens) are coded for in the region of the MHC that also controls expression of MLC antigens. As a result of these observations, a search for correlation between diseases and specific associated MLC antigens was begun. Stastny extensively evaluated MLC typing in patients with RA, and identified a significantly increased frequency of a specific antigen (38). In a subsequent study, after controlling for drug therapy, antilymphocyte antibody, and rheumatoid factor titers, he demonstrated 73% of patients with RA to be poor responders to this MLC antigen and concluded that this was because of a sharing of MLC determinants (41). According to McDevitt and his associates, 40% of RA patients are nonresponders to the MLC antigen DW10, as compared to 10% of controls (42). The implications of these findings are provocative. Pathogenetically, such an association might represent an identity of the MLC antigen with the agent responsible for RA. This could result in the latter's persistence due to failure to recognize it as nonself. Alternatively, there could be a linkage between the MLC antigen and a specific immune response gene. This hypothesis is particularly attractive in autoimmune diseases in which a dominant gene could determine the expression of a deleterious immune response.

In the absence of an in vitro culture system to assay B cell function in humans, attempts to identify B cell defects in RA patients can only be explored indirectly. Most studies are concerned with circulating immunoglobulin levels or antibody responses to immunization. It should be appreciated, however, that deficiencies or excesses could reflect T cell as well as B cell abnormalities, since optimal antibody production by B cells requires effective T-B interaction. Total serum immunoglobulin levels in patients with RA are increased (43,44), but this may well represent the nonspecific stimulatory effect of chronic inflammation, rather than specific hyperreactivity of the humoral immune system. Naturally occurring antibodies, such as the isohemagglutinins (anti-A and anti-B), are not elevated in rheumatoid subjects, but possibly are decreased (45,46). When exogenous antigens, such as *Brucella abortus* or tetanus toxoid, are administered and the specific antibody responses measured, most investigators have noted no marked difference of rheumatoid subjects from normal or matched control groups (18,47–49). Some earlier studies demonstrated increased antibody production in patients with RA (50,51), but the results were not controlled for age and sex differences. Bandilla et al. identified a reduced primary IgM antibody response to relatively weak antigenic stimuli (44), and suggested this might be due to antigenic competition (17). Thus, there is little evidence that rheumatoid patients have a significantly excessive or deficient humoral response to exogenous antigens. On the other hand, the response to endogenous antigens (i.e., autoantibodies to self-antigens such as thyroglobulin) appears to exceed that of age- and sex-matched controls (18).

In conclusion, when all the studies evaluating the functional capacity of the immune system in patients with RA are considered, it appears that there are occasional abnormalities, but no gross aberrances. Unfortunately, subtle but potentially characteristic defects in RA lymphocyte function will not be elucidated without the development of more sophisticated experimental techniques and refinement of study designs. Individual investigations are seldom comparable because of a number of inconsistencies. Parameters of disease activity are often not defined or analyzed, either in study patients or controls. Seropositive (i.e., those with serum rheumatoid factor) and seronegative patients are frequently admixed. Treatment regimens are seldom recorded, despite the knowledge that virtually all drugs used to treat RA can suppress in vitro immune responses such as PHA- and antigen-induced mitogenesis (52,53). Finally, the most important information may only be uncovered by longitudinal analysis of the same patients, but these are the most difficult studies to perform.

THE JOINT IN RHEUMATOID ARTHRITIS

Although systemic in nature, rheumatoid arthritis is primarily a disease characterized by articular inflammation and destruction. It is not surprising, therefore, that the bulk of the investigation in the past decade has focused on the rheumatoid joint. Indeed, because it is an anatomically confined space with a limited capacity for removing reactant materials, the articular cavity has provided a unique opportunity to study acute and chronic inflammation in man. Such investigations have led to the suggestion that rheumatoid joint disease is, at least in part, an extravascular immune complex disease (54). The interaction of antigen and antibody in synovial tissues and fluid initiates the complement sequence, generating a number of biologically active products. Some of these cause increased vascular permeability, allowing an influx of serum proteins and cellular blood elements into the site where the complexes reside. Polymorphonuclear leukocytes are attracted by complement-derived chemotactic factors, and the complexes are attached to their cell surfaces by receptors for IgG and C3. Engulfment follows, with a concomitant release of large quantities of hydrolytic enzymes. It is these lysosomal enzymes that are responsible for much of the inflammation and some of the tissue damage (55).

But immune complexes alone cannot explain all the articular changes in RA. Clearly, both cellular hypersensitivity and granulation tissues play an important role in the proliferative and destructive aspects of rheumatoid joint disease (56). In the interest of clarity, the discussion that follows will divide the joint into its component parts: the lining synovial membrane; the articular cavity and synovial fluid; and the cartilage, ligaments, and tendons. Inflammatory and destructive events will be discussed separately, but the discerning reader will appreciate that they all occur simultaneously, in varying proportions, in different areas of the joint.

The Synovial Membrane

Most observations of the joint lining have been made in chronic and well-established disease. Synovial biopsy specimens taken in the first two months of disease demonstrate evidence of microvascular injury, as manifested by gaps between endothelial cells, extravasation of erythrocytes, small vessel thrombosis, and endothelial cell injury. Polymorphonuclear cells predominate, infiltrating the superficial synovium and perivascular locations. Mononuclear cells are observed in the synovial effusions, which is in direct contrast to the findings later in the disease (57,58).

As time passes, the rheumatoid synovitis becomes more characteristic, demonstrating a hypertrophied, edematous, and inflamed synovial lining surface, protruding into the joint space as slender villous projections. Normally few in number, the lining cells become multilayered, occasionally reaching a depth of 10 to 20 cells with multinucleated giant cells interspersed among them. Most typical, however, is the intense infiltration of the synovium by mononuclear cells, largely lymphocytes and plasma cells. These are frequently collected into aggregates or follicles, particularly around the small blood vessels, but true germinal centers are rarely seen (59,60). The predominant cell in these nodules is a lymphocyte, but about the periphery are typical plasma cells that by immunofluorescent analysis are found to contain deposits of immunoglobulins (61).

Electron micrographs of densely infiltrated areas confirm that the predominant cells are mainly small lymphocytes, less than 5% transformed blast-like cells. In some places, plasma cells are the most numerous; in others (transitional areas), lymphocytes, plasma cells, and a larger percentage of blast cells exist together (62). Fluoresceinated rabbit antihuman T cell antiserum applied to frozen sections of human rheumatoid synovium stains the majority of the cells within the lymphoid infiltrates (63). The technique of cytoadherence, applied to the study of rheumatoid synovial membranes, yields conflicting data. When suspensions of sheep erythrocytes (E) or erythrocytes coated with antibody and the third component of complement (EAC) are layered over frozen serial sections of rheumatoid synovium, these respective T and B lymphocyte markers adhere to areas corresponding to those of lymphoid infiltration. Van Boxel and Paget (64) claim that the major lymphocyte is a T cell, whereas Sheldon and Holborow (65) concluded that B lymphocytes predominate. There is general agreement, however, that the majority of viable lymphocytes extracted from rheumatoid synovial membrane are T cells, and the proportion of B lymphocytes is usually below that of levels normally found in the blood (64,66–68). It remains to be ascertained whether the presence of T lymphocytes results from a nonspecific attraction into an inflammatory focus or a specific response to antigenic materials in the synovium.

There is ample evidence that the rheumatoid synovium contains large amounts of immunoglobulin, much of it locally synthesized (69,70). IgG and IgM, singly or in combination, are regularly demonstrated by immunofluorescence in synovial lining cells, in blood vessels, and in the interstitial connective tissue of the synovial membrane.

The predominant immunoglobulin in the plasma cells in the deeper layers of the membrane is IgG. Munthe and Natvig demonstrated that the IgG within many of these plasma cells had anti-gamma globulin (rheumatoid factor) activity (71). Theoretically, IgG rheumatoid factor is difficult to detect, because it complexes with itself. This problem was circumvented by pepsin digestion of the tissue sections, which removes the antigenic (Fc) portion of the IgG molecule but leaves the reactive F $(ab)_2$ fragments intact. Before pepsin treatment, there was no binding of fluorescein-labeled aggregated IgG to the plasma cells, but afterward, binding to a large proportion of the IgG-containing cells was observed. Native IgG blocked the reaction, but it was not abolished by reduction and alkylation of the aggregated IgG, implying that these were true anti-IgG reactions. The results were similar in tissues from either seronegative or seropositive patients—namely, 20 to 60% of the IgG plasma cells showed anti-gamma globulin activity (71). It thus appears that plasma cells in the rheumatoid synovium make an IgG rheumatoid factor that combines with similar IgG molecules ("self-associating IgG") within the cell. Although these complexes do not activate or bind complement within the plasma cell cytoplasm, they might have important complement-fixing activities after secretion from the cells. It is somewhat surprising to note, however, that the results obtained are similar in patients with seronegative and seropositive joint disease, since the latter are generally accepted to have more aggressive and destructive arthritis and more profound intra-articular complement consumption. Perhaps a better understanding of the antibodies from the remaining 40 to 50% of IgG-producing plasma cells or the role of IgM rheumatoid factors will shed light on these differences.

The Articular Cavity and Synovial Fluid

Normal synovial fluid has been characterized as a dialysate of plasma to which hyaluronate has been added (73). In the normal joint the amount and type of protein are carefully regulated. Plasma proteins with a high molecular weight or asymmetrical shape, such as fibrinogen, are not detected in normal synovial fluid. However, synovial inflammation permits introduction of increased amounts of both large- and small-molecular-weight proteins into the synovial fluid.

Proteins of the complement system have been studied in detail because of the observation that complement levels in RA effusions are significantly lower than in companion serum samples or synovial fluids from other forms of inflammatory joint disease (74,75), suggesting local activation by immune complexes. Subsequent investigations focused on the complement proteins because of their potential as mediators of articular inflammation.

According to current understanding, the complement system is comprised of a group of serum proteins whose sequential interaction generates a number of biologically important factors. Most of these are derived from the terminal components (C5–C9). Activation of the terminal portion of the sequence can be accomplished by at least two discrete mechanisms. The first, known as the "classical pathway," is initiated by the binding of C1 through its C1q subunit to a site on the Fc portion of IgM or most IgG molecules. Binding of C1 results in its conversion to an enzyme whose two natural substrates are the fourth (C4) and second (C2) complement components. Their interaction causes the formation of a new bimolecular complex of fragments of C2 and C4 ($\overline{\text{C4b, 2a}}$), which becomes membrane-bound and is capable of cleaving the third component (C3), and subsequently activates the terminal components (76).

Another pathway has recently been recognized that can bypass the early components and leads directly to the cleavage of C3. This "alternate pathway" (or properdin system) is readily activated by complex polysaccharides, such as inulin or zymosan; bacterial lipopolysaccharides or endotoxin; some immune complexes; aggregates of IgA; and a "nephritic factor" isolated from serum of patients with chronic membranoproliferative glomerulonephritis. The known components of this pathway include a recently described initiating factor (related to nephritic factor); properdin; factor D or C3 proactivator convertase

(C3PAse); factor A, which is probably native C3; and factor B or C3 proactivator (C3PA). The precise mechanisms involved in the alternate pathway are still being defined, but it appears to include an activating substance and the assembly of a C3 converting enzyme from the interaction of initiating factor, factor B, factor D, native C3, and magnesium. The C3 converting enzyme deposits C3b on the surface of the activating substance, where it combines with factor B to form an exceedingly labile enzyme ($\overline{C3b, B}$) with C3 and C5 convertase activity. Properdin appears to act by stabilizing this enzyme (77).

A summary of the findings for the various complement components in rheumatoid synovial fluids is shown in Table 2. In the majority of RA joint fluids, the C1 hemolytic activity is not significantly reduced (78), but inferential evidence for the activation of C1 comes from the observation of a parallel reduction of its two natural substrates, C4 and C2. Ruddy and Austen found that the mean C4 hemolytic activity per gram of synovial fluid protein of seropositive RA patients was 700 ± 200 units as compared to 4300 ± 500 units in fluids from seronegative patients and 7800 ± 1100 units in fluids from patients with degenerative arthritis. Measurement of synovial fluid C2 activity yielded analogous results (78). C3 levels in synovial fluids are generally decreased proportional to total hemolytic complement (78–80). The reduction of these early complement components is what would be expected if there was activation of the classical pathway by aggregated gamma globulin or immune complexes.

There is also evidence of activation of the alternate complement pathway in rheumatoid synovial fluids. The average C3PA concentration in the effusions of seropositive rheumatoid arthritis patients is significantly less than in the fluids from patients with infectious arthritis or nonrheumatoid inflammatory joint disease (54). Ruddy et al. found a similar reduction of factor B concentration and properdin levels in seropositive RA joint fluids (81). Immunoelectrophoretic evidence of C3A was found in three of nine RA effusions and three of six joint fluids from patients with infectious arthritis, but was absent from nine other fluids of patients with inflammatory nonrheumatoid arthritis and disorders in the osteoarthritis group. Addition of inulin to rheumatoid fluids to test for

Table 2. Complement Components Identified in Rheumatoid Synovial Fluids

Protein	Levels[a]
C1	N or ↓
C4	↓↓
C2	↓
C3	↓
C9	N or ↓
$C\overline{567}$	P
C5a	P
C1 INH	N
C3 PA	↓
C3 A	P
C3d	P
C4α	P

[a]N = normal, expected amount; ↓ = decreased, less than expected; P = present.

residual alternate pathway activity caused no conversion of C3PA to C3A, whereas it did cause this in fluids from other joint diseases (54).

Reaction products from the terminal components of the complement sequence have been identified in rheumatoid synovial fluids. Cleavage products of C3b have been detected by immunoelectrophoresis in synovial fluids from patients with a variety of joint diseases, but a significant correlation exists between their presence and the diagnosis of RA, particularly seropositive RA (79,80). Approximately two-thirds of rheumatoid synovial fluids contain substances that are chemotactic for granulocytes: a macromolecular complex (C567) and a low-molecular-weight cleavage product of C5 (C5a) (82). Finally, the suggestion that the complement sequence goes to completion is supported by the finding of a relative depletion of C9. Serum levels of C9 are increased almost twice normal in patients with both seropositive and seronegative RA; however, the synovial fluid C9 levels of seronegative patients are significantly higher than those from seropositive patients (83).

Do rheumatoid effusions contain immune complexes, and what is their relationship to complement depletion? Almost coincident with the finding of depressed complement in rheumatoid joint fluids, Hollander and his associates reported that these effusions contained white blood cells whose cytoplasm was filled with numerous dense particles (84). Immunofluorescent staining disclosed that they were composed, at least in part, of immunoglobulins and complement components. IgG and C3 were present in phagocytic cells from both seronegative and seropositive effusions, whereas IgM and anti-gamma globulin inclusions were limited to cells from the joints of seropositive RA patients. Generally, the representation of a single complement component within the inclusion is inversely proportional to its concentration in the accompanying fluid (85) (Table 3).

Synovial fluids also contain an ill-defined material called rheumatoid biologically active factor (RBAF) that releases histamine from perfused guinea pig lungs; this is a recognized property of immune complexes. RBAF-positive fluids have a lower mean complement level (35.7 ± 3.9 units) than the RBAF-negative

Table 3. Correlates of Depressed Synovial Fluid Complement

Granulocyte Inclusions	
IgM	+
C components	+
Anti-IgG	+
Immune Complexes	
IgG-anti-IgG (7S)	+
IgG-anti-IgG (19S)	?
DNA-anti-DNA	+
sNP-anti-sNP	?
Cryoprecipitates	+
RBAF	+

ones (57 ± 7.3, $p < 0.01$); this finding is consistent with the observation that RBAF in synovial fluid is associated with complement-fixing activity (86).

A number of other techniques have directly demonstrated immune complexes in joint fluids. These include analytical ultracentrifugation (87), sodium sulfate fractionation (88), cryoprecipitation (89–91), and precipitation with either C1q (92) or polyclonal or monoclonal rheumatoid factors (87,88,93). Hannestad made the original observation that a precipitate formed when certain rheumatoid synovial fluids were reacted in gel with sera containing high titers of IgM rheumatoid factor. He suggested that the reactant material behaved like aggregated IgG (94). Winchester and his associates found similar complexes to be composed of IgG rheumatoid factor and autologous IgG and noted a direct relationship between the amount of IgG-anti-IgG complexes in the joint fluid and the decrease in total hemolytic complement (87,88). Precipitation of these complexes with C1q did not require participation of IgM rheumatoid factor. On the other hand, addition of serum from patients with seropositive RA to joint fluids containing IgG complexes enhanced the anticomplementary effect of the joint fluid, suggesting that the serum IgM rheumatoid factor increased complement consumption.

Deoxyribonucleic acid and soluble nucleoprotein are regularly found in exudates from all inflamed joints. This prompted speculation that nuclear antigens, derived from disintegrating granulocytes, might complex with antinuclear antibodies to aggravate or perpetuate the articular inflammation (95). Support for this idea comes from the observation that 8 of 31 (26%) rheumatoid synovial fluids contained antibody to nuclear antigens, as compared to only 1 of 23 inflammatory nonrheumatoid effusions (96).

RA fluids contain large amounts of cold-precipitable (4°C) proteins; these are seldom found in other inflammatory joint effusions. The cryoprecipitates consist, in the main, of immunoglobulins—predominantly IgG and IgM—complement components, and fibrinogen or fibrin degradation products. Deoxyribonucleic acid has been detected in the majority (89,90). Cryoprecipitates can fix complement and contain anti-gamma globulin antibody, predominantly of the IgM class, and show antinuclear activity (90,91). Marcus and Townes studied solubilized cryoprecipitates by sucrose density gradient ultracentrifugation and found anticomplementary activity in fractions heavier than 19S. These same fractions contained variable amounts of DNA and rheumatoid factor, but the complement fixation appeared distinct from the anti-gamma globulin activity (89).

A number of other antibodies of potential pathogenetic significance have been recognized in inflammatory joint effusions. They are of interest because their antigens are constituents of articular tissues or by-products of the inflammatory process. These include antibodies to collagen, cartilage, fibrinogen and fibrin degradation products, and partially digested IgG (pepsin agglutinators) (91). Evidence that they are present more often in RA effusions is lacking.

Immunoglobulins and complement components have been demonstrated in hyaline articular cartilage and menisci from 90% of patients with classical seropositive RA and 67% of seronegative patients (97). The authors have proposed that such immune complexes are sequestered in a location where their gradual release acts as a chronic inflammatory stimulus. These observations are of interest in light of Henson's finding that neutrophils encountering minute amounts of immune complexes along a nonphagocytosable surface discharge lysosomal enzymes despite an inability to ingest the complexes (98). Thus, neutrophils could be continually discharging their enzymes in proximity to articular cartilage in response to sequestered complexes that cannot be removed by conventional phagocytic mechanisms. It remains to be determined whether this situation is peculiar to RA or is a generalized phenomenon contributing to all chronic synovitis.

Since the synovial membrane in RA is heavily populated by lymphocytes, plasma cells, and mononuclear cells, it is not surprising that substances produced by sensitized lymphocytes are present in rheumatoid synovial effusions. These factors, collectively known as lymphokines, affect the behavior of other cells (see Chapters 4 and 5). There are factors in the fluid that lead to the accumulation and stimulation of macrophages, and factors that act on lymphocytes to cause them to proliferate and differentiate (99,100). Addition of synovial fluids or supernatants from cultures of rheumatoid synovial tissues causes human peripheral blood lymphocytes to synthesize immunoglobulins (101). It is not clear that this B cell stimulating factor is derived exclusively from T cells, because it is known that antigen-antibody complexes can induce blastic transformation. The significance of these observations, therefore, awaits further characterization of the factors with reference to known lymphokines generated in vitro, and the demonstration that these by-products of lymphocyte activation are limited to rheumatoid joint fluids. Of interest, however, is the observation that an experimental arthritis of rabbits can be produced by the intra-articular injection of lymphokine-containing fluids (102).

Cartilage and Other Articular Connective Tissues

Whereas there is a consensus that the acute inflammatory phase of rheumatoid arthritis results from immune reactions, there is less agreement about the mechanisms responsible for the chronic proliferative lesions leading to the destruction of cartilage, bone, and periarticular structures. An appreciation of the characteristics of the tissues involved is helpful in understanding this process.

Cartilage and other articular connective tissues are comprised primarily of a ground substance (proteoglycans) and collagen. The former consists of repeating disaccharide subunits linked covalently to a protein core. Initial evidence of injury to cartilage is a loss of metachromatic staining because of a leaching out of the proteoglycans (103). Cartilage that has lost ground substance has a diminished capacity to resist deformation and is at risk for permanent damage through mechanical disruption. Proteoglycan loss is reversible, and complete recovery is possible. But once collagen, which forms the structural skeleton, is lost, cartilage disintegration becomes irreversible (104).

In RA the cartilage appears to be injured by a dual process, from without by enzymes in the synovial fluid and from above and below by granulation tissue. A number of potentially damaging enzymes released from phagocytic synoviocytes and polymorphonuclear leukocytes are in the fluid that continually bathes the cartilage surfaces. These include acid and neutral proteases that can split proteoglycan from its protein matrix and collagenases (105–107). Collagen, when in its triple helical configuration, resists degradation by nonspecific proteases. However, specific collagenases derived from polymorphonuclear leukocytes and rheumatoid synovial cells can cleave the collagen polypeptide chains into two fragments, exposing them to further degradation by proteolytic enzymes (108). Both the collagenolytic and proteolytic enzymes are active at neutral pH and body temperature. The observation of proteoglycan depletion and cartilage injury at sites distant from the advancing margin of the proliferating synovial membrane (see below) is additional confirmation of the importance of enzymes derived from white blood cells (103).

An important feature of the pathology of rheumatoid arthritis is the formation of pannus, a vascular granulation tissue composed of proliferating fibroblasts, numerous small blood vessels, and variable numbers of inflammatory cells (59,60). This aggressive material seems to be responsible for the ultimate destruction of joints in rheumatoid arthritis. Studies of early RA lesions show proliferation of synovial lining cells beginning at the joint margin where periosteum, perichondrium, and synovium attach (57,60). As the disease progresses, pannus spreads and begins to adhere to the cartilage surface. Three types have been described (109). The first, a cellular pannus, has the appearance of synovium and infiltrates the cartilage with proliferating blood vessels and perivascular mononuclear cells. Collagen and proteoglycans seem to be dissolved in the region immediately surrounding the nests of cells. A second type of pannus resembles a granulation tissue composed of monocytic cells and fibroblasts. Multiple filopodia extend from these cells into the cartilage matrix, and degradation proceeds around them. Another variety of pannus is composed of a dense avascular, acellular, fibrous tissue tightly adherent to cartilage.

It seems likely that the first type of pannus, which has the appearance of an "activated" synovial membrane, produces cartilage destruction by enzymatic degradation (108,109). The second, "cellular" form of pannus may operate in the same way, but its similarity to granulation tissue seen at other sites of injury suggests the alternate possibility that this cellular and fibrous infiltrate is the result of cartilage injury, rather than the cause. The third type of pannus probably acts as a mantle interfering with cartilage nutrition (60). Although the three types of pannus can be found simultaneously in the same joint, it is not clear whether they represent a sequential phenomenon or each develops independently.

THE IMMUNOPATHOLOGY OF THE EXTRA-ARTICULAR MANIFESTATIONS OF RHEUMATOID ARTHRITIS

Although characteristically a joint disease, RA can affect a number of other tissues. Lesions of the nerves, heart, lung, and eyes have long been recognized. These extra-articular manifestations probably occur with considerable frequency, but are usually occult and of limited clinical significance. Occasionally, however, the extra-articular events dominate the clinical picture. Terms like "rheumatoid disease" and "malignant rheumatoid arthritis" have been used to describe this form of the illness. Two pathologic features account for most of the tissue lesions—namely, vascular injury and rheumatoid nodules. Evidence that at least a portion of these lesions is caused by immune complexes will be reviewed in this section.

A spectrum of vascular lesions accompanies RA. The majority are "silent" and are only discovered at postmortem examination. They take many forms: capillaritis and venulitis, felt to be important in the development of rheumatoid nodules and synovitis; a bland intimal proliferation commonly affecting digital and mesenteric vessels; subacute lesions of arterioles and venules in scattered locations; and, finally, an acute, widespread, necrotizing arteritis of small- and medium-sized arteries that may, at times, be indistinguishable from polyarteritis nodosa. The most severe form of rheumatoid vasculitis, designated "rheumatoid arteritis," characteristically produces polyneuropathy, skin necrosis and ulceration, digital gangrene, and visceral infarction (110). It may present in an explosive fashion and terminate in death after a few weeks or months.

Fortunately, the full-blown picture is rare, but any of the above manifestations can appear insidiously, over a period of months to years, and pose little threat to life. When present, the neuropathy takes the form of an acute sensorimotor mononeuritis (mononeuritis multiplex) with foot or wrist drop and a patchy sensory loss in one or more extremities (111). Ischemic skin lesions appear in crops as small brown spots, not unlike splinter hemorrhages, in the nail beds, nail folds, and digital pulp. Large ischemic ulcerations can develop in the lower extremities, particularly over the malleoli. Fatal intestinal and myocardial infarctions have been reported. Patients with the acute form of rheumatoid arteritis are commonly febrile, sometimes with temperatures to 104°F or more, and polymorphonuclear leukocytosis is common. Many will have concomitant episcleritis, scleromalacia, pleuritis, myocarditis, and/or pericarditis. The prognosis for life in the fulminant form of vasculitis is exceedingly poor, and the terminal picture is usually complicated by the superimposition of malnutrition, infection, congestive heart failure, and/or gastrointestinal bleeding.

The cause of the various vascular lesions and their relationship to one another has not been defined, but a number of observations suggest that they result from injury induced by immune complexes, especially those containing antibodies to IgG. These include: (1) the generally held view that patients with the largest amount of serum IgM rheumatoid factor have more systemic manifestations of the disease (112,113); (2) the correlation of depressed serum hemolytic complement activity, decreased concentration of several components (C4, C2), and hypercatabolism of C3 with the clinical signs of vasculitis (113–115); and (3) immunofluorescent deposits of IgG, IgM, and complement (C3) in the vasonervorum of patients with rheumatoid neuropathy, and immunoglobulins and rheumatoid factor in vessel walls of vasculitis patients (116).

Immune complex-like materials were identified in the circulation of patients with RA as early as 1957. Kunkel and his associates demonstrated, by analytical ultracentrifugation, a high-molecular-weight material (22S) in the serum of rheumatoid patients. Acid or 6M urea dissociation revealed 7S and 19S components, with the latter containing anti-Ig activity (117). Subsequently, the same workers demonstrated large amounts of unusual gamma globulin complexes with sedimentation rates ranging from 9S to 17S in patients with advanced RA

(118). These complexes, which are readily dissociated to 7S units, have been designated as "intermediate complexes."

A precise definition of the role of these presumed complexes in the pathogenesis of RA was not possible because of the lack of sensitive, reproducible, quantitative methods. Some of these problems have recently been obviated by the development of a number of techniques for accurately measuring complexes.

Winchester et al. first showed that monoclonal IgM rheumatoid factors can be used to demonstrate small complexes or aggregates of IgG in the serum of approximately 50% of patients with RA (87). This method detects aggregates that escape precipitation by polyclonal rheumatoid factors or C1q. A radioimmunoassay based on the ability of test samples to inhibit the interaction of iodinated aggregated IgG with monoclonal rheumatoid factor detected immune complex-like material in the serum of 12 of 51 (27%) RA patients examined, and correlates with more severe disease, greater functional impairment, and more advanced joint destruction. Serum C4 levels were inversely correlated with the amount of inhibiting material, but no relationship existed with rheumatoid factor titers. Three-fourths of the patients had extra-articular manifestations, including Sjögren's syndrome, leg ulcers, Felty's syndrome, neuropathy, and pulmonary fibrosis (93).

A sensitive assay for soluble antigen-antibody complexes is their capacity to liberate histamine from the perfused guinea pig lung. The histamine-releasing activity found in RA serum is removed by antisera to human IgG, but not IgA or IgM. Activity persists following reduction and alkylation, and unlike conventional complexes, is not completely dissociable at low pH (119). Broder et al. named this soluble, complex-like material rheumatoid biologically active factor (RBAF) and found it in the serum of 38 of 127 (30%) carefully studied patients with RA. RBAF is correlated with disease activity and impaired function, and there is an overall statistical correlation of its presence with a composite of extra-articular manifestations of RA, although no one feature (e.g., arteritis, neuropathy, etc.) is present with increased frequency in these patients. Rheumatoid factor titers and RBAF are not correlated (119,120).

Quantitative cryoprecipitation of sera from an unselected group of 38 patients with RA revealed that 12 (31%) had significant amounts of cryoglobulins. Two-thirds of the cryoprecipitable protein was composed of IgG and IgM, with the relative amount of IgM to IgG greater than found in serum. Complement components were detected in six precipitates and antinuclear antibody in seven (121). Systemic vasculitis, present in three of the original 38 patients, was associated with the largest amount of cryoglobulin. Subsequently, five more patients with vasculitis were studied, all of whom had detectable cryoglobulins (122). Their immunologic characteristics are shown in Table 4. The cryoglobulin IgG and IgM were polyclonal. Density gradient analysis demonstrated the majority of the cryoglobulin antiglobulin activity to reside in the 19S IgM fraction. A monoclonal rheumatoid factor did not detect 7S-anti-IgG complexes in the cryoprecipitates, but acid eluates from some cryoglobulins absorbed with insoluble IgG revealed an antiglobulin of the IgG class. Serial studies performed on vasculitis patients treated with cyclophosphamide disclosed a close relationship between clinical evidence of vasculitis and the presence of cryoglobulins. The

Table 4. Immunologic Characteristics of Patients with Rheumatoid Vasculitis

	Cryoglobulins							Serum		
Patient	Protein mg/ml	IgG mg/ml	IgM mg/ml	C1q[a]	C3[a]	ANA[b]	Anti-globulins[c]	Anti-globulins[c]	ANA[b]	C3 (mg/100 ml)
D.A.	0.66	0.125	0.50	+	0	0	512	160	<10	180
M.H.	0.19	0.12	0.08	0	+	0	160	2,560	<10	140
L.T.	0.61	0.165	0.22	0	0	0	160	640	50	92
W.H.	0.30	0.10	0.11	0	0	0	10	320	10	155
J.S.	0.32	0.14	0.08	+	+	4	40	2,560	400	120
R.M.	0.52	0.27	0.15	0	0	0	80	5,120	10	120
J.S.	0.21	0.08	0.03	+	+	0	40	10,240	10	105
D.M.	0.15	0.07	0.05	0	0	0	40	2,560	<10	120

[a]Recorded as present (+) or absent (0).
[b]Reciprocal of antinuclear antibody titer.
[c]Reciprocal of bentonite flocculation titer.
Source: Weisman and Zvaifler (122).

findings were interpreted as evidence that the widespread vascular complications of RA are mediated, at least in part, by circulating immune complexes (122).

Other forms of rheumatoid factor have been described in the rheumatoid vasculitis. Theofilopoulous and his associates (123) detected IgG rheumatoid factor in 10 of 15 (67%) patients with rheumatoid vasculitis, but in only 3 of 33 without vasculitis. Eighty percent of the vasculitis patients also had 7S IgM in their serum, whereas only 18% of the nonvasculitis patients had this unusual immunoglobulin. Stage and Mannik also found an increased frequency of 7S IgM in vasculitis patients (124).

In summary, it appears that one-quarter to one-third of patients with RA have circulating soluble complexes detectable by a variety of techniques. Anti-gamma globulins of the IgG and IgM classes and IgG are integral parts of these soluble complexes. The presence of these materials seems to correlate with the severity of RA and the presence of extra-articular manifestations, in particular, vasculitis. Whether they are responsible for these changes, or are merely markers for severe rheumatoid disease, remains a moot question.

THE SIGNIFICANCE OF IgM RHEUMATOID FACTORS

Rheumatoid factors (RF) are generally defined as a group of antibodies with specificity for antigens located in the Fc portion of IgG. As originally described, RF was a 19S IgM antibody, but subsequently anti-IgG activity has been shown in IgG, IgA, and in low-molecular-weight (7S) IgM also. The significance of IgG-anti-IgGs in the circulation and the joint space is discussed at length elsewhere in this chapter. An understanding of the 19S IgM antibody is important, however, because it is the antibody detected in most conventional tests for RF and because its presence in the serum is a hallmark for RA. This section, therefore, will examine some of the information on the formation and potential biologic significance of this class of RF.

Theoretically, RF might develop as (1) a nonspecific response to synovitis or vasculitis or (2) a secondary response to whatever causes RA (i.e., like antibody to cardiolipin in syphilis); or (3) RF is a direct result of the primary etiologic events and may mediate the pathogenesis of the disease (analogous to Rh antibodies and erythroblastosis fetalis) (125). There is little evidence to support the first suggestion, and the presence of otherwise typical RA in some patients who are seronegative (negative serologic tests for RF) speaks against it. The other possibilities cannot be excluded until we know the cause of RA. None of these theories, however, addresses the question of why patients with RA develop antibodies to a normal constituent of plasma (IgG). The answer to that question is important, not only for RA, but for a number of human diseases. Similar antibodies are present in the serum of persons with liver disease, Sjögren's syndrome, SBE, syphilis, infectious hepatitis, infectious mononucleosis, a number of viral illnesses, leishmaniasis, schistosomiasis, trypanosomiasis, sarcoidosis, tuberculosis, leprosy, cancer, myocardial infarction, and many others. The common immunologic feature that most of these diseases share with RA is chronic antigenic stimulation and/or the presence of immune complexes in the circulation. This is consistent with the experimental models for studying the production of RF. In the classic experiments of Abruzzo and Christian, prolonged immunization of rabbits with dead *Escherichia coli* resulted in the formation of a 19S RF (126,127). Rabbits chronically stimulated with ferritin or enzyme-treated autologous gamma globulin produce 7S and 19S rheumatoid factor (128). Although repetitive immunization with ferritin alone is effective, higher titers of RF are obtained if ferritin-antibody complexes are injected. Therefore, both clinical and experimental data suggest that RF is generated as a normal response to an IgG that has complexed with its specific antigen.

The mechanism by which autologous IgG is recognized as immunogenic remains a source of controversy. Because RF binds more avidly to IgG altered by heat aggregation or complexed with antigen than to native IgG, it is generally assumed that the stimulus for RF production is the recognition of new determinants created by alteration of the molecule. However, the affinity of some RFs for native, autologous Fc domains implies that other mechanisms are operative (129,130). An alternative explanation of the preference of RF for aggregated IgG comes from observations on polyvalent antigen-antibody interactions. In the case of IgM RF, there are five binding sites per molecule, and aggregated immunoglobulin would have multiple antigenic determinants. Theoretically, simultaneous interaction of more than one antibody and antigenic site on the same particle would result in an appreciable increase in the overall binding affinity of the reaction (131). Thus, RF should prefer to bind to aggregates rather than monomeric IgG. Indeed, when monomeric (7S) subunits of RF or Fab fragments of monovalent RF are used to eliminate the contribution of polyvalency, there is a similar binding to monomeric and polymeric (aggregated) IgG (132,133). This implies that the development of new IgG determinants is not necessary.

These findings may also bear on the induction of RF. Presumably there are lymphocytes with an IgM-RF receptor. Ordinarily, these receptors would only bind weakly to the antigenic determinants on monomeric, autologous IgG molecules. Exposure of the receptor to aggregates or antigen-antibody complexes, however, would result in high-affinity polyvalent interactions, binding to the cell membrane, and the stimulation of anti-IgG production (133). If RF is an antibody to a normal ("self") protein, then its induction might occur through an abrogation of immunologic tolerance. Presumably, clones of B cells with specificity for autologous native Fc sites exist, but are nonoperative because of tolerant T cells. Examples of tolerance limited to T cells have been demonstrated for a multiplicity of antigens (134). Therefore, the production of RF would require either (1) a source of T cell cooperation or (2) that the IgG be presented directly to B cells as a T-independent antigen. Conceivably, an antigen-antibody complex might serve as a hapten-carrier conjugate with the T cell recognizing either the antigen or the antigen plus the antibody-combining site as foreign and cooperating with a B cell recognizing the Fc portion of the IgG. Alternatively, polyvalent immune complexes may be capable of eliciting a T-independent B cell response. B cells with receptors for aggregated IgG or immune complexes are well known (134). Both postulated mechanisms require that native IgG behave as neither an immunogen nor a tolerogen, which is consistent with the observed low affinity of RF for native as compared to aggregated or complexed IgG.

What would be the benefit to the host of an antibody that reacts with immune complexes? Presumably, the attachment of IgM molecules to such complexes would increase their size, decrease their solubility, and enhance their elimination from the bloodstream (135). Thus, RF could be viewed as a host response aimed at minimizing the potentially harmful effects of circulating antigen-antibody complexes. The association of high titers of IgM RF with many of the systemic features of RA would, at first glance, be inconsistent with such a protective role for RF. In these circumstances, however, we may be observing instances in which the protective mechanism is overwhelmed. High titers of RF may merely reflect an excessive immunologic stimulus, i.e., large amounts of immune complexes. The finding of circulating immune complexes in most patients with rheumatoid vasculitis is consistent with this view. On the other hand, IgM RF is clearly associated with detrimental effects on the joints in RA. This apparent contradiction is probably best explained by anatomic considerations. In the articular cavity, large, insoluble complexes can only be removed by phagocytic mechanisms with the resultant release of lysosomal enzymes into an anatomically confined space; whereas in the circulation, the same complexes would be efficiently eliminated by the reticuloendothelial system.

The possibility that RF is beneficial under some circumstances and harmful in others is not surprising when one considers the remarkable diverse effects that RF has on a number of in vitro immunologic reactions. This is most impressive with reactions that depend on the Fc region of the IgG molecules. Complement fixation by IgG antibodies, for example, can be either enhanced or decreased by IgM RF, depending on reaction temperatures, the order of addition of reagents, or the amount of IgG (136–138). RF interferes with opsonization of bacteria (139), but has variable effects on complement-mediated phagocytosis of antibody-coated erythrocytes (140) or antigen-antibody complexes by polymorphonuclear leukocytes (141–142). In contrast, when joint fluids from seronegative RA patients are incubated with normal white blood cells, no cytoplasmic inclusions are detected. But following the addition of isolated IgM rheumatoid factors, discrete cytoplasmic inclusions develop that stain for IgG, IgM, and C3 (143). Similarly, RF generally inhibits antibody-dependent cell-mediated cytotoxicity (ADCC) reactions, presumably by combining with antibody and blocking access to the Fc receptor of the effector (killer) cell (144). Incubation of the effectors with RF before their addition to target cells, however, results in a remarkable enhancement of killing (145). Thus, if RF has pathogenetic significance in vivo, then its expression will probably vary from time to time under different conditions in various locations, even in the same person.

The occurrence of RF in serum from patients with viral diseases has been alluded to. Recent evidence suggests that this is more than just a response to complexes of viral antigen and antibodies. RF may have a more specific biologic function, namely viral protection. In some circumstances, the attachment of antibody to virus does not result in neutralization of the virus. Thus, persistent infectious virus-antibody complexes are regularly found in the circulation of several laboratory animal models (i.e., New Zealand mice, Aleutian mink) with disorders that mimic human diseases. This is also true for some primate viruses, such as vaccinia and herpes simplex. In vitro neutralization of these infective complexes can be accomplished by addition of IgM RF and the first few components of complement, whereas complement alone is insufficient (146–148). In contrast, RF can interfere with complement-mediated immune lysis of vaccinia virus-infected cells (149).

Reports of the effect of RF on tumor immunity are now beginning to appear. The cytotoxicity of human lymphoid cells on ovarian carcinoma target cells is inhibited by RF (150). This is best explained if target lysis is generated by ADCC and the RF is reacting with the tumor-specific antibody. Extensive investigations by the Hellstroms (151) and others have shown that in vitro tumor-specific immunity is inhibited in vivo by serum blocking factors. These circulating factors are felt to represent free antigen and antigen-antibody complexes. Preliminary clinical data suggest that recurrences of bladder cancer are positively correlated with RF titer and serum blocking activity (152). Although this, too, could represent inhibition of an ADCC mechanism, an alternative explanation is that the RF titer reflects the quantity of circulating complexes, and that it is these that are responsible for blocking activity. If this were true, RF could be of potential benefit in tumor immunity by enhancing elimination of complexes. Of interest is the observation that death from cancer is significantly less in RA patients than in control populations (153). Furthermore, RF might be important in the neutralization of oncogenic viruses, since infectious virus-antibody complexes have been identified in murine sarcoma and leukemia (154).

Before concluding, we suggest that it must be recognized that any theory proposing that the stimulus for RF formation is immune complexes must deal with the fact that some diseases have circulating complexes and relatively little IgM RF. Wager, in reviewing serology from 27 patients with systemic lupus erythematosus (SLE) (155), remarked on the generally low titer of RF, as compared to patients with RA, and hypothesized (as others have before) that this is, in part, responsible for the dramatic systemic manifestations of SLE. Why patients with SLE do not often develop an IgM RF response is unclear, although Bokisch and co-workers, in evaluating RF production in rabbits, demonstrated that a complex relationship between the animal's genetic background and the immunizing antigen ultimately determines whether or not rheumatoid factors are produced (156,157). Although the aggressiveness of SLE in the absence of RF conforms well with the notion of a protective role of RF, the benignity of a disease such as hypergammaglobulinemic purpura, with associated circulating immune complexes and absent IgM RF, is puzzling. Because the pathogenicity and fate of immune complexes are dependent on a multitude of factors, such as valency of the antigen, degree of lattice formation of the complex, subclass of IgG, ability to bind C1q, etc., it will only be when more information about these factors is available that we will begin to understand how they stimulate the production of RF.

REFERENCES

1. Micheli, A., and Bron, J., *Ann. Rheum. Dis.* **33**, 435 (1974).
2. Tannenbaum, H., and Schur, P. H., *J. Rheumatol.* **1**, 392 (1974).
3. Williams, R. C., DeBord, J. R., Mellbye, O. J., Messner, R. P., and Lindstrom, F. D., *J. Clin. Invest.* **52**, 283 (1973).
4. Zeiders, R. S., Johnson, J. S., Edgington, T. S., and Vaughan, J. H., *Arthritis Rheum.* **16**, 478 (1973).
5. Utsinger, P. D., and Bluestein, H. G., *J. Rheumatol.* **1** (Suppl.), 75 (1974).
6. Fröland, S. S., Natvig, J. B., and Husby, G., *Scand. J. Immunol.* **2**, 67 (1973).
7. Papamichail, M., Brown, J. C., and Holborow, E. J., *Lancet* **2**, 850 (1971).
8. Mellbye, O. J., Messner, R. P., DeBord, J. R., and Williams, R. C., *Arthritis Rheum.* **15**, 371 (1972).
9. Vernon-Roberts, B., Currey, H. L. F., and Perrin, J., *Ann. Rheum. Dis.* **33**, 430 (1974).
10. Winchester, R. J., Siegal, F. P., Bentwich, Z. H., and Kunkel, H. G., *Arthritis Rheum.* **16**, 138 (1973).
11. Messner, R. P., *Arthritis Rheum.* **17**, 339 (1974).
12. Williams, R. C., Lies, R. B., and Messner, R. P., *Arthritis Rheum.* **16**, 597 (1973).
13. Winchester, R. J., Winfield, J. B., Siegal, F., Wernet, P., Bentwich, Z., and Kunkel, H. G., *J. Clin. Invest.* **54**, 1082 (1974).
14. Waxman, J., Lockshin, M. D., Schnapp, J. J., and Doneson, I. N., *Arthritis Rheum.* **16**, 499 (1973).
15. Bitter, T., in *Rheumatoid Arthritis: Pathogenetic Mechanisms and Consequences in Therapeutics* (W. Muller, H. G. Harweth, and K. Fehr, eds.), Academic Press, New York, 1971, p. 305.
16. Whaley, K., Glen, A. C. A., MacSween, R. N. M., Deodhar, S. L., Dick, W. C., Nuki, G., Williamson, J. A., and Buchanan, W. W., *Clin. Exp. Immunol.* **9**, 721 (1971).
17. Adler, F. L., *Prog. Allergy* **8**, 41 (1964).
18. Muller, W., in *Rheumatoid Arthritis: Pathogenetic Mechanisms and Consequences in Therapeutics* (W. Muller, H. G. Harweth, and K. Fehr, eds.), Academic Press, New York, 1971, p. 297.
19. Leventhal, B. G., Waldorf, D. S., and Talal, N., *J. Clin. Invest.* **46**, 1338 (1967).
20. Epstein, W. L., and Jessar, R. A., *Arthritis Rheum.* **2**, 178 (1959).
21. Paty, J. G., Sienknecht, C. W., Townes, A. S., Hannisian, A. S., and Masi, A. T., *Arthritis Rheum.* **17**, 324 (1974).
22. Reynolds, M. D., and Abdou, N. I., *J. Clin. Invest.* **52**, 1627 (1973).
23. Georgescu, C. M., Gheorghiu, M., and Gociu, M., *Scand. J. Rheumatol.* Suppl. **8** (abstr.), 14–23 (1975).
24. Lockshin, M. D., Eisenhauer, A. C., Kohn, R., Weksler, M., Block, S., and Mushlin, S. B., *Arthritis Rheum.* **18**, 245 (1975).
25. Menard, H. A., Harm, T., and Peltier, A., *Ann. Rheum. Dis.* **33**, 361 (1974).
26. Yu, D. T. Y., and Peter, J. B., *Arthritis Rheum.* **4**, 25 (1974).
27. Tapanes, F., Armas, P., Perez, G., Zschaek, D., Abadi, I., Feo, E., Bianco, N., and Suarez, R., *Scand. J. Rheumatol.* Suppl. **8** (abstr.), 14–95 (1975).
28. Kacaki, J. N., Bullock, W. E., and Vaughan, J. H., *Lancet* **1**, 1289 (1969).
29. Runge, L. A., and Mills, J. A., *Arthritis Rheum.* **14**, 631 (1971).
30. Reynolds, M. D., and Abdou, N. I., *J. Clin. Invest.* **52**, 1627 (1973).
31. Kinsella, T. D., *J. Clin. Invest.* **53**, 1108 (1974).

32. Fröland, S. S., and Gaarder, P. I., *Scand. J. Immunol.* **2**, 385 (1973).
33. Brostoff, J., Howell, A., and Roitt, I. M., *Clin. Exp. Immunol.* **15**, 1 (1973).
34. Eibl, M. M., and Sitko, C., *Ann. Rheum. Dis.* **34**, 117 (1975).
35. Weisbart, R. H., Bluestone, R., and Goldberg, L. S., *Clin. Exp. Immunol.* **20**, 409 (1975).
36. Weisbart, R. H., Bluestone, R., and Goldberg, L. S., *Arthritis Rheum.* (abstr.) **19**, 828 (1976).
37. Thorsby, E., *Transplant. Rev.* **18**, 51 (1974).
38. Stastny, P., *Tissue Antigens* **4**, 571 (1974).
39. Astorga, G. P., and Williams, R. C., *Arthritis Rheum.* **12**, 547 (1969).
40. Hedberg, H., Kallen, B., Low, B., and Nilsson, D., *Clin. Exp. Immunol.* **9**, 201 (1971).
41. Stastny, P., *J. Clin. Invest.* **57**, 1148 (1976).
42. McDevitt, H., personal communication.
43. Barden, J., Mullinax, F., and Waller, M., *Arthritis Rheum.* **10**, 228 (1967).
44. Bandilla, K. K., Pitts, N. C., and McDuffie, F. C., *Arthritis Rheum.* **13**, 214 (1970).
45. Meyer, G. J., and Muller, W., *Z. Rheumaforsch.* **28**, 35 (1969).
46. Rawson, A. J., Abelson, N. M., and McCarty, D. J., *Arthritis Rheum.* **4**, 463 (1961).
47. Shearn, M. A., Epstein, W. V., and Engleman, E. P., *Proc. Soc. Exp. Biol. Med.* **113**, 1001 (1963).
48. Waller, M. H., Ellman, M., and Toone, E. C., *Acta Rheum. Scand.* **12**, 250 (1966).
49. Rhodes, K., Scott, A., Markham, R. L., and Monk-Jones, M. E., *Ann. Rheum. Dis.* **28**, 104 (1969).
50. Meiselas, L. E., Zingale, S. B., Lee, S. L., Richman, S., and Siegel, M., *J. Clin. Invest.* **40**, 1872 (1961).
51. Greenwood, R., and Barr M., *Ann. Phys. Med.* **5**, 258 (1960).
52. Opelz, G., Terasaki, P. I., and Hirata, A. A., *Lancet* **2**, 478 (1973).
53. Panush, R. S., *Arthritis Rheum.* (abstr.) **18**, 418 (1975).
54. Zvaifler, N. J., *Arthritis Rheum.* **17**, 297 (1974).
55. Weissmann, G., *N. Engl. J. Med.* **286**, 41 (1972).
56. Pearson, C. M., Paulus, H. E., and Machleder, H. I., *Ann. N.Y. Acad. Sci.* **256**, 150 (1975).
57. Kulka, J. P., Bocking, D., Ropes, M. W., and Bauer, W., *Arch. Pathol.* **59**, 129 (1955).
58. Schumacher, H. R., and Kitridou, R. C., *Arthritis Rheum.* **15**, 465 (1974).
59. Gardner, D. L., *The Pathology of the Connective Tissue Diseases*, Williams and Wilkins, Baltimore, 1965.
60. Hamerman, D., Barland, P., and Janis, R., in *The Biological Basis of Medicine*, vol. 3 (E. E. Bittar and N. Bittar, eds.), W. B. Saunders, Philadelphia, 1969, p. 269.
61. Fish, A. J., Michael, A. F., Gewurz, H., and Good, R. A., *Arthritis Rheum.* **9**, 267 (1966).
62. Kobayashi, I., and Ziff, M., *Arthritis Rheum.* **16**, 471 (1973).
63. Williams, R. C., in *Rheumatoid Arthritis as a Systemic Disease*, W. B. Saunders, Philadelphia, 1974.
64. Van Boxel, J. A., and Paget, S. A., *N. Engl. J. Med.* **293**, 517 (1975).
65. Sheldon, P. J., and Holborow, E. J., *Scand. J. Rheumatol.* Suppl. **8** (abstr.), 14–08 (1975).
66. Abrahamsen, T. G., Natvig, J. B., Fröland, S. S., and Pahle, J., *Scand. J. Immunol.* **4**, 823 (1976).
67. Wangel, A. G., Klockars, M., and Wegelius, O., *Scand. J. Rheumatol.* Suppl. **8** (abstr.), 14–07 (1975).
68. Loewi, G., Lance, E. M., and Reynolds, J., *Ann. Rheum. Dis.* **34**, 524 (1975).
69. Smiley, J. D., Sachs, C., and Ziff, M., *J. Clin. Invest.* **47**, 624 (1968).
70. Sliwinski, A. J., and Zvaifler, N. J., *J. Lab. Clin. Med.* **76**, 304 (1970).
71. Munthe, E., and Natvig, J. B., *Clin. Exp. Immunol.* **12**, 55 (1972).
72. Munthe, E., and Natvig, J. B., *Scand. J. Immunol.* **1**, 217 (1972).
73. Sandson, J., and Hamerman, D., *J. Clin. Invest.* **43**, 1372 (1964).
74. Pekin, T. J., and Zvaifler, N. J., *J. Clin. Invest.* **43**, 1372 (1964).
75. Hedberg, H., *Acta Rheum. Scand.* **10**, 109 (1964).
76. Müller-Eberhard, H. J., *Harvey Lect. Ser.* **66**, 75 (1972).
77. Medicus, R., Schreiber, R. D., Goetze, O., and Müller-Eberhard, H. J., *Proc. Natl. Acad. Sci.* (U.S.A.) **73**, 612 (1976).
78. Ruddy, J., and Austen, K. F., *Arthritis Rheum.* **13**, 713 (1970).
79. Zvaifler, N. J., *J. Clin. Invest.* **48**, 1532 (1969).
80. Hedberg, H., Lundh, B., and Laurell, A. B., *Clin. Exp. Immunol.* **6**, 707 (1970).
81. Ruddy, S., Fearon, D., and Austen, K. F., *Arthritis Rheum.* **18**, 289 (1975).
82. Ward, P. A., and Zvaifler, N. J., *J. Clin. Invest.* **50**, 606 (1971).

83. Ruddy, S., Everson, L. K., Schur, P. H., and Austen, K. F., *J. Exp. Med.* **134**, 259s (1971).
84. Hollander, J. L., McCarty, D. J., Astorga, G., and Castro-Murillo, E., *Ann. Intern. Med.* **62**, 271 (1965).
85. Britton, M. C., and Schur, P. H., *Arthritis Rheum.* **14**, 87 (1971).
86. Russell, M. L., Gordon, D. A., and Broder, S., *J. Rheumatol.* **1**, 153 (1974).
87. Winchester, R. J., Agnello, V., and Kunkel, H. G., *Clin. Exp. Immunol.* **6**, 689 (1970).
88. Winchester, R. J., *Ann. N.Y. Acad. Sci.* **256**, 73 (1975).
89. Marcus, R., and Townes, A. S., *J. Clin. Invest.* **50**, 282 (1971).
90. Cracchiolo, A., Goldberg, L. S., Barnett, E. V., and Bluestone, R., *Immunology* **20**, 1067 (1971).
91. Zvaifler, N. J., *Adv. Immunol.* **16**, 265 (1973).
92. Agnello, V., Winchester, R. J., and Kunkel, H. G., *Immunology* **19**, 909 (1970).
93. Luthra, H. S., McDuffie, F. M., Hunder, G. G., and Samayoa, E. A., *J. Clin. Invest.* **56**, 458 (1975).
94. Hannestad, K., *Clin. Exp. Immunol.* **2**, 511 (1967).
95. Zvaifler, N. J., *Arthritis Rheum.* **8**, 289 (1965).
96. Robitaille, P., Zvaifler, N. J., and Tan, E. M., *Clin. Immunol. Immunopathol.* **1**, 385 (1973).
97. Cooke, T. D., Hurd, E. R., Jasin, H., Bienenstock, J., and Ziff, M., *Arthritis Rheum.* **18**, 541 (1975).
98. Henson, P., *J. Immunol.* **107**, 1547 (1971).
99. Stastny, P., Rosenthal, M., Andreis, M., and Ziff, M., *Arthritis Rheum.* **18**, 737 (1975).
100. Maini, R. N., Hersfall, A., Raffe, L., Hanson, J., and Dumonde, D. C., *Scand. J. Rheumatol.* Suppl. **8** (abstr.), 14–11 (1975).
101. Stastny, P., Rosenthal, M., Andreis, M., Cooke, D., and Ziff, M., *Ann. N.Y. Acad. Sci.* **256**, 117 (1975).
102. Andreis, M., Stastny, P., and Ziff, M., *Arthritis Rheum.* **17**, 537 (1974).
103. Hamerman, D., Janis, R., and Smith, C., *J. Exp. Med.* **126**, 1005 (1967).
104. Harris, E. D., Jr., Parker, H. D., Radin, E. L., and Krane, S. M., *Arthritis Rheum.* **15**, 497 (1972).
105. Dingle, J. T., in *Tissue Proteinases* (A. J. Barrett and J. T. Dingle, eds.), North Holland, Amsterdam, 1971, p. 313.
106. Oronsky, A. L., Ignarro, L., and Perper, R. J., *J. Exp. Med.* **138**, 461 (1973).
107. Harris, E. D., Jr., DiBona, D. R., and Krane, S. M., *J. Clin. Invest.* **48**, 2104 (1969).
108. Krane, S. M., *Arthritis Rheum.* **17**, 306 (1974).
109. Kobayashi, I., and Ziff, M., *Arthritis Rheum.* **18**, 475 (1975).
110. Schmid, F. R., Cooper, N. S., Ziff, M., and McEwen, C., *Am. J. Med.* **30**, 56 (1961).
111. Hart, F. D., Golding, J. R., and MacKenzie, D. H., *Ann. Rheum. Dis.* **16**, 471 (1957).
112. Epstein, W. V., and Engleman, E. P., *Arthritis Rheum.* **2**, 250 (1959).
113. Mongan, E. S., Cass, R. M., Jacox, R. F., and Vaughan, J. H., *Am. J. Med.* **47**, 23 (1969).
114. Franco, A. E., and Schur, P. H., *Arthritis Rheum.* **14**, 231 (1971).
115. Weinstein, A., Peters, K., Brown, D., and Bluestone, R., *Arthritis Rheum.* **15**, 49 (1972).
116. Conn, D. L., McDuffie, F. C., and Dyck, P. J., *Arthritis Rheum.* **15**, 135 (1972).
117. Franklin, E. C., Holman, H. R., Müller-Eberhard, H. J., and Kunkel, H. G., *J. Exp. Med.* **105**, 425 (1957).
118. Kunkel, H. G., Franklin, E. C., and Müller-Eberhard, H. J., *J. Clin. Invest.* **38**, 424 (1959).
119. Gordon, D. A., Bell, D. A., Baumal, R., and Broder, I., *Clin. Exp. Immunol.* **5**, 57 (1969).
120. Gordon, D. A., Stein, J. L., and Broder, I., *Am. J. Med.* **54**, 445 (1973).
121. Weisman, M., and Zvaifler, N. J., *Rheumatology* **6**, 1 (1975).
122. Weisman, M., and Zvaifler, N. J., *J. Clin. Invest.* **56**, 725 (1975).
123. Theofilopoulos, A. N., Burtonboy, G., LoSpalluto, J. J., and Ziff, M., *Arthritis Rheum.* **17**, 272 (1974).
124. Stage, D. E., and Mannik, M., *Arthritis Rheum.* **14**, 440 (1971).
125. Christian, C. L., *Arthritis Rheum.* **4**, 86 (1961).
126. Abruzzo, J. L., and Christian, C. L., *J. Exp. Med.* **114**, 791 (1961).
127. Christian, C. L., *J. Exp. Med.* **18**, 827 (1963).
128. Williams, R. C., and Kunkel, H. G., *Proc. Soc. Exp. Biol.* **112**, 554 (1963).
129. Schur, P., and Kunkel, H. G., *Arthritis Rheum.* **8**, 468 (1965).
130. Allen, J. C., and Kunkel, H. G., *Arthritis Rheum.* **9**, 758 (1966).
131. Crothers, D. M., and Metzger, H., *Immunochemistry* **9**, 341 (1972).

132. Normansell, D. E., *Immunochemistry* **8**, 593 (1971).
133. Eisenberg, R., *Immunochemistry* **13**, 355 (1976).
134. Weigle, W. O., *Adv. Immunol.* **16**, 61 (1973).
135. Mannik, M., and Arend, W. P., *J. Exp. Med.* **134**, 19s (1971).
136. Heimer, R. F., Levin, F. M., and Kahn, M. F., *J. Immunol.* **91**, 866 (1963).
137. Zvaifler, N. J., *Ann. N.Y. Acad. Sci.* **168**, 146 (1969).
138. Schmid, F. R., Roitt, I. M., and Rocha, M. J., *J. Exp. Med.* **132**, 673 (1970).
139. Messner, R. P., Laxdal, T., Quie, P. G., and Williams, R. C., *J. Clin. Invest.* **47**, 1109 (1968).
140. McDuffie, F. C., and Brumfield, H. W., *J. Clin. Invest.* **51**, 3007 (1972).
141. Parker, R. L., and Schmid, F. R., *J. Immunol.* **88**, 519 (1962).
142. Ward, P. A., and Zvaifler, N. J., *J. Immunol.* **111**, 1777 (1973).
143. Hurd, E. R., Lo Spallruto, J., and Ziff, M., *Arthritis Rheum.* **13**, 724 (1970).
144. Diaz-Jouner, E., Bankhurst, A. D., Messner, R. P., and Williams, R. C., *Arthritis Rheum.* **19**, 142 (1976).
145. Vaughan, J. H., personal communication.
146. Notkins, A. I., *J. Exp. Med.* **134**, 41s (1971).
147. Gipson, T. G., Daniels, C. A., and Notkins, A. I., *J. Immunol.* **112**, 2087 (1974).
148. Hoofnagle, J. H., Markenson, J. A., Gerety, R. J., Daniels, C. A., and Barker, L. F., *Bacteriol. Proc.* **73**, 198 (1973).
149. Gipson, T. G., and Daniels, C. A., *Clin. Immunol. Immunopathol.* **4**, 16 (1975).
150. Hay, F. C., and Nincham, L., in *Progress in Immunology* **II**, vol. 5, North Holland, Amsterdam, 1974, p. 307.
151. Hellstrom, K. E., and Hellstrom, I., *Adv. Immunol.* **18**, 209 (1974).
152. Pyrhonen, S., Timonen, T., Heikkinen, A., Penttinen, K., Alfthan, O., Sakseilo, E., and Wager, O., *Eur. J. Cancer* (in press).
153. Isomaki, H. A., Mutrie, O., and Koota, K., *Scand. J. Rheumatol.* **4**, 205 (1976).
154. Hirsch, M. S., Allison, A. C., and Harvey, J. J., *Nature* (London) **223**, 739 (1969).
155. Wager, O., *Scand. J. Rheumatol.* **5** (Suppl. **12**), 67 (1975).
156. Bokisch, V. A., and Bernstein, D., *Arthritis Rheum.* **15**, 104 (1972).
157. Bokisch, V. A., Bernstein, D., and Krause, R., *J. Exp. Med.* **136**, 799 (1972).

Chapter Thirteen

Disorders of Phagocytic Effector Cells

THOMAS P. STOSSEL

Department of Pediatrics, Harvard Medical School and Massachusetts General Hospital, Boston, Massachusetts

Although the importance of phagocytes for human host defense was appreciated nearly a century ago (1), the realization that abnormalities of phagocytes predispose to infection occurred recently. Most studies of phagocytes prior to the last decade asked how phagocytes recognize invading microbes and how prior confrontation with pathogens enhances this recognition (2,3). The discovery of antibody deficiency states (Chapter 7) initiated the search for other derangements of host defense against infection, but despite the knowledge that antibody was important for the function of phagocytes, the role of the phagocyte in these syndromes was not emphasized. Knowledge that a disease characterized by recurrent and severe pyogenic infections, chronic granulomatous disease of childhood (4), was the result of defective microbicidal activity of phagocytes (5) brought the phagocyte again into the foreground of the defense against pyogenic infection in a clinical context.

This chapter reviews the pathogenetic mechanisms and clinical consequences of disorders involving the major phagocytic effector cells, the neutrophilic polymorphonuclear leukocytes (neutrophils), and the mononuclear phagocytes (monocytes and macrophages). Phagocytes do not operate in vacuo but depend on serum factors for optimal function, many of which are generated by humoral or cell-mediated immunologic reactions. Since the mechanisms and defects of serum generation of chemotactic substances and of factors that render microorganisms tasty to phagocytes, opsonins, have been discussed in earlier chapters, this aspect of phagocytic function and its disorders will not be covered in detail.

Supported by USPHS Grant HL-19429.

THE PHAGOCYTE DEFICIENCY SYNDROMES

The most frequent cause of susceptibility to infection related to disorders of effector phagocytes is a diminution in the number of phagocytic cells. Phagocyte deficiency may arise from derangement of any aspect of the normal life cycles of these cells, as briefly reviewed below.

Life Cycle of the Neutrophil

Neutrophils arise ultimately from a pluripotential stem cell in the bone marrow, and progeny of this stem cell become "committed" to differentiation into neutrophils (6). The committed stem cell gives rise to a series of morphologically identifiable neutrophil precursors, which ripen in the bone marrow. The earliest of these forms, the myeloblasts, promyelocytes, and especially the myelocytes, constitute a mitotic pool, capable of dividing, and therefore serve to amplify the cohorts of developing neutrophils. Cytoplasmic granules synthesized by these early precursors, called primary or azurophilic granules, are diluted by subsequent mitotic events, and therefore are barely visible in the mature neutrophil (7). More mature neutrophil precursors, the metamyelocyte, band form, and segmented neutrophil, do not divide but demonstrate condensation of their nuclear chromatin, synthesize cytoplasmic granules that stain poorly with Wright's stain (hence the term "neutrophil"), and acquire attributes that characterize their behavior in the mature state, namely motility, deformability, and ability to ingest particulate objects (8,9). The entire maturation process occurs in about a week's time. Under normal circumstances, only mature segmented neutrophils and a few band forms enter the blood, where they circulate with a half-time of about six hours.* Thereafter, it is presumed that the neutrophils enter various tissues, where their survival is short, although relatively little information is available concerning this point.

The complex life cycle of the neutrophil presents many points for regulation. Infection, inflammation, or tissue necrosis, even when relatively localized, elicits peripheral blood neutrophils in vivo, suggesting that humoral mechanisms are involved in the evolution of the neutrophil response. A microbial substance, bacterial endotoxin, has many effects on the neutrophil cycle, which include redistribution of neutrophils within the vascular compartment, enhancement of neutrophil production, maturation and release from the bone marrow. Cross-transfusion experiments have suggested that these inflammatory signals act through humoral mechanisms (14,15), and at least one of the humoral factors may be derived from the serum complement system (16). In recent years, techniques have been developed for cultivating neutrophil progenitors in vitro (17). A glycoprotein required for maintenance of neutrophil cultures, colony stimulat-

---

*The most widely accepted estimates of neutrophil survival are based on autotransfusion studies with di-isopropylfluorophosphate-^{32}P-labeled neutrophils in man or experimental animals (10,11), or on pulse-labeling experiments with ^{3}H-thymidine in animals (12), and are consistent with emerging data from homologous neutrophil transfusions into pancytopenic individuals. Some argue that the neutrophil survivals are artifactually short, and that neutrophils sojourn considerably in the circulation when labeled with ^{51}Cr (13). The dispute awaits resolution.

ing factor, has been extensively studied. This material is excreted in the urine and is produced by a wide variety of cell types, including monocytes, macrophages, lymphocytes, and tumor cells (18,19). It is evidently distinct from other factors that stimulate neutrophil release from the bone marrow (20), other factors that promote neutrophil growth in vitro (21,22), and inhibitors of neutrophil production (chalones) (23,24). Neutrophil maturation also appears to be influenced by nonhumoral factors, such as cell density (25,26).

Life Cycle of the Monocyte

The monocyte, like the neutrophil, arises from a pluripotent stem cell of the bone marrow. It exists as a promonocyte in the marrow for approximately one to two days and emerges as a monocyte in the peripheral blood, where it circulates for an equivalent interval (27). On the basis of studies both in vivo and in vitro, it is generally accepted that monocytes enter the tissues and, whether lodged in normal or inflamed organs, evolve into macrophages (28). Furthermore, the monocytes are the precursors of all the macrophages constituting the "reticuloendothelial" or mononuclear phagocyte system, although macrophages may persist for prolonged periods in situ (29,30). Considerable knowledge exists concerning the differentiation of monocytes into macrophages in vitro (31). Like the neutrophils, the blood monocytes increase in number in response to inflammation, especially to chronic inflammation (32–34). However, little is known about what regulates the life cycle of mononuclear phagocytes in the organism.

Neutropenia

Neutropenia is arbitrarily defined as a neutrophil count of less than $1,500/mm^3$. However, this is a statistical definition, and certain populations may have mean neutrophil counts that are considerably below the "normal" mean without apparent ill effect (35–37). The current poor understanding of the neutrophil life cycle and its regulation has forced the taxonomy of neutropenic states to rely on statistical, clinical, and morphologic description, resulting in the accumulation of a vast number of ill-defined syndromes. For the purposes of this discussion, a few entities will be described in which some knowledge of the pathogenesis of the neutropenic state exists. Other forms of neutropenia are "lumped" under the rubric of chronic idiopathic neutropenia, pending the necessary information for subdividing them.

Cyclic Neutropenia. Cyclic neutropenia, a genetic disease of man (38) and of the gray collie dog (39), transmitted as an autosomal dominant trait with variable penetrance (40), is actually cyclic hematopoiesis (41,42). Careful enumeration of the blood elements has shown that all undergo regular oscillations. The neutrophil, because of its long maturation time and short life span, demonstrates the most dramatic fluctuations, characterized by regular 21-day zeniths and nadirs. The monocytes have the next most prominent cycle and peak during the dip in the neutrophil count. The rise and fall in the platelet and erythrocyte concentrations, because of the damping effect of their longer life spans, are subtle. The finding of cyclic hematopoiesis and the transmission and cure of the disease in gray collie dogs by bone marrow transplantation (43,44) establish cyclic neutropenia as a disease of the pluripotent stem cell. The ultimate cause of the intermittent stem cell activity in this disease is unknown.

Chronic Neutropenia. Syndromes characterized by noncyclical persistent neutropenia without other hematologic deficiencies comprise a heterogenous group of disorders from a pathogenetic standpoint. Congenital neutropenia, which may be inherited either as an autosomal dominant or recessive trait, presents with markedly variable mean neutrophil counts, bone marrow morphology, and clinical severity (45). Monocytosis or eosinophilia, or both, may or may not be present. Because of the relative benignity of most cases of congenital neutropenia (see below), many adult patients with "idiopathic neutropenia" may in fact have congenital neutropenia that was only detected in mature life.

The pathogenesis of congenital or chronic idiopathic neutropenia is not easily amenable to study with current techniques, is probably variable, and is hence poorly understood. Indeed, it is not known whether most of these diseases result from diminished neutrophil production, ineffective neutropoiesis, marrow neutrophil dysfunction, increased peripheral neutrophil destruction, or a combination of these factors. Most claims to support any of these mechanisms have been based on impressions obtained from bone marrow morphology or from imprecise and difficult assays of bone marrow neutrophil function (45–47). Neutrophil kinetic studies in patients with chronic idiopathic neutropenia (which can only be done in mildly affected patients) have demonstrated normal or shortened neutrophil survival times (48–50). In vitro bone marrow neutrophil cloning and maturation assays have produced conflicting results, some patients' marrows yielding subnormal numbers of neutrophil colonies, others generating colonies that failed to mature, and some, colonies that behaved like controls (94,51–55). It is not known whether the discrepancies reflect sampling difficulties, methodologic inconsistencies, or true heterogeneity among the patients sampled.

The basis of chronic neutropenia in an indeterminate subset of patients is the presence of antibodies directed against neutrophils. To deduce from the well-established entities, autoimmune hemolytic anemia and (idiopathic) autoimmune thrombocytopenic purpura, it seemed logical that autoimmune neutropenia must exist as well. However, only the recent development of reliable techniques for detecting antineutrophil antibodies and the definition of neutrophil antigens has permitted stronger evidence to accrue in support of this diagnosis as the basis of neutropenia in certain cases (56–58). Except for the presence of serum antibody specific for neutrophils, and responses to corticosteroids or splenectomy by some patients, the clinical and hematologic profiles of these patients do not differ from those of others with nonimmune "idiopathic" neutropenia. Transplacental passage of maternal antibodies directed against fetal neutrophils causes transient neonatal neutropenia in infants of mothers sensitized to the baby's neutrophils (59).

Neutropenia Associated with Other Diseases. Patients with a variety of illnesses, including hypersplenism, rheumatoid arthritis, congenital antibody deficiency syndromes, certain inborn metabolic errors, and congenital pancreatic insufficiency, may also have neutropenia of varying severity. In most of these disorders, the basis of the neutropenia is unknown, excepting hypersplenism, in which sequestration of the neutrophils in the enlarged organ is the underlying cause (45). Some cases of neutropenia subsequently evolve into acute myelogenous leukemia or aplastic anemia and then acquire the more serious prognosis associated with these disorders.

The Clinical and Pathologic Consequences of Neutropenia. Neutropenia of any cause amounts to a diminution in the number of phagocytes that enter the tissues most rapidly. Even in cases of persistent and profound congenital neutropenia, pus appears in infected lesions. However, the number of neutrophils arriving into inflammatory sites is diminished in proportion to the diminution in the peripheral neutrophil count (60). Most patients with chronic neutropenia unassociated with other illnesses have relatively little increased susceptibility to infection, suggesting that the "normal" neutrophil turnover is much higher than absolutely required for protection against pyogenic infection. However, some patients with chronic neutropenia have severe and frequent infections, and it would be of importance to know why. The number of blood monocytes does not seem to determine the different clinical courses, because the most frequently infected patients may have large quantities of peripheral monocytes that appear to have normal function (45). It may be that these patients simply have the lowest neutrophil counts at all times and have less capacity to mobilize neutophils in response to infection. However, all patients with neutropenia have decreased bone marrow neutrophil reserves, as assessed by current techniques (48).

Conclusions concerning the importance of neutrophils derived from clinical histories must be tempered by the fact that susceptibility to infection is a complex interaction between the adequacy of all host defenses and the frequency and virulence of pathogens encountered. Some of these questions could best be answered by graded microbial challenge of experimental animals rendered neutropenic, but this has not yet been done.

When infection occurs in the setting of chronic neutropenia, the commonest pathogen is *Staphylococcus aureus.* Gram-negative enteric organisms follow in frequency. The sites infected are most often the skin and lungs. Mucosal sores and gingivitis arise frequently. Rarely, intestinal perforation has been reported. The pattern suggests that the major role of neutrophils is to keep the exposed surfaces of the body from uncontrolled invasion by low-grade pathogens.

Panphagocytopenia. Bone marrow failure of any etiology is the important cause of diminution in both neutrophils and monocytes. Unlike isolated neutropenia, bone marrow failure renders patients or experimental animals highly susceptible to infection by virulent or opportunistic microorganisms, and the risk of infection is proportional to the diminution in circulating neutrophils (61).

Why these patients are more susceptible involves many factors. Neutrophils, monocytes, and even normal lymphocytes are lacking, and the neutropenia may be more profound than in the syndromes of isolated neutropenia. Patients with aplastic anemia, carcinoma metastatic to the bone marrow, or acute leukemia may have tissue hemorrhages that predispose to bacterial invasion. Antitumor chemotherapy and irradiation, in addition to inducing pancytopenia, may damage mucosal barriers. Finally, as discussed below, phagocytes may function abnormally in leukemic or other neoplastic states.

The persistence of functioning tissue macrophages despite profound and prolonged monocytopenia in clinical disorders of bone marrow failure and in experimental models is a tribute to the longevity of the macrophage (62,63).

THE PHAGOCYTE DYSFUNCTION SYNDROMES

Disorders of the Humoral Arm of Phagocyte Function

Neutrophils and monocytes depend on serum-derived chemotactic factors to find invading microorganisms and depend on opsonins, also originating in serum, to coat many microbes and render them recognizable for ingestion. Therefore, it is not surprising that the abnormalities of serum described in Chapters 8 and 9 may impair responses of phagocytes, and that the affected patients or animals have recurrent infections. Noteworthy is the fact that infections observed in the setting of deficiencies of the serum proteins known to be of major importance for chemotactic and opsonic activity, antibody and C3, are associated with recurrent infections by high-grade encapsulated pathogens, pneumococci, streptococci, and *Hemophilus influenzae*. This pattern of susceptibility differs from that encountered in the neutropenia syndromes but is identical to that associated with the asplenic state (64). The primary role of these serum factors may be to promote clearance of a limited spectrum of pathogens by mononuclear phagocytes in filtering organs. This pathogenetic speculation must be tempered by the same caveat mentioned previously concerning the establishment of biologic principles from clinical information alone.

Disorders of Cellular Responses to Humors and Pathogens

The Physiology of Responses by Neutrophils and Mononuclear Phagocytes. Neutrophils and monocytes encountering a gradient of chemotactic factors locomote toward the source of the gradient. The morphology and pharmacology of this vectorial locomotion have been described (65,66), but little is known about its fundamental mechanisms. Neutrophils, monocytes, and macrophages ingest opsonized microorganisms by surrounding them with pseudopodia. The pseudopodia fuse, resulting in the enclosure of the microbes within sacs of inverted plasma membrane. At the same time, cytoplasmic granules of the phagocytes fuse with the sac or phagosome and discharge their contents into it. The disappearance of the granules during fusion is the basis of this phenomenon's being termed "degranulation" (67).

Evidence is accumulating that the morphologic responses of phagocytes described depend in part on the interaction of cytoskeletal elements. These elements include the protein actin, which composes thin filaments that are prominent in pseudopods of neutrophils and macrophages (68). Under certain conditions in vitro, an "actin-binding protein" of neutrophils and macrophages causes actin to form a gel that is subsequently contracted by myosin. Under the same conditions, these molecules interact in the identical manner in extracts of neutrophils and macrophages (69). If relevant to the activities of the phagocytes in vivo, these phenomena would provide a molecular explanation for the consistency changes and movement of peripheral cytoplasm which characterize the activities of phagocytes during locomotion, and ingestion. The presence of a filamentous gel may act as a barrier to granule fusion with membranes. The reversible assembly of this gel would provide a mechanism for regulating granule fusion and degranulation.

Concomitant with ingestion, and even with locomotion, the phagocytes metabolize oxygen to generate products that are toxic to microorganisms. These oxygen metabolites include the superoxide anion, hydrogen peroxide, hydroxyl radicals, and singlet oxygen (70). It is not known how these agents kill microbes, but their action is rapid and precedes detectable degradation of most microbial macromolecules (71). The toxic action of oxygen products is potentiated by substances entering the phagosome by degranulation. These include the enzyme myeloperoxidase, which is present in neutrophils and monocytes and which in the presence of halide ions, chloride or iodide, increases the microbicidal action of hydrogen peroxide (72). Macrophages that lack peroxidase may utilize other mechanisms to potentiate the activity of oxygen metabolites. These include lysozyme, which hydrolyzes the 1,4-glycosidic linkage of cell walls of susceptible organisms, products of lipid peroxidation, or catalase (72,73). Oxygen-independent mechanisms possibly used by phagocytes to kill microorganisms include acid that accumulates in the phagosome (74), and granule-based substances, bactericidal cationic proteins (75), and lactoferrin (76). These agents have relatively weak antimicrobial activity. The reactants of these various antimicrobial systems are clearly concentrated within phagosomes of phagocytes (67,77) but may also operate outside the cells. Hydrogen peroxide, superoxide anions, products of lipid peroxidation, and contents of cytoplasmic granules all appear in the medium bathing phagocytes exposed to opsonized objects or certain humoral agents (73,78–80). The localization of these substances prevents somewhat their acting deleteriously on the phagocyte itself. But the oxygen metabolites are highly diffusible and do enter the cytoplasm of phagocytes, where they are detoxified by the enzyme superoxide dismutase (which rapidly converts superoxide to hydrogen peroxide), catalase, and reactions coupled to the hexosemonophosphate shunt which destroy hydrogen peroxide (72,98).

The triggering site for the morphologic and biochemical responses of phagocytes is the plasma membrane, but little is known about its function. The many stimuli that activate phagocytes to move, secrete, ingest, and metabolize oxygen are presumed to act on molecular entities, "receptors," but these are defined only phenomenologically at present.

The Chédiak-Higashi Syndrome. This autosomal recessive genetic disease was initially recognized as a disorder of leukocyte morphology in which neutrophils, monocytes, and lymphocytes contained giant cytoplasmic granules (Fig. 1) (81,82). The syndrome is a generalized dysfunction of cells characterized by fusion of cytoplasmic granules. Albinism, involving the hair, skin, and ocular fundi, is the result of pathologic aggregation of melanosomes. Increased suscep-

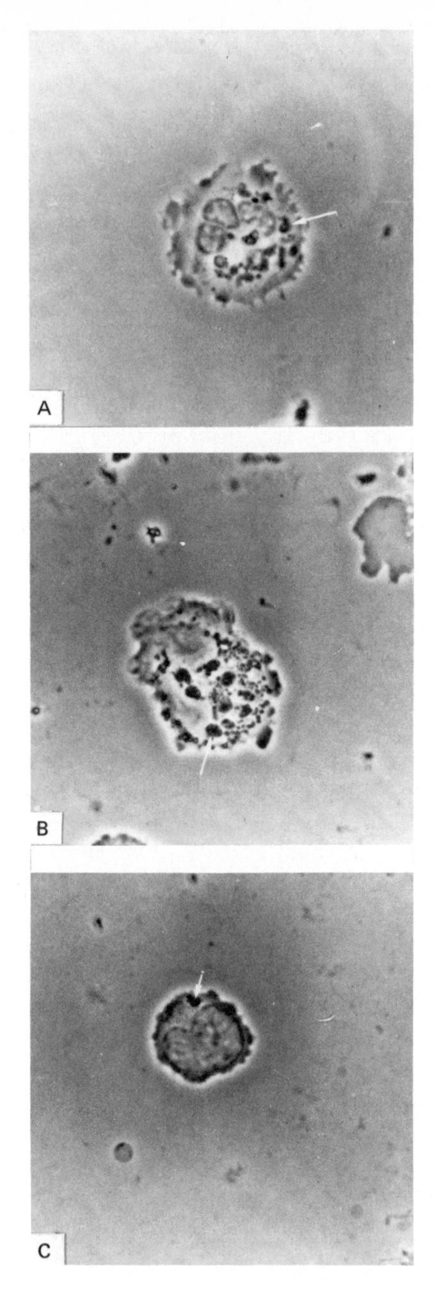

Figure 1. Phase photomicrographs of Chédiak-Higashi syndrome leukocytes. A, neutrophil; B, eosinophil; C, lymphocyte. (Reprinted from *Birth Defects,* Original Article Series, vol. 8, no. 3, 1972, with permission.)

tibility of the patients to infection can, in part, be explained by defective degranulation of giant neutrophil and monocyte lysosomes. Similar genetic syndromes have been discovered in mice, mink, cattle, and killer whales (83).

Other features of the human disease are not currently amenable to such clear-cut structure-function correlation. These include neutropenia, thrombocytopenia, recurrent unexplained fever, peripheral neuropathy, and a lymphohistiocytic proliferation in the liver, spleen, and bone marrow which intensifies the pancytopenia. This proliferation is associated with frequent bacterial and viral infections, fever, and prostration and usually results in death. At autopsy, the "lymphohistiocytic" infiltrates in the liver, spleen, and lymph nodes are not clearly neoplastic. This constellation has been termed the "accelerated phase" of the Chédiak-Higashi syndrome.

Patients with the Chédiak-Higashi syndrome have light skin, silvery hair, and photophobia. Other signs and symptoms that vary considerably include solar sensitivity, infections, neuropathy, and concomitants of the "accelerated phase." The diagnosis is easily established by the presence of large inclusions in all nucleated blood cells, which are seen with the Wright's stain, and which are brought out by peroxidase histochemical stains.

The infections are caused by gram-positive and gram-negative bacteria and by fungi, and involve the skin, respiratory tract, and mucous membranes. The most common organism is *Staphylococcus aureus*. The neuropathy may be sensory or motor in type. Ataxia may also be a predominant feature. The onset of the "accelerated phase" may occur at any age and varies considerably. Hepatosplenomegaly develops, and patients have high fevers in the absence of demonstrable bacterial sepsis. The pancytopenia worsens at this stage and may result in hemorrhage and exacerbation of the susceptibility to infection. Overwhelming sepsis resulting in death follows.

The basic abnormality underlying the Chédiak-Higashi syndrome is unknown. Neutrophils act as if in a state of chronic surface stimulation. They spontaneously aggregate surface molecules into "caps," ingest particles, and release enzymes associated with specific granules into the extracellular medium, at supernormal rates, and demonstrate hyperactive oxygen metabolism (84–86). The giant cytoplasmic granules of the neutrophil contain myeloperoxidase and acid phosphatase, and for this reason it has been assumed that they are primary granules. However, they might rather be "secondary lysosomes," formed from chronic membrane interiorization and granule fusion, beginning early in neutrophil development (87,88). In spite of the rapid ingestion of particles and active oxygen metabolism, the Chédiak-Higashi neutrophils demonstrate a delay in killing of ingested microorganisms. This delay reflects slow delivery of myeloperoxidase into the phagocytic vacuole, because the giant granules, which have accumulated much of the cell's myeloperoxidase, fuse poorly with phagosomes (85,86). In addition to abnormal degranulation, the neutrophils respond poorly to chemotactic stimuli (89). The reason for this deficiency is not clear. Many of the functional derangements of neutrophils in this syndrome have also been found in monocytes (90). Recently, parasympathomimetic agents have been shown to normalize some of the cytologic abnormalities of Chédiak-Higashi syndrome fibroblasts, neutrophils, and monocytes of humans and mice in vitro and of mice in vivo (91).

Since fusion of granules with phagosomes in neutrophils and macrophages occurs only during active ingestion, it appears that membrane activation and granule fusion are linked events (92,93). Although speculative, a unifying explanation for the manifold cellular aberrations of the Chédiak-Higashi syndrome is that chronic membrane activation leads to uncontrolled granule fusion, as well as other effects.

Neutrophil Actin Dysfunction. A male infant had repeated infections with gram-positive and gram-negative bacteria from birth but failed to produce pus (94). The infections involved the skin and gastrointestinal tract and were characterized by collections of bacteria in necrotic tissue, mononuclear cell infiltrates, and fluid. Entero-entero and enterocutaneous fistulas formed which healed poorly. The patient's blood contained large numbers of morphologically normal neutrophilic polymorphonuclear leukocytes and band forms. Although the patient's serum was active in generating chemotactic factors and opsonins, his neutrophils did not migrate toward inflamed sites in vivo or toward a source of chemotactic factor in vitro. They ingested at a markedly depressed rate. The metabolic activities of the neutrophils were intact, as evidenced by normal to high adenosine triphosphate (ATP) levels, rates of lactate production, and rates of reactions associated with oxygen metabolism. Oxygen metabolism of the neutrophils was activated in response to ingestible particles, and for the impaired ingestion, markedly increased quantities of granule enzymes were extruded into the extracellular medium and into phagosomes. Monocytes of the patient functioned normally.

An explanation for the abnormalities of neutrophil function was provided by the finding that monomeric actin in homogenates of the patient's neutrophils did not polymerize into filaments under conditions that polymerized normal neutrophil actin. The basis of the defective polymerizability of the actin was not determined, but the fact that a bone marrow graft resulted in normally functioning neutrophils indicated that the cause was genetic in origin. The failure of actin to assemble into filaments was consistent with the putative role assigned to reversible polymerization of this protein as the cause for formation of pseudopods for locomotion and ingestion and as a barrier regulating granule fusion with the membrane. The failure to create pseudopods would explain the impaired motility of the patient's cells, while the failure to produce a barrier to granule fusion would explain the increased granule enzyme secretion in response to a given quantity of ingested particles (Fig. 2).

The discovery of this patient and of the basis of the defect in locomotion and ingestion supports that attractive idea that contractile proteins are essential for many aspects of normal neutrophil function. Furthermore, this patient had the equivalent of functional absolute neutropenia. The clinical and pathologic picture resembled the severe end of the spectrum of chronic neutropenia and supports the formulation presented previously for the role of neutrophils in immunity against pyogenic infection.

Abnormal Neutrophil Responses Associated with Defects of Energy Metabolism

Many activities of phagocytes are accompanied by increased metabolic activity. Lactate production, glucose consumption, and glycogenolysis increase during ingestion and chemotactic locomotion by neutrophils, and ingestion increases

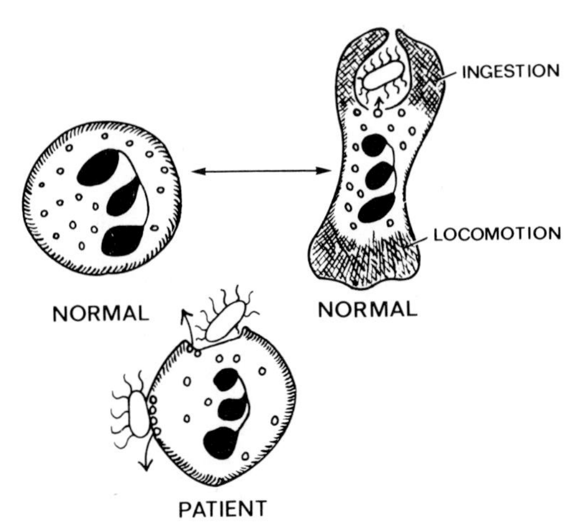

Figure 2. Model of neutrophil function of normal neutrophil and neutrophil of a patient with neutrophil actin dysfunction. The cell at upper left represents a normal resting cell with its cortical filamentous network. Actin microfilament polymerization reversibly generates pseudopodia for ingestion and locomotion. Degranulation results from partial dissipation of the cortical microfilaments. The lower cell represents the patient's neutrophil, in which postulated failure of actin to polymerize prevents ingestion and locomotion but allows for more rapid granular fusion with membranes in response to the signal produced by particle contact.

lactate production by mononuclear phagocytes (68,95,96). Metabolic poisons inhibit the motile functions of phagocytes (66,68,95), which, taken together with the foregoing, indicates that energy in the form of ATP is needed for these functions. The emerging role of contractile proteins in these activities is consistent with the need for chemical energy. Some clinical conditions support these ideas.

Dogs and humans receiving intravenous hyperalimentation, without supplementation by phosphate, develop hypophosphatemia (97). Peripheral blood leukocytes from these patients and animals become ATP-depleted. The neutrophils evolve a deficiency in their ability to locomote toward a chemotactic gradient and to ingest. The ATP content of the leukocytes and the functional abnormalities of the neutrophils can be reversed by adenosine or phosphate. The results highlighted the importance of energy in the form of ATP for the motile responses of polymorphonuclear leukocytes.

Neutrophils of patients with deficiency of a glycolytic pathway enzyme, phosphoglycerate kinase, utilize mitochondrial metabolism to maintain their ATP levels for functional activities (98). The neutrophils of the patients with this enzyme deficiency, which affects erythrocytes as well, function normally (99), and the patients with this disorder, which is inherited as an X-syntenic trait, have hemolytic anemia, but have not been shown to be susceptible to pyogenic infection. However, a state of neutrophil ATP deficiency and hypofunction manifested by an impaired ability to ingest can be created in vitro by poisoning the mitochondria of the deficient neutrophils with potassium cyanide (98).

Phagocyte "Paralysis" Syndromes. Given the extreme complexity of phagocyte responses and the vast number of pharmacologic agents that have been shown to inhibit these responses (66,68), it is not surprising that many reports have appeared describing patients whose phagocytes had impairments of chemotactic responsiveness, ingestion, metabolic activities, or combinations thereof. In most of these accounts, the basis of the abnormalities has not been defined. Abnormal neutrophil responses have been observed in various patients with systemic illnesses. Patients with rheumatoid arthritis (100), uremia (101), multiple myeloma (102,103), systemic lupus erythematosus (104), hepatic cirrhosis (105,106), thermal burns (107), and severe bacterial or viral infections (108–110) have been said to have phagocytes with diminished chemotactic responsiveness, adhesiveness, or ability to ingest, in addition to serum abnormalities. Investigators have reported cases of severe eczema associated with eosinophilia, hypergammaglobulinemia E, recurrent skin infections, and defective chemotactic responsiveness of the neutrophils (111,112). Although the cause of all the defects is unknown, immune complexes or circulating endotoxins, which characterize some of these diseases, could adsorb to the neutrophil membranes, causing general activation of the cell. As in the Chédiak-Higashi syndrome, in which the activated neutrophils are deficient in directed locomotion, neutrophils exposed to these agents have high resting rates of oxygen metabolism and granule enzyme release.

Hyperosmolarity clearly impairs neutrophil function. Therefore, it is logical that patients with diabetic ketoacidosis or poorly controlled hyperglycemia might have neutrophils that do not perform adequately. However, diminutions in neutrophil chemotactic responsiveness have also been reported of leukocytes from patients with diabetes mellitus in which the experiments were performed in media of normal osmolarities (114,115).

Corticosteroid therapy, especially with high and sustained doses, has been shown to inhibit neutrophil migration, adhesiveness, and ability of various phagocytes to ingest (116–119), although corticosteroid administration on the alternate-day basis was reported not to interfere with neutrophil movement (119). If corticosteroid treatment resulted in neutrophils with diminished functional capacities, the well-known effect of the medication in raising the total body granulocyte pool and granulocyte production might be explained as a compensatory attempt by the marrow in response to decreased neutrophil efficiency in the tissues. Indeed, a diminution in granulocyte egress from the blood has been observed in kinetic studies of patients receiving corticosteroids (10). Since corticosteroids have long been known to diminish the clearance of sensitized cells by intact animals, an attractive theory is that the drug acts in part by decreasing the ingestion capacity of mononuclear phagocytes.

The phagocytic clearance of pathogens may also be impaired in hemolytic diseases, especially in disorders secondary to abnormal hemoglobins (119a). The mechanisms of this impairment are diverse. Some patients with hemolysis have deficiencies of serum complement components (119b). In sickle cell anemia, phagocytosis by splenic macrophages is sometimes subnormal, possibly because the cells become engorged with damaged red cells (119c); eventually splenic infarction eliminates this organ as an effective filter.

Chronic Granulomatous Disease. Chronic granulomatous disease of childhood (CGD) is a genetic disorder in which polymorphonuclear leukocytes and monocytes ingest but do not kill catalase-positive microorganisms, because the cells fail to generate oxygen metabolites that normally kill these microbes. The disease is therefore defined biochemically by phagocytes which, when activated with ingestible particles or other stimuli, do not demonstrate an enhancement of the reactions associated with oxygen metabolism: oxygen consumption, hydrogen peroxide formation, superoxide production, singlet oxygen formation (as determined by chemoluminescence), or hexosemonophosphate shunt activity (72,120). Nitroblue tetrazolium, a reagent that is reduced to an insoluble purple formazan by superoxide anion, is used most often in clinical practice to diagnose CGD (121).

In CGD, an oxidase enzyme system that reduces oxygen to hydrogen peroxide and other molecules is either absent or is not activated by membrane stimulation. The choice between these alternatives is undecided, because neither the activation mechanism nor the responsible oxygen-metabolizing enzymes have been definitively identified.

In fact, CGD as a biochemical entity (phagocytes that do not metabolize oxygen) may be heterogenous from a molecular standpoint. The genetics of CGD support this idea. In some families, CGD is clearly transmitted as an X-syntenic disorder (122). In others, it appears to be sporadic, or else is inherited as an autosomal recessive trait (123,124). Attempts to differentiate the patients biochemically have been inconclusive. Some investigators reported finding diminished hydrogen peroxide-mediated reduced glutathione (GSH)-oxidizing activity in leukocytes of female patients with CGD (124). Others were unable to confirm the findings in different female patients (125). Although it has been possible to document subnormal bactericidal and oxygen-metabolizing activity in leukocytes of putative female carriers of the X-syntenic variety of CGD, it has not been shown that leukocytes from relatives of other CGD patients have abnormal functional or metabolic capacities.

Although most patients with CGD have leukocytes with normal glucose-6-phosphate dehydrogenase activity, a few individuals have been described with clinical findings of CGD and with leukocytes totally or else almost totally lacking glucose-6-phosphate dehydrogenase activity (127). As in other CGD patients, the leukocytes of these patients failed to activate their oxygen metabolism in response to membrane stimulation. The observations support the concept that reduced pyridine nucleotides, which are regenerated by activity of glucose-6-phosphate dehydrogenase, are involved in the production of oxygen metabolites by phagocytes; and that "CGD" can be the final common pathway of a number of different molecular defects.

As described above, normal phagocytes accumulate hydrogen peroxide (and other oxygen metabolites) in the phagosome containing ingested microorganisms. Hydrogen peroxide plus myeloperoxidase, delivered to the phagosome by degranulation, kills the incorporated microbe. The quantity of hydrogen peroxide produced by the normal phagocyte is sufficient to overcome the activity of catalase, a hydrogen peroxide-catabolizing enzyme, associated with many aerobic microorganisms including *Staphylococcus aureus,* most gram-negative enteric bacteria, *Candida albicans,* and *Aspergillus* species. However, when these organisms gain entry to CGD phagocytes, they are not exposed to hydrogen peroxide because the phagocyte does not produce it; and hydrogen peroxide that is generated by the microbes themselves is destroyed by the accompanying catalase. The catalase-positive microbes can multiply intracellularly, can be protected in their intracellular location from most circulating antibiotics, can be transported to distant sites, and can be released to establish new foci of infection (128). The granulomatous nature of the infected lesions of CGD is reminiscent of infections by organisms that survive intracellularly in normal phagocytes, such as mycobacteria. Macrophages in hematoxylin-eosin-stained sections of tissue of patients with CGD may contain a golden pigment that is thought to reflect abnormal accumulation of ingested material (129). Its relation to the biochemical disorder of CGD is unknown. When CGD phagocytes ingest pneumococci or streptococci, they kill them, because these organisms do not contain catalase. They therefore accumulate hydrogen peroxide around themselves, which, together with peroxidase, delivered to the phagosomes of CGD neutrophils, kills the bacteria. These species thus effectively "commit suicide" in the CGD phagosomes.

The pathogenetic mechanisms just described fit with the epidemiologic pattern of infections of CGD patients and with results of studies employing bacterial mutants. Patients with CGD are susceptible to infection with catalase-positive, but not catalase-negative, microorganisms (10). Phagocytes of patients with CGD can kill pneumococci that produce hydrogen peroxide, but not mutant pneumococci, which are incapable of producing it in net amounts (130).

Although the most impressive functional disorder of CGD phagocytes is their failure to activate their oxygen metabolism in response to membrane stimulation, other functional abnormalities have been reported. Some (10,131–133) but not all (86,134–136) investigators have described quantitative deficiencies of degranulation or ingestion by CGD neutrophils. Impaired chemotactic responsiveness by neutrophils has also been noted (137,138). Whether these findings and discrepancies are due to the variable consequences of chronic infection itself or reflect the heterogeneity of CGD is not clear at this time.

The clinical presentation of CGD is highly variable, and not all of its manifestations are explicable in terms of the known aspects of its pathogenesis. The onset of clinical signs and symptoms may occur at any age, ranging from early infancy to adulthood. The attack rate and severity of infections are exceedingly variable. By far the leading pathogen for these patients is *Staphylococcus aureus,* although, as described above, any catalase-positive microorganisms may be involved. *Serratia marcescens* and *Salmonella* species seem to appear quite frequently. Infections are characterized histopathologically by microabscess and granuloma formation; the pigmented histiocytes described in the previous section are helpful in making the diagnosis. These patients may suffer from sequelae of a chronically infected state: these include the anemia of chronic disease and systemic manifestations possibly related to the presence of circulating immune complexes.

A peculiar manifestation associated with CGD is the finding that several mothers of patients in whom X-linked inheritance was documentable had an illness resembling systemic lupus erythematosus (139). Most carriers of CGD are clinically well, although one woman was reported to suffer from recurrent salmonellosis (140). Fewer of this woman's neutrophils may have been metabolically normal than those of most carriers of CGD, suggesting a greater than usual amount of the X-inactivation predicted by the Lyon hypothesis.

Some male patients with CGD have a rare Kell blood group phenotype on their erythrocytes, and neutrophils and are unusually susceptible to sensitization with Kell antigens (141).

Myeloperoxidase Deficiency. Absence of the enzyme myeloperoxidase from the granules of neutrophils and monocytes, but not eosinophils, is inherited as an autosomal recessive trait (142,143). The functional features of this deficiency were studied in detail in one affected family (143,144). The enzyme was inactive both functionally and immunochemically. The lack of myeloperoxidase, an enzyme that potentiates the microbicidal potency of hydrogen peroxide in the phagosome, causes a microbicidal deficiency of the neutrophils that is detectable in vitro, but is not as severe as that observed in the CGD neutrophil. It has been postulated that myeloperoxidase-deficient neutrophils accumulate more hydrogen peroxide and other oxygen products than normal neutrophils, and that this increased peroxide concentration improves the bactericidal activity of the affected neutrophils (72). The patients with this genetic disorder have not been unusually susceptible to pyogenic infections.

Deficiency of neutrophil myeloperoxidase has also been observed as an acquired disorder in patients with hematologic abnormalities such as refractory anemias or myeloproliferative disorders (145–147).

Miscellaneous Disorders of Bactericidal Function. Tests of phagocytic bactericidal function have been performed in various disease states, and abnormalities reported. In many if not most of these reports, it is not possible to determine the cause or the significance of the findings. Such abnormalities have been found in patients receiving craniospinal irradiation for acute lymphoblastic leukemia (148), in patients in remission from various leukemias (149), and in patients with protein-calorie malnutrition (150), paraproteinemia (151), rheumatoid arthritis (152), recurrent staphylococcal infections (153,154), chronic myelogenous leukemia (155), and lymphomas (156).

REFERENCES

1. Metschnikoff, E., *Ann. Inst. Pasteur* **1**, 321 (1887).
2. Mudd, S., McCutcheon, M., and Lucké, B., *Physiol. Rev.* **14**, 210 (1934).
3. Rowley, D., *Adv. Immunol.* **2**, 241 (1962).
4. Bridges, R. A., Berendes, H., and Good, R. A., *Am. J. Dis. Child.* **97**, 387 (1959).
5. Good, R. A., Quie, P. G., Windhorst, D. B., et al., *Semin. Hematol.* **5**, 215 (1968).
6. Cline, M. J., Craddock, C. G., Gale, R. P., et al., *Ann. Intern. Med.* **81**, 801 (1974).
7. Bainton, D. F., *Br. J. Haematol.* **29**, 17 (1975).
8. Lichtman, M. A., and Weed, R. I., *Blood* **39**, 301 (1972).
9. Altman, A., and Stossel, T. P., *Br. J. Haematol.* **27**, 241 (1974).
10. Athens, J. W., Haab, O. P., Raab, S. O., et al., *J. Clin. Invest.* **40**, 989 (1961).
11. Deubelbeiss, K. A., Dancey, J. T., Harker, L. A., et al., *J. Clin. Invest.* **55**, 833 (1975).
12. Vincent, P. C., Chanana, A. D., Cronkite, E. P., et al., *Blood* **43**, 371 (1974).
13. Dresch, C., Faille, A., Rain, J. D., et al., *Nouv. Rev. Fr. Hematol.* **15**, 31 (1975).
14. Quesenberry, P., Morley, A., Stohlman, F., et al., *N. Engl. J. Med.* **286**, 227 (1972).
15. Boggs, D. R., Marsh, J. C., Chervenick, P. A., et al., *Proc. Soc. Exp. Biol. Med.* **127**, 689 (1968).
16. McCall, C. E., DeChatelet, L. R., Brown, D., et al., *Nature* **249**, 841 (1974).
17. Bradley, T. R., and Metcalf, D., *Aust. J. Exp. Biol. Med. Sci.* **44**, 287 (1966).
18. Robinson, W. A., and Mangalik, A., *Semin. Hematol.* **12**, 7 (1975).
19. Chervenick, P. A., and LoBuglio, A. F., *Science* **178**, 164 (1972).
20. Broxmeyer, H., Van Zant, G., Zucali, J. R., et al., *Proc. Soc. Exp. Biol. Med.* **145**, 1262 (1974).
21. Rothstein, G., Hügl, E. H., Chervenick, P. A., et al., *Blood* **41**, 73 (1973).
22. Price, G. B., McCulloch, E. A. M., and Till, J. E., *Blood* **42**, 341 (1973).
23. MacVittie, T. J., and McCarthy, K. F., *Exp. Hematol.* **2**, 182 (1974).

24. Rytömaa, T., *Br. J. Haematol.* **24**, 141 (1973).
25. Niskanen, E., Tyler, W. S., Symann, M., et al., *Blood* **43**, 23 (1974).
26. Marmor, J. B., Russell, J. L., Miller, A. M., et al., *Blood* **46**, 39 (1975).
27. Meuret, G., *Monozytopoese beim Menschen,* J. F. Lehmanns-Verlag, Munich, 1974.
28. Ebert, R. H., and Florey, H. W., *Br. J. Exp. Pathol.* **20**, 342 (1939).
29. Godleski, J. J., and Brain, J. D., *J. Exp. Med.* **136**, 630 (1972).
30. Van Furth, R., Langevoort, H. L., and Schaberg, A., in *Mononuclear Phagocytes in Immunity, Infection and Pathology* (R. Van Furth, ed.), Blackwell Scientific Publications, Oxford, 1975.
31. Gordon, S., and Cohn, Z. A., *Int. Rev. Cytol.* **36**, 171 (1973).
32. Volkman, A., and Collins, F. M., *J. Exp. Med.* **139**, 264 (1974).
33. Adams, D. O., *Am. J. Pathol.* **76**, 17 (1974).
34. Van Furth, R., Diesselhoff-den Dulk, and Mattie, H., *J. Exp. Med.* **138**, 1314 (1973).
35. Shaper, A. G., and Lewis, P., *Lancet* **2**, 1021 (1971).
36. Caramihai, E., Karayalcin, G., Aballi, A. J., et al., *J. Pediatr.* **86**, 252 (1975).
37. Djaldetti, M., Joshua, H., and Kalderon, M., *Bull. Res. Coun. Israel* **9E**, 24 (1960).
38. Reimann, H. A., and DeBerardinis, C. T., *Blood* **4**, 1109 (1949).
39. Lund, J. E., Padgett, G. A., and Ott, R. L., *Blood* **29**, 452 (1967).
40. Morley, A. A., Carew, J. P., and Baikie, A. G., *Br. J. Haematol.* **13**, 719 (1967).
41. Guerry, D., IV, Dale, C. C., Omine, M., et al., *J. Clin. Invest.* **52**, 3220 (1973).
42. Dale, D. C., Alling, D. W., and Wolff, S. M., *J. Clin. Invest.* **51**, 2197 (1972).
43. Dale, C. C., and Graw, R. G., Jr., *Science* **183**, 83 (1974).
44. Weiden, P. L., Robinett, B., Graham, T. C., et al., *J. Clin. Invest.* **53**, 950 (1974).
45. Kauder E., and Mauer, A. M., *J. Pediatr.* **69**, 147 (1966).
46. Zuelzer, W. W., *N. Engl. J. Med.* **270**, 699 (1964).
47. Miller, M. E., Oski, F. A., and Harris, M. B., *Lancet* **1**, 665 (1971).
48. Biship, C. R., Rothstein, G., Ashenbrucker, H. E., et al., *J. Clin. Invest.* **50**, 1678 (1971).
49. Wriedt, K., Kauder, E., and Mauer, A. M., *N. Engl. J. Med.* **283**, 1072 (1970).
50. Deinhard, A. S., and Page, A. R., *Br. J. Haematol.* **28**, 333 (1974).
51. Mintz, U., and Sachs, L., *Blood* **41**, 745 (1973).
52. Barak, Y., Paran, M., Levin, S., et al., *Blood* **38**, 74 (1971).
53. L'Esperance, P., Brunning, R., and Good, R. A., *Proc. Natl. Acad. Sci.* (U.S.A.) **70**, 669 (1973).
54. Greenberg, P. L., and Schrier, S. L., *Blood* **41**, 753 (1973).
55. Senn, J. S., Messner, H. A., and Stanley, E. R., *Blood* **44**, 33 (1974).
56. Boxer, L. A., and Stossel, T. P., *J. Clin. Invest.* **53**, 1534 (1974).
57. Boxer, L. A., Greenberg, M. S., Boxer, G. J., et al., *N. Engl. J. Med.* **293**, 748 (1975).
58. Lalezari, P., Jian, A.-F., Yegen, L., et al., *N. Engl. J. Med.* **293**, 744 (1975).
59. Lalezari, P., and Radel, E., *Semin. Hematol.* **11**, 281 (1974).
60. Dale, D. C., Wolff, S. M., *Blood* **38**, 138 (1971).
61. Bodey, G. P., Buckley, M., Sathe, Y. S., et al., *Ann. Intern. Med.* **64**, 328 (1966).
62. Halpern, B. N., *Physiopathology of the Reticuloendothelial System,* C. S. Thomas, Springfield, Ill., 1957.
63. Golde, D. W., Finley, T. N., and Cline, M. J., *N. Engl. J. Med.* **290**, 875 (1974).
64. Bisno, A. L., and Freeman, J. C., *Ann. Intern. Med.* **72**, 389 (1970).
65. McCutcheon, M., *Physiol. Rev.* **26**, 319 (1946).
66. Becker, E. L., and Henson, P. M., *Adv. Immunol.* **17**, 93 (1973).
67. Hirsch, J. G., and Cohn, Z. A., *J. Exp. Med.* **112**, 1005 (1960).
68. Stossel, T. P., *Semin. Hematol.* **14**, 83 (1975).
69. Stossel, T. P., *Fed. Proc.* **36**, 2181 (1977).
70. Babior, B. M., *N. Engl. J. Med.* **298**, 659 (1978).
71. Elsbach, P., *N. Engl. J. Med.* **289**, 846 (1973).
72. Klebanoff, S. J., *Semin. Hematol.* **12**, 117 (1975).
73. Stossel, T. P., Mason, R. J., and Smith, A. L., *J. Clin. Invest.* **54**, 638 (1974).
74. Jensen, M. S., and Bainton, D. F., *J. Cell Biol.* **56**, 379 (1973).
75. Zeya, H. I., and Spitznagel, J. K., *J. Bacteriol.* **91**, 755 (1966).
76. Masson, P. L., Heremans, J. E., and Schonne, E., *J. Exp. Med.* **130**, 643 (1969).
77. Root, R. K., and Stossel, T. P., *J. Clin. Invest.* **53**, 1207 (1974).
78. Root, R. K., Metcalf, J., Oshino, N., et al., *J. Clin. Invest.* **55**, 945 (1975).
79. Babior, B. M., Kipnes, R. S., and Curnutte, J. T., *J. Clin. Invest.* **52**, 741 (1973).

80. Weissmann G., Zurier, R. B., and Hoffstein, S., *Am. J. Pathol.* **68**, 539 (1972).
81. Chediak, M., *Rev. Hematol.* **7**, 362 (1952).
82. Higashi, O., *Tokohu J. Exp. Med.* **59**, 315 (1954).
83. Blume, R. S., and Wolff, S. M., *Medicine* **51**, 247 (1972).
84. Oliver, J. M., Zurier, R. B., and Berlin, R. D., *Nature* **253**, 471 (1975).
85. Root, R. K., Rosenthal, A. S., and Balestra, D. J., *J. Clin. Invest.* **51**, 649 (1972).
86. Stossel, T. P., Root, R. K., and Vaughan, M., *N. Engl. J. Med.* **286**, 120 (1972).
87. White, J. G., *Blood* **29**, 435 (1967).
88. Oliver, C., and Essner, E., *Lab. Invest.* **32**, 17 (1975).
89. Clark, R. A., and Kimball, H. R., *J. Clin. Invest.* **50**, 2645 (1971).
90. Gallin, J. I., Klimerman, J. A., Padgett, G. A., et al., *Blood* **45**, 863 (1975).
91. Oliver, J. M., Krawiec, J. A., and Berlin, R. D., *J. Cell Biol.* **69**, 205 (1976).
92. Stossel, T. P., Pollard, T. D., Mason, R. J., et al., *J. Clin. Invest.* **50**, 1745 (1971).
93. Stossel, T. P., Mason, R. J., Pollard, T. D., et al., *J. Clin. Invest.* **51**, 604 (1972).
94. Boxer, L. A., Hedley-Whyte, E. T., and Stossel, T. P., *N. Engl. J. Med.* **293**, 1093 (1974).
95. Karnovsky, M. L., *Prog. Immunol.* **4**, 83 (1974).
96. Goetzl, E. J., and Austen, K. F., *J. Clin. Invest.* **53**, 591 (1974).
97. Craddock, P. R., Yawata, Y., VanSanten, L., et al., *N. Engl. J. Med.* **290**, 1403 (1974).
98. Baehner, R. L., Feig, S. A., Segel, G. B., et al., *Blood* **38**, 833 (1971).
99. Strauss, R. G., McCarthy, D. J., and Mauer, A. M., *J. Pediatr.* **85**, 431 (1974).
100. Turner, R. A., Schumacher, H. R., and Myers, A. R., *J. Clin. Invest.* **52**, 1632 (1973).
101. Baum, J., in *The Phagocytic Cell in Host Resistance* (J. A. Bellanti and D. H. Dayton, eds.), Raven Press, New York, 1975, p. 283.
102. Penny, R., and Galton, D. A. G., *Br. J. Haematol.* **12**, 633 (1966).
103. Spitler, L. E., Spath, P., Petz, L., et al., *Br. J. Haematol.* **29**, 279 (1975).
104. Brandt, L., and Hedberg, H., *Scand. J. Haematol.* **6**, 548 (1969).
105. Maderazo, E. G., Ward, P. A., and Quintiliani, R., *J. Lab. Clin. Med.* **85**, 621 (1975).
106. Tan, J. S., Strauss, R. G., Akabatu, J., et al., *Am. J. Med.* **57**, 251 (1974).
107. Warden, G. D., Mason, A. D., Jr., and Pruitt, B. A., Jr., *J. Clin. Invest.* **54**, 1001 (1974).
108. McCall, C. E., Caves, J., Cooper, M. R., et al., *J. Infect. Dis.* **124**, 68 (1971).
109. Smith, C. W., Hollers, J. C., Dupree, E., et al., *J. Lab. Clin. Med.* **79**, 878 (1972).
110. Van Epps, D. E., Palmer, D. L., and Williams, R. C., Jr., *J. Immunol.* **113**, 189 (1974).
111. Van Scoy, R. E., Hill, H. R., Ritts, R. E., Jr., et al., *Ann. Intern. Med.* **82**, 765 (1975).
112. Clark, R. A., Root, R. K., Kimball, H. R., et al., *Ann. Intern. Med.* **78**, 515 (1973).
113. Sbarra, A. J., Shirley, W., and Baumstark, J. S., *J. Bacteriol.* **85**, 306 (1963).
114. Miller, M. E., and Baker, L., *J. Pediatr.* **81**, 980 (1972).
115. Hill, H. R., Sauls, H. S., Dettloff, J. L., et al., *Clin. Immunol. Immunopathol.* **2**, 395 (1974).
116. Cohn, Z. A., *Yale J. Biol. Med.* **35**, 29 (1962).
117. Boggs, D. R., Athens, J. W., Cartwright, G. E., et al., *Am. J. Pathol.* **44**, 763 (1964).
118. Handin, R. I., and Stossel, T. P., *Blood* **51**, 771 (1978).
119. Dale, D. C., Fauci, A. S., and Wolff, S. M., *N. Engl. J. Med.* **291**, 1154 (1974).
119a. Kaye, D., and Hook, E. W., *J. Immunol.* **91**, 518 (1963).
119b. Johnston, R. B., Jr., Newman, S. L., and Struth, A. G., *N. Engl. J. Med.* **288**, 803 (1973).
119c. Pearson, H. A., Spencer, R. P., and Cornelius, E. A., *N. Engl. J. Med.* **281**, 923 (1969).
120. Baehner, R. L., Murrmann, S. K., Davis, J., et al., *J. Clin. Invest.* **56**, 571 (1975).
121. Baehner, R. L., and Nathan, D. G., *N. Engl. J. Med.* **278**, 971 (1968).
122. Windhorst, D. B., Page, A. R., Holmes, B., et al., *J. Clin. Invest.* **47**, 1026 (1968).
123. Dupree, E., Smith, C. W., and MacDougall, N. L. Y., *J. Pediatr.* **81**, 770 (1972).
124. Azimi, P. H., Bodenbender, J. G., Hintz, R. L., et al., *J.A.M.A.* **206**, 23 (1968).
125. Holmes, B. H., Park, B. H., Malawista, S. E., et al., *N. Engl. J. Med.* **283**, 217 (1970).
126. Nathan, D. G., and Baehner, R. L., *Prog. Hematol.* **7**, 235 (1970).
127. Cooper, M. R., DeChatelet, L. R., McCall, C. E., et al., *J. Clin. Invest.* **51**, 769 (1972).
128. Johnston, R. B., Jr., and Baehner, R. L., *Pediatrics* **48**, 730 (1971).
129. Landing, B. H., and Shirkey, H. S., *Pediatrics* **20**, 431 (1957).
130. Pitt, J., and Bernheimer, H. P., *Infect. Immunol.* **9**, 48 (1974).
131. Stossel, T. P., *Blood* **42**, 121 (1973).
132. Eschenbach, C., *Pediatr. Res.* **4**, 493 (1970).
133. Gold, S. B., Hanes, D. M., Stites, D. P., et al., *N. Engl. J. Med.* **291**, 332 (1974).

134. Baehner, R. L., Karnovsky, M. J., and Karnovsky, M. L., *J. Clin. Invest.* **47**, 187 (1968).
135. Kauder, E., Kahle, L. L., Moreno, H., et al., *J. Clin. Invest.* **47**, 1753 (1968).
136. Ulevitch, R. J., Henson, P., Holmes, B., et al., *J. Immunol.* **112**, 1383 (1974).
137. Ward, P. A., and Schlegel, R. A., *Lancet* **2**, 344 (1969).
138. Usui, T., Amano, D., Amano, T., et al., *Ann. Paediat. Japon.* **19**, 22 (1973).
139. Schaller, J., *Ann. Intern. Med.* **76**, 747 (1972).
140. Moellering, R. C., Jr., and Weinberg, A. N., *Ann. Intern. Med.* **73**, 595 (1970).
141. Marsh, W. L., Øyen, R., Nichols, M. E., et al., *Br. J. Haematol.* **29**, 247 (1975).
142. Grignaschi, V. J., Sperperatp, A. M., Etcheverry, M. J., et al., *Rev. Asoc. Med. Argent.* **77**, 218 (1963).
143. Lehrer, R. I., and Cline, M. J., *J. Clin. Invest.* **48**, 1478 (1969).
144. Salmon, S. E., Cline, M. J., Schultz, J., et al., *N. Engl. J. Med.* **282**, 250 (1970).
145. Higashi, O., Katsuyama, N., and Satodate, R., *Tokohu J. Exp. Med.* **87**, 77 (1965).
146. Arakawa, T., Wada, Y., Hayashi, T., et al., *Tokohu J. Exp. Med.* **87**, 52 (1965).
147. Lehrer, R. I., Goldberg, L. S., Apple, M. A., et al., *Ann. Intern. Med.* **76**, 447 (1972).
148. Baehner, R. L., Neiburger, R. G., Johnson, D. E., et al., *N. Engl. J. Med.* **289**, 1209 (1973).
149. Souillet, G., Germain, D., Carraz, M., et al., *Rev. Inst. Pasteur de Lyon* **6**, 87 (1975).
150. Seth, V., and Chandra, R. K., *Arch. Dis. Child.* **47**, 282 (1972).
151. Douglas, S. D., Lahav, M., and Fudenberg, H. H., *Am. J. Med.* **49**, 274 (1970).
152. Rodey, G. E., Park, B. H., Ford, D. K., et al., *Am. J. Med.* **49**, 322 (1970).
153. Davis, W. C., Douglas, S. D., and Fudenberg, H. H., *Ann. Intern. Med.* **69**, 1237 (1968).
154. Mandell, G. L., *Arch. Intern. Med.* **130**, 754 (1972).
155. Odeberg, H., Olofsson, T., and Olsson, I., *Br. J. Haematol.* **29**, 427 (1975).
156. Cline, M. J., *J. Clin. Invest.* **52**, 2185 (1973).

Chapter Fourteen

Human Complement Deficiencies

CHESTER A. ALPER AND FRED S. ROSEN

Center for Blood Research, Division of Immunology, Department of Medicine, Children's Hospital Medical Center, and Department of Pediatrics, Harvard Medical School, Boston, Massachusetts

Although the first autosomally inherited deficiency of a serum protein was that of a complement component in guinea pigs discovered almost 60 years ago (1), most of the known complement deficiency states in man and experimental animals have been identified within the past 10 years. Several factors have permitted the recent explosion of knowledge in this area. Most important has been remarkable recent progress in our basic knowledge of the complement system, including the identification, characterization, and purification of individual proteins. Antisera are now available to almost all complement proteins, so that immunochemical as well as functional means are available to study patients and experimental animals and to identify deficiency states.

The study of humans and animals with hereditary deficiency of complement proteins has provided invaluable information on the role of complement in host defense and in the pathogenesis of disease, on reaction mechanisms within the complement system, on predisposing noncomplement genetic factors linked to complement genes in certain diseases, and on molecular mechanisms in protein synthesis. Although this review will stress inherited complement deficiency states in man, some attention will be given to deficiencies in experimental animals and to apparently acquired deficiencies of complement proteins in certain patients.

Complement takes part in the phlogistic response in a number of ways, and a variety of biologic activities are elaborated at different points during complement activation, as seen in Fig. 1. The role of some of these activities, such as increased vascular permeability, chemotaxis, and enhancement of phagocytosis, in the inflammatory response is clear. Others, such as conglutination, appear to be chiefly curiosities and research tools. It is evident from Fig. 1 that a number of

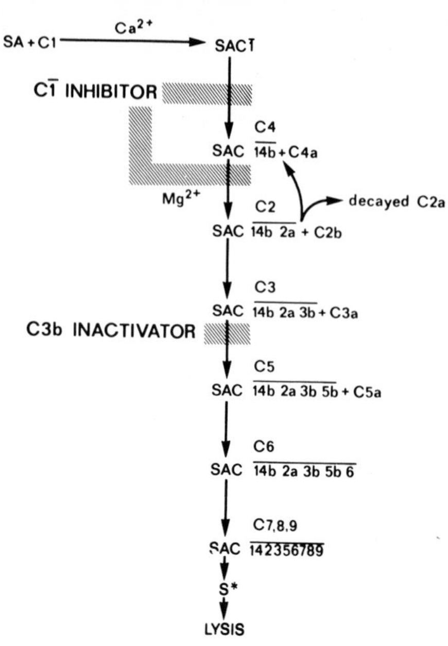

Figure 1. Scheme of complement activation via the classical pathway. SA is an antigenic site combined with antibody.

complement-mediated functions are developed at more than one stage of complement activation. For example, the small fragments of C3 and C5 have similar physiologic activities. Moreover, immune adherence is exhibited by particles bearing bound C4, C3, or both. The only complement-mediated function requiring all classical and common pathway components is cell lysis, including bactericidal activity (which may also proceed via the alternative and common pathways).

INHERITED DEFICIENCIES OF HUMAN COMPLEMENT PROTEINS

Most genetic defects in human complement are rare. Such deficiencies may affect one of the components or one of the two known inhibitors of the system, C1̄ inhibitor and C3b inactivator. All save one of the known defects in man are inherited as autosomal codominant traits with severe deficiency in homozygotes and approximately half-normal levels in heterozygotes. The single but important exception to this mode of inheritance is hereditary angioedema. Subjects affected with this disorder are all heterozygotes who have either much less than half the normal serum level of normal C1̄ inhibitor or normal or elevated serum concentrations of dysfunctional protein without appreciable normal protein.

The most common of the genetic deficiencies of complement in man would appear to affect C2. Several dozen homozygous C2-deficient subjects are now known, whereas deficiencies of other components have been found in less than half a dozen individuals. Because of the dramatic symptoms of hereditary angioneurotic edema, several hundred affected kindred have been identified. Precise incidence or mutation rate estimates are unavailable for any complement protein deficiency state.

Hereditary Angioneurotic Edema

Hereditary angioneurotic edema was recognized during the last century (2,3), but the molecular basis of the disease, a genetically determined deficiency of the $C\bar{1}$ inhibitor, was not defined until 1963 (4). The defect is transmitted as an autosomal dominant. The serum of most affected patients contains between 5 and 30% of the normal concentration of $C\bar{1}$ inhibitor.

Patients with this disease are prone to recurrent episodes of swelling. The edema fluid accumulates rapidly in the affected part, which becomes tense but not discolored; no itching, no pain, and no redness are associated with the edema. Laryngeal edema may be fatal because of airway obstruction and consequent pulmonary edema. If the intestinal tract is involved, most often the jejunum, severe abdominal cramps and bilious vomiting ensue. Diarrhea, which is clear and watery in character, occurs when the colon is affected. The attacks last 48 to 72 hours. Although they are often unheralded, they may occur subsequent to trauma, menses, excessive fatigue, and mental stress. Attacks of angioedema are infrequent in early childhood; the disease exacerbates at adolescence and tends to subside in the sixth decade of life. In children especially, a mottling of the skin reminiscent of erythema marginatum may be frequently noticed and not necessarily be associated with attacks of angioedema (5).

During attacks of angioedema, activated C1 ($C\bar{1}$) can be demonstrated in plasma, an event that cannot be detected in normal plasma (6). C4 and C2, the natural substrates of $C\bar{1}$, are consumed so that their serum concentration falls precipitously as the attack progresses. There is little change in the terminal complement components. Highly purified $C\bar{1}$ or $C\bar{1}s$, when injected intradermally into normal skin or into patients, induces angioedema (7). This reaction does not occur in people genetically deficient in C2, or in guinea pigs genetically deficient in C4, thus suggesting that the interaction of $C\bar{1}$ with C4 and C2 generates one or more factors that enhance vascular permeability (7). The effect is on the postcapillary venule (8).

A polypeptide kinin-like substance that has vasopermeability-inducing properties has also been generated in the plasma of the patients in vitro (9). The generation of this peptide is inhibited by soybean-trypsin inhibitor, purified $C\bar{1}$ inhibitor, heparin, and antibody to C4 and C2, but not by antibody to C3. In addition to enhancing vascular permeability, the peptide contracts estrous rat uterus and causes histamine release from mast cells (8). However, antihistaminics or histamine-depleting substances such as 48/80 do not inhibit the angioedema induced by $C\bar{1}s$ or the peptide (7). Very recently, mixtures of purified C1s, plasmin, C4, and C2 have generated the peptide. With large inputs of C2, C4 was not necessary. Although patients with angioneurotic edema have massive histaminuria, antihistamine drugs neither prevent nor diminish attacks of angioedema (5).

The autosomal dominant inheritance of hereditary angioneurotic edema presents an interesting puzzle. Obviously, affected individuals are heterozygous for the abnormality. Despite this, their serum contains very little $C\bar{1}$ inhibitor (average, 17% of normal) (10). Liver biopsy specimens can be shown to contain no hepatic parenchymal cells detectably engaged in synthesis of $C\bar{1}$ inhibitor, whereas 3 to 5% of normal hepatic cells give positive fluorescence with a fluorescein-labeled antibody to C1 inhibitor (11).

The $C\bar{1}$ inhibitor, or α_2-neuraminoglycoprotein, is the most highly glycosylated glycoprotein of serum. It contains over 40% carbohydrate, almost half of which is neuraminic acid (12–14). It has a molecular weight of 106,000 but behaves like a 7S protein on gel filtration. It is a single polypeptide chain of three repeating subunits in linear array. In addition to its capacity to inactivate $C\overline{1s}$, it inhibits $C\overline{1r}$, plasmin, kallikrein, factor XIa of the clotting system, and activated Hageman factor (15). However, these other inhibitory activities can be replaced by α_2-macroglobulin or antithrombin III. It remains the unique inhibitory substance in serum for $C\bar{1}$. Both plasmin and trypsin cleave the $C\bar{1}$ inhibitor and render it inactive (16), as does acidity; the protein loses its functional inhibitory activity when exposed to a pH below 7.0 (12).

In 15% of affected kindred, sera of patients contain normal or elevated amounts of an immunologically cross-reacting (CRM^+), nonfunctional protein (17,10). The CRM^+, nonfunctional $C\bar{1}$ inhibitors differ among the different kindred with respect to (1) their electrophoretic mobilities (Fig. 2), (2) their capacity to bind $C\overline{1s}$, and (3) their capacity to inhibit esterolysis by $C\overline{1s}$ of *N*-acetyl-tyrosine ethyl ester. However, all CRM^+ $C\bar{1}$ inhibitors fail to inhibit destruction of C4 by $C\bar{1}$ (10). The clinical course of the disease is the same in CRM^+ and CRM^- patients, and the CRM^+ proteins are inherited as autosomal dominant traits.

Approximately 50% of patients with hereditary angioneurotic edema will have a complete cessation of symptoms by taking a methyltestosterone linguet daily (18). Recent studies (19,20) with synthetic androgens have shown even more striking suppression of attacks and, remarkably, a rise in $C\bar{1}$ inhibitor serum levels in deficient patients. In those patients with increased levels of dysfunctional protein, the latter have fallen in concentration with the appearance of normal $C\bar{1}$ inhibitor. C4 and C2 levels in serum of patients under treatment have increased toward normal. Epsilon-aminocaproic acid and its analogue, tranexamic acid, are also effective as prophylactic therapy (21,22). It is now

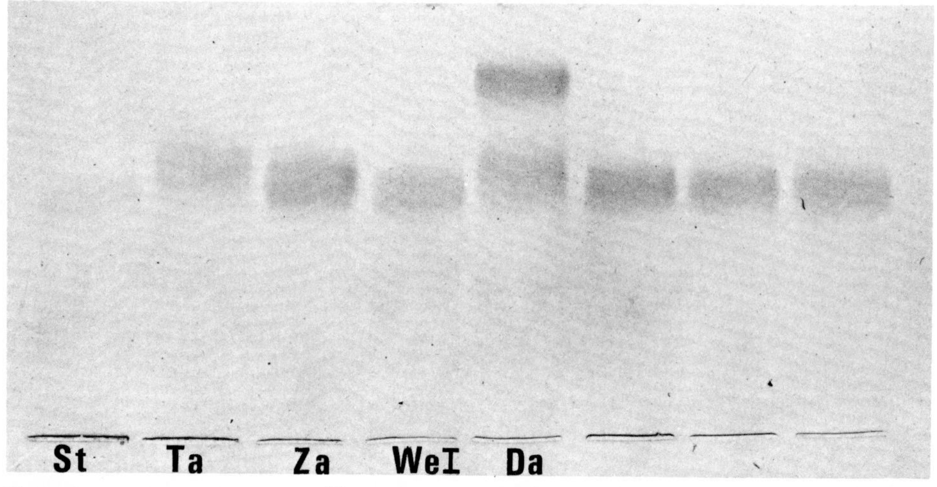

Figure 2. An immunofixation of $C\bar{1}$ inhibitor after agarose gel electrophoresis at pH 8.6. The serum samples are (from left to right) from a CRM^- patient, from four CRM^+ patients, and a normal subject. The normal serum is untreated, incubated with $C\overline{1s}$, and incubated with antigen-antibody precipitate.

known that plasmin is required for the production of the C2-kinin, and this fact explains the efficacy of plasminogen inhibitors in the therapy of this disease (23). Although plasma infusions have been attempted in the therapy of acute attacks of angioedema (24), this procedure has no merit in light of present knowledge and may in fact be dangerous since substrate for $C\bar{1}$ is being infused along with inhibitor.

C3b Inactivator Deficiency

Two patients with inherited deficiency of C3b inactivator have been reported. The original patient, who is now 30 years old, also has Klinefelter's syndrome (25). He has a lifelong history of severe infections with such organisms as *Diplococcus pneumoniae, Hemophilus influenzae,* and β-hemolytic streptococci. These infections have included septicemia, pneumonia on several occasions, meningitis, sinusitis, and otitis media. The second patient is an 11-year-old girl (26) who has had several episodes of meningitis but no other serious infections. The first patient has been studied extensively, but the abnormalities noted appear to be identical to those observed in the second case and our discussion will deal with findings in his case.

The C3b inactivator serves as an inhibitor of the alternative pathway of complement activation by cleaving C3b and destroying its ability to activate factor D and by destroying factor $\bar{D}$ already formed. Owing to the absence of this inhibitor, there is continuous activation of the alternative pathway in vivo and consumption of factor B and C3. C5 and properdin are only minimally affected.

The patient's serum is deficient in complement-mediated functions, such as hemolytic activity for antibody-sensitized sheep red cells, bactericidal activity for smooth gram-negative organisms, opsonic activity for antibody-sensitized pneumococci and endotoxin particles, and chemotaxis (25). These abnormalities could not be corrected by the addition of purified C3.

Measurement of the classical components of complement revealed a markedly lowered concentration of C3. On crossed immunoelectrophoresis of freshly drawn plasma with edetic acid (EDTA) (to inhibit activation in vitro), it could be seen that of the total immunochemically detected C3, which was about 20% of the normal mean, about 75% was present in this patient's blood as the conversion product, C3b. Thus, the patient's native C3 concentration was only about 5% of normal. Functional titration of C3 gave the latter figure. That C3 was being cleaved in vivo was confirmed by metabolic studies with purified, radioisotope-labeled C3. The fractional catabolic rate for C3 in this patient was about five times normal, and 40% of the labeled protein was converted to C3b within two hours following the injection. Of the remaining classical components, only C5 was lowered, to about 40% of the normal mean concentration. These observations were interpreted as evidence for nonclassical pathway activation of C3 with only a modest attack on C5, the next component in the complement sequence (25).

The patient's serum had a markedly lowered concentration of factor B (about 5% of the normal level), and most of this circulated as the conversion fragments, Ba and Bb. When purified factor B was added to his serum and incubated, there was prompt cleavage of factor B in vitro, indicating the presence of factor $\overline{\mathrm{D}}$ (27). In fact, factor $\overline{\mathrm{D}}$ was first recognized as an enzyme capable of cleaving factor B and characterized physicochemically in 1971 (27) as a result of studies of this patient.

Infusion of 500 ml of normal plasma caused prompt conversion of C3b to C3c, disappearance of C3 conversion products within a few hours, a rise of native C3 concentration to half-normal by five days, a gradual restoration of complement-mediated functions, and a rise in C5 to normal (28). Factor B rose transiently to a maximum within the first day and then fell again, but C3 and most complement-mediated functions remained partially restored for 17 days. The C3 could be shown to be the patient's since it was C3 S, whereas that in the donor plasma was C3 FS. A second metabolic study with purified, labeled C3 showed a normalization of the fractional catabolic rate to about twice normal. These observations suggested that C3 and factor B were being attacked and consumed in vivo, and that the patient's missing inhibitor of the alternative pathway (later shown to be the C3b inactivator) was being supplied by the plasma (29,30). This was later confirmed when all the effects of whole plasma were mimicked by an infusion of purified C3b inactivator (31).

That the C3b inactivator deficiency was the patient's primary defect and that the other protein deficiencies were secondary and on the basis of consumption were suggested by the fact that the concentration of the C3b inactivator declined exponentially after the plasma infusion, whereas C3, factor B, and C5 rose gradually (29). Properdin concentration, which was initially slightly low, also rose following the infusion of either plasma or C3b inactivator, but a metabolic study with labeled properdin failed to show increased catabolism in the patient's resting state (32).

Confirmation that the patient was probably homozygous for C3b inactivator deficiency was obtained by the study of the concentration of this protein in the serum of his family (30). His mother, three of his six siblings, and two nephews had approximately 40 to 50% of the normal concentration of this protein (Fig. 3). His father's serum could not be tested.

C1r Deficiency

Deficiency of C1r has been found in two families. A 16-year-old Puerto Rican boy (33,34) with a lupus-like syndrome of malar rash, arthralgia, and subacute focal membranous glomerulitis was found to be C1r-deficient. His lupus erythematosus (LE) cell test was negative. A 24-year-old sister was reported to have recurrent fever, arthralgia, and a malar rash. She was also C1r-deficient. Three siblings of the propositus died at an early age of overwhelming infection or lupus-like disease. Five other siblings were alive and well. It is of interest that in the homozygous C1r-deficient individuals, serum concentrations of C1s were approximately half-normal. The C1r deficiency has been demonstrated in the propositus and his sister by functional and immunochemical tests (35). C1r levels in the healthy siblings and parents of the propositus were intermediate or normal, and their total hemolytic C1 activity was in the normal range.

In another family (36), an 11-year-old girl with chronic glomerulonephritis lacked detectable C1r. In her serum, too, C1s levels were half-normal.

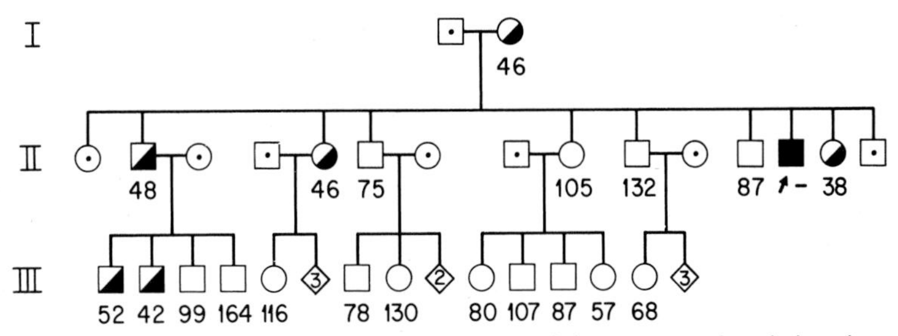

Figure 3. Family tree of a patient (↗) with C3b inactivator deficiency. Numbers below the symbols are C3b inactivator levels as per cent normal serum (normal range = 57 to 132%). *Diamonds* are untested siblings. *Half-blackened symbols* indicate heterozygous deficient persons. *Dots within a symbol* indicate an untested individual.

Unambiguous determination of heterozygotes for C1r deficiency may not be possible. This clearly limits attempts to define linkage of C1r deficiency to other genetic loci.

C4 Deficiency

The serum of an 18-year-old girl with a lupus-like syndrome was found to be totally deficient in C4 by functional and immunochemical criteria (37). Although she had a typical malar rash and arthralgia, her LE cell test was negative. The serum of the patient's mother contained half-normal levels of C4. Other family members are possible heterozygotes (37).

A second C4-deficient subject has been identified (38,39). This patient is a 5-year-old boy with typical systemic lupus erythematosus. He has had fever, myalgia, arthritis, and, more recently, nephrotic syndrome. Renal biopsy showed diffuse proliferative glomerulonephritis. By both functional and immunochemical testing, heterozygous deficient family members could be identified. However, the normal range for C4 in serum is very wide, and the lower limit of this range (mean less two standard deviations) is well below 50% of the mean normal level. Thus, the unambiguous identification of heterozygous deficient individuals, even in a family with known homozygous deficient subjects, is impossible by measuring serum C4 concentration only.

If, as has been suggested (40), there is inherited structural polymorphism in C4, then an additional means of identifying some heterozygotes and distinguishing them from normals within families of C4-deficient subjects is available. Such analysis has been performed, and is said to have shown $C4^{-}$ gene (40), analogous to $C3^{-}$ found in C3 deficiency (see that section). However, the nature of the genetic polymorphism of C4 needs to be confirmed.

C2 Deficiency

Inherited deficiency of C2 is probably the commonest of genetic complement deficiency states. One healthy C2-deficient blood donor was found in a survey of 10,000 blood donors in Manchester, England (41). Glass and co-workers (42) found 1.2% of random individuals to be heterozygous for C2 deficiency, in approximate keeping with the Manchester findings.

A large number of reports of individuals homozygous for C2 deficiency have appeared in the literature (for reviews see Alper and Rosen, 43, or Agnello, 44). The defect is transmitted as an autosomal recessive trait, but heterozygotes are easily detected by their having half the normal serum C2 concentration as determined by functional or immunochemical measurements.

C2 is synthesized by fixed and wandering macrophages (45). Such macrophages are normal in C2-deficient individuals with regard to their phagocytic function. However, culture of macrophages from the blood of C2-deficient individuals reveals the failure of these cells to synthesize and secrete C2 (46).

The propositi in the first four kindred discovered to have C2 deficiency and four homozygous affected siblings were all found to be healthy individuals. In fact, in two cases the discovery was made in immunologists whose blood was being used for routine hemolytic or immune adherence tests. Subsequently, four more kindred were discovered because the propositae presented with systemic lupus erythematosus (SLE). The propositi in three further kindred presented with Schönlein-Henoch purpura, and yet another, with polymyositis. These findings suggested that C2 deficiency may be associated with a high incidence of connective tissue disease. This subject is dealt with in more detail below.

Serum from homozygotes for C2 deficiency lacks certain complement-mediated functions: hemolytic activity, bactericidal activity, and immune adherence (47). It appears probable that the deficiency gene for C2 is an allele of the structural locus for this protein. Some 4% of random individuals have inherited structural variants of C2 (48–50), and in one individual who has a half-normal concentration in serum of C2, the only gene product found is one of these variants (50). Studies of the family of this individual have not been reported, but this suggests that the C2 deficiency gene is a silent allele at the structural C2 locus.

C3 Deficiency

Hereditary deficiency of C3 was first detected in heterozygotes who had approximately 50% of the normal level of this protein (51). Affected persons were entirely healthy, although minor defects in complement-mediated functions could be detected in their serum. Serum hemolytic complement was variably slightly reduced, and the enhancement of phagocytosis of antibody-sensitized pneumococci was subnormal (52).

Analysis of the inheritance patterns of partial C3 deficiency revealed that affected persons had inherited a silent C3 gene, $C3^{-}$, that produced no detectable protein. This gene was allelic to the common structural genes, $C3^{F}$ and $C3^{S}$ (53).

Several years later, a 15-year-old Afrikaner girl was found to have no detectable C3 in her serum (54). She had had numerous episodes of infection by pyogenic bacteria, including pneumonia (14 episodes), septicemia, otitis media, and bacterial meningitis. By immunochemical estimation, her serum C3 level was less than 0.25 mg/100 ml (normal range, 100 to 200 mg/100 ml). On functional analysis, 13 U (units) of C3 per ml were detected, which may or may not have been attributable to C3. Thus, this patient had less than 0.1% of the normal serum concentration of C3. All other complement components were present in normal or near-normal concentrations in her serum.

Most complement-mediated functions, such as hemolytic activity, opsonization of endotoxin particles (54), and bactericidal activity, were markedly depressed or absent from this patient's serum. Of considerable interest was the failure of a leukocytosis to occur in this patient in the face of severe, systemic gram-positive bacterial infection (54). In contrast to these deficits, immune adherence was near normal in her serum (55), as were her humoral antibody response and the capacity of her serum to produce passive hemolysis of guinea pig erythrocytes on incubation with purified cobra venom factor. These observations confirm the requirement of C3 for whole-serum hemolytic complement activity, bactericidal activity, opsonization, and leukocyte mobilization. They confirm that immune adherence requires only the first three complement components, C1, C4, and C2. They also indicate that C3 is not required for normal antibody production or for passive hemolysis induced by cobra venom factor (55).

To determine the mode of inheritance of C3 deficiency, over 100 of the patient's relatives were studied (Fig. 4). The patient's parents, who were first cousins, had half-normal C3 levels, as did four of five of her siblings and a large number of collateral relatives. Furthermore, from C3 typing it was clear that the patient was homozygous for $C3^-$, a gene indistinguishable from that found earlier only in heterozygotes (51). A remarkable finding was that an unrelated woman, who was also heterozygous for C3 deficiency, married a normal member of the proposita's family and transmitted $C3^-$ to her two children. This suggests that $C3^-$ is relatively common in the Afrikaner population, a possibility also supported by the finding of a second Afrikaner child, unrelated to the heterozygotes in this family, who apparently also was homozygous for C3 deficiency. This child unfortunately died of bacterial infection (56).

Three other patients with severe deficiency of C3 have been found. A 4-year-old girl had a history of severe infections with *H. influenzae, D. pneumoniae,* and *Escherichia coli.* She had no detectable serum C3 by radial immunodiffusion or hemolytic assay (57). Her serum was found to be defective in opsonization, bactericidal activity, and hemolytic complement activity. Immune adherence was normal. There was delayed neutrophil migration into a Rebuck skin window, but the patient had a normal neutrophilia when infected, in contrast to the first C3-deficient patient, in whom leukocytosis did not occur during infection. Family studies were not possible in this case, but it appears likely that she was homozygous C3-deficient.

Another patient with C3 deficiency has been identified (58), a 3-year-old child whose serum contained about 1% of the normal concentration of C3. The parents, who were distantly related, had reduced serum C3 concentrations, as did two paternal uncles and a sibling. C3 typing was uninformative since all persons tested were S- or SS. The complement abnormalities in this patient were similar to those reported earlier for the other C3-deficient subjects. This patient, in contrast to the other three, has not had severe infections but had an episode of fever, rash, and arthralgia, which suddenly terminated coincident with the infusion of normal plasma.

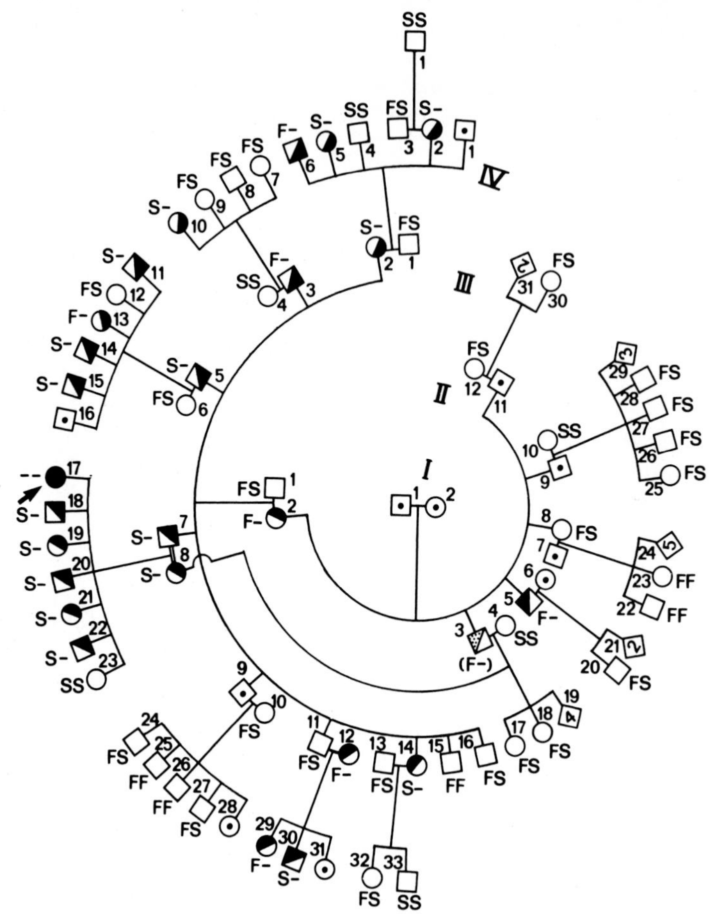

Figure 4. The family tree of a patient homozygous for C3 deficiency. Symbols as in Fig. 3. The letters next to each symbol indicate C3 type. The homozygote is indicated by the arrow. Half-blackened symbols represent heterozygous deficient individuals. Males are squares and females circles.

Finally, homozygous C3 deficiency was found in a 6-year-old girl of English extraction who also had agenesis of the corpus callosum (59). This patient had had pneumonia at age 5 months and frequent infections since that time, including presumed septic arthritis, and recurrent otitis media and pharyngitis. There was a definite but blunted leukocytosis in response to infection. The concentration of C3 in the serum of this patient was initially 50 μg/ml and over 300 U/ml or 1 to 2% of normal, but two years later was only 17 ng/ml, as measured by radioimmunoassay (59). By the same technique, two other homozygous C3-deficient patients were found to have 24 (54) and 58 ng/ml (58).

C5 Deficiency

Inherited deficiency of C5 has been found in two half-siblings in a single black family (60). The proposita had systemic lupus erythematosus, and her serum had no hemolytically or immunochemically detectable C5. Her half-sister was healthy, and her serum had 2% of the normal level of C5 by functional assay. Nine heterozygotes were found in the immediate family of the proposita (61).

Hemolytic, chemotactic, and bactericidal activity, as well as the ability to support lysis of paroxysmal nocturnal hemoglobinuria (PNH) erythrocytes, was grossly deficient in serum deficient in C5. These functions were restored by the addition of purified C5. Opsonic activity for *Staphylococcus aureus, Candida albicans,* and Baker's yeast was entirely normal in C5-deficient serum (60).

C6 Deficiency

An absence of C6 was found by functional and immunochemical tests in an 18-year-old black woman with gonococcal arthritis. Heterozygosity was detected in the parents and five of nine siblings of the proposita (62). The hemostatic function of the blood of the proposita was normal (63). This observation was of considerable interest because of the retarded coagulation of blood from C6-deficient rabbits (64). (In that species, complement accelerates release of platelet factor III.) The proposita in this kindred also has mild Raynaud's phenomenon.

The serum was deficient in hemolytic and bactericidal activity and lysis of PNH cells. These deficiencies were restored to the serum by purified human C6. Chemotactic activity was normal, thereby casting doubt on the role of $C\overline{567}$ as a major chemotactic influence in man.

A second patient with inherited deficiency of C6 has been reported (65). This 6-year-old boy lacks detectable serum C6, and he had meningococcal meningitis.

C7 Deficiency

Homozygous C7 deficiency has been found in three families, two of which have been reported in detail (66,67). In one of the latter, the propositus was healthy, and in the other, the proposita had severe Raynaud's phenomenon. In one of the families, the parents, children, brother, and niece of the proposita have half-normal serum C7 levels (66). Deficient hemolytic activity was restored to the C7-deficient serum by purified human C7.

C8 Deficiency

A black woman with prolonged disseminated gonococcal infection was found to be C8-deficient following the demonstration of absent hemolytic and bactericidal activity in her serum (68). A number of individuals in the family, including her parents and children, were found to have half-normal C8 levels (68). Preliminary evidence suggests that the C8 deficiency gene is a "silent" allele of the structural gene (69).

In a second family from North Africa (70), the mode of inheritance of C8 deficiency was obscure because the parents were normal; but of their eight children, three were severely deficient, three were normal, and two had intermediate C8 levels in serum. Three lateral relatives also had intermediate C8 levels.

A third C8-deficient subject, a black woman with systemic lupus erythematosus, has not been reported in detail as yet (71). She has not had apparent increased susceptibility to infection. Her serum, like that of the first C8-deficient patient, exhibited deficiency only of hemolytic complement and bactericidal activity among complement-mediated functions.

BIOLOGIC SIGNIFICANCE OF COMPLEMENT DEFICIENCY STATES IN MAN

Complement deficiencies in man (and in experimental animals, a topic not dealt with here but reviewed elsewhere, in ref. 43) have provided valuable evidence for the role of complement in vivo. The serum of patients genetically deficient in single complement proteins has proved to be a powerful tool in dissecting mechanisms of complement action and the participation of that component in a variety of complement-mediated functions. More recently, such sera have been used to explore genetic polymorphism in complement proteins in man and experimental animals.

In general, persons deficient in specific complement proteins have one or more kinds of disorders (if they have symptoms at all): "allergic"-vascular, increased susceptibility to bacterial infection, and collagen vascular. These associations will be dealt with separately.

"Allergic"-Vascular Manifestations

Although a few subjects with C2 deficiency suffered classic atopy (47), allergy as such does not appear to have an increased incidence in complement-deficient subjects. On the other hand, persons with hereditary angioedema ($C\overline{1}$ inhibitor deficiency) and C3b inactivator deficiency have clear-cut vascular permeability changes related to their basic genetic abnormalities. In both disorders there is unbridled activation of complement, either of its classical or its alternative arm.

As was mentioned earlier, the uninhibited action of $C\overline{1}$ on C4 and C2 is attended by cleavage of these substrates, and the elaboration of a vasoactive peptide that has been isolated from patients' plasma and partly characterized (9). Recently, this material has been generated in vitro from mixtures of purified $C\overline{1}$, C4, C2, and plasmin (23). With sufficient input of C2, C4 can be eliminated, providing further evidence for the earlier conclusion that the vasoactive peptide is derived from C2 (7). The requirement for plasmin in the in vitro generation system is almost certainly important in vivo, since $C\overline{1}$ inhibitor inhibits plasmin and synthetic inhibitors of plasminogen activation, such as ε-aminocaproic acid or tranexamic acid, can provide effective prophylaxis against attacks of angioedema in this disease. Although patients with hereditary angioedema have hyperhistaminuria (72), perhaps from some elaboration of C3a in vivo, they do not have urticaria.

In contrast, there is massive histaminuria in C3b inactivator deficiency (28), and the first patient to be described with this disorder had intermittent urticaria, particularly after a shower or when given normal plasma (and hence C3 as substrate). It is reasonable to attribute these abnormalities to the elaboration in vivo of large amounts of C3a from uninhibited alternative pathway activation with attendant C3 cleavage.

Increased Susceptibility to Infection

There appear to be two groups of complement-deficient patients with undue susceptibility to infection: those with deficits of C3 directly, or of C3 and factor B secondary to C3b inactivator deficiency; and those with deficiencies of later-acting or common pathway proteins, particularly C6 and C8. The organisms involved in C3-deficient patients are chiefly the pyogens: the streptococcus, the pneumococcus, the meningococcus, and *H. influenzae.* These bacteria are much the same as those that afflict agammaglobulinemics. Although severe deficits in most complement-mediated functions can be demonstrated in serum from these patients, it appears that a deficit in opsonization is central to their reduced host resistance. It is dangerous to be too simplistic, however, since one C3-deficient subject had had no serious infections by the age of 4 years (58). Clearly, other factors, including environment, play their part in any specific instance.

Both known C6-deficient subjects have had disseminated neisserial infection, meningitis in one instance, gonococcal arthritis in the other. This has also been the case for one of three known C8-deficient persons. On the other hand, neither of the two C7-deficient patients has had unusual infections. Since the only known defect in host resistance in serum from any of these subjects is in the bactericidal reaction, it would seem logical to ascribe their increased susceptibility to this deficit.

Collagen Vascular Disease

Table 1 summarizes the clinical associations of reported cases with inherited complement deficiency states. There is a striking incidence of systemic lupus erythematosus, "lupus-like" disease, and a variety of phenomena probably not the same but all suspected of having an immunologic basis. These associations are with deficiencies of late-acting components of complement as well as of early components. Because C2 deficiency is so common, most attention has been directed to this deficiency. Agnello (44) has summarized and analyzed the current information on the relationship between homozygous C2 deficiency and disease. As can be seen in Table 1 (from his publication), of 38 homozygous C2-deficient subjects, 23 have disease, chiefly of suspected immunologic type. Fourteen had systemic lupus erythematosus or discoid lupus erythematosus, and of these, the female to male ratio was 6:1, whereas the overall female to male ratio in the non-SLE C2-deficient subjects was nearly 1:1.

This association between lupus and C2 deficiency may have one or more of several explanations. The gene for C2 deficiency (and the structural locus for C2) is on the sixth human chromosome, closely linked with the HLA region (73). The *C2* locus is 2 to 4 centimorgans from HLA-B and even closer to HLA-D. In other words, the genes at the *C2* locus are inherited together with those for HLA

Table 1. HLA Types and Clinical Findings in Kindred of Hereditary C2 Deficiency[a]

Kindred No.	Homozygous Individuals		Clinical Findings
	Age	Sex	
1	45	M	Normal
	43	F	Normal
	40	M	Normal
2	40	M	Normal
3	7	F	Normal
4	19	M	Normal
	12	M	Normal
	10	F	Normal
5	55	F	SLE with discoid
6	18	M	SLE with discoid
7	24	F[b]	Anaphylactoid purpura
8	31	F	Normal
	37	M	Discoid LE
9	11	M[b]	Anaphylactoid purpura
10	18	M	Normal
11	25	F	Idiopathic membranous GN
12	22	F	SLE with discoid
	65	F	Discoid LE
13	50	M	Normal
	60	M	Dermatomyositis
14	10	M	Normal
	13	F	Anaphylactoid purpura
15	44	F[b]	Chronic vasculitis
16	17	F	SLE
17	2	M	Normal
	24	M	Hodgkin's disease
18	23	F	SLE
19	37	F	Discoid LE
20	62	F	Discoid LE
21	1½	F	Frequent infections
	7	F	Frequent infections
22	48	F	SLE
	57	F	Normal
23	24	F	Discoid LE
	12	M	Normal
24	22	F	SLE
25	26	F	SLE
26	16	F	Probable SLE

[a]Adapted from ref. 44.
[b]Presumed to be hereditary deficiency; family studies not possible.

with only minimal (2 to 4%) recombination. Furthermore, there is marked linkage disequilibrium between the C2 deficiency gene *(C2D)* and *HLA A10 B18* (73), and even more striking linkage disequilibrium between *C2D* and *HLA Dw2* (74,75) and Bf^{S} (76). In other words, among random, apparently unrelated individuals, *C2D* is found linked to specific nearby genes. This disequilibrium could be the result of selective pressure keeping them together or could result from the fact that the C2 deficiency mutation occurred fairly recently in human evolution. That the latter is the case is suggested by the fact all the cases of C2 deficiency uncovered to date have been white. In contrast, many of the homozygotes for deficiency of later-acting components, such as C5, C6, or C8, are black.

In any event, it is possible that an unusual immune response gene linked with *C2D* is somehow involved in an increased incidence of lupus in C2-deficient subjects. This possibility is enhanced by the evidence that lupus may result from viral infection. Further evidence for this hypothesis was obtained in a study of C2-deficient heterozygotes wherein it was found that although the incidence among normal individuals was 1.2%, the incidence in patients with lupus was significantly greater (two to three times) (77).

Homozygous deficiency of complement proteins, particularly early-acting components, may predispose to lupus because of the deficiency per se. A possible mechanism is the requirement for complement in the solubilization of immune complexes (78). This would help explain the observed high incidence of lupus in C4 deficiency (37,38), hereditary angioedema (79), and C1r deficiency (33). Since the system only through C3 appears to participate in this function (80), it cannot be invoked to explain lupus in association with deficiencies of C5 (60) and C8 (71).

Finally, there is the problem of bias in the ascertainment and reporting of cases of complement deficiencies that favors a higher incidence of disease in general and collagen vascular disease in particular. Total hemolytic complement was measured initially only in specialized laboratories, so that it is not surprising that the first few cases of C2 deficiency were found among immunologists. As the test became a relatively common routine procedure, those tested tended to have or be suspected of having "immunologic disease" and, in particular, lupus. The association may therefore reflect the incidence of these diseases in the tested population.

That there is a real association is suggested by the studies in heterozygous deficient subjects (77) mentioned above. It is also suggested by a brief consideration of numbers. Assuming the incidence of lupus (both systemic and discoid varieties) to lie between 1 and 0.1% of the general population in the United States and the incidence of homozygous C2 deficiency is 1 in 10,000, there are approximately 20,000 homozygotes for C2 deficiency in the United States, of whom 20 to 200 would be expected to have lupus by chance alone. To have already identified 14 such subjects suggests that the number who have both C2 deficiency and lupus is much greater than the random association would predict. Thus, it appears likely that C4 (also HLA-linked; refs. 37,39) and C2 deficiency (and perhaps other complement deficiencies) predispose to lupus, but the exact relationship and possible explanations need further exploration.

REFERENCES

1. Moore, H. D., *J. Immunol.* **4**, 425 (1919).
2. Quincke, H., *Monatsh. Prakt. Dermatol.* **1**, 129 (1882).
3. Osler, W., *Am. J. Med. Sci.* **95**, 362 (1882).
4. Donaldson, V. H., and Evans, R. R., *Am. J. Med.* **35**, 37 (1963).
5. Donaldson, V. H., and Rosen, F. S., *Pediatrics* **37**, 1017 (1966).
6. Donaldson, V. H., and Rosen, F. S., *J. Clin. Invest.* **43**, 2204 (1964).

7. Klemperer, M. R., Donaldson, V. H., and Rosen, F. S., *J. Clin. Invest.* **47**, 604 (1968).
8. Willms, K., Rosen, F. S., and Donaldson, V. H., *Clin. Immunol. Immunopathol.* **4**, 174 (1975).
9. Donaldson, V. H., Ratnoff, O. D., Dias da Silva, W., et al., *J. Clin. Invest.* **48**, 642 (1969).
10. Rosen, F. S., Alper, C. A., Pensky, J., et al., *J. Clin. Invest.* **50**, 2143 (1971).
11. Johnson, A. M., Alper, C. A., Rosen, F. S., et al., *Science* **173**, 553 (1971).
12. Pensky, J., Levy, L. R., and Lepow, I. H., *J. Biol. Chem.* **236**, 1674 (1961).
13. Schultze, H. E., Heide, K., and Haupt, H., *Naturwissenschaften* **49**, 133 (1962).
14. Pensky, J., and Schwick, H. G., *Science* **163**, 698 (1969).
15. Ratnoff, O. D., Pensky, J., Ogston, D., et al., *J. Exp. Med.* **129**, 315 (1969).
16. Harpel, P. C., and Cooper, N. R., *J. Clin. Invest.* **55**, 593 (1975).
17. Rosen, F. S., Charache, P., Donaldson, V., et al., *Science* **148**, 957 (1965).
18. Spaulding, W. B., *Arch. Intern. Med.* **53**, 739 (1960).
19. Gelfand, J. A., Sherins, R. J., Alling, D. W., et al., *Clin. Res.* **24**, 446A (abstr.) (1976).
20. Rosse, W. F., Logue, G. L., and Silberman, H. R., *Clin. Res.* **24**, 482A (abstr.) (1976).
21. Lundh, B., Laurell, A. B., Wetterqvist, H., et al., *Clin. Exp. Immunol.* **3**, 733 (1968).
22. Sheffer, A. L., Austen, K. F., and Rosen, F. S., *N. Engl. J. Med.* **287**, 452 (1972).
23. Donaldson, V. H., Rosen, F. S., and Bing, D. H., *Trans. Assoc. Am. Physicians* **90,** 174 (1977).
24. Pickering, R. J., Kelly, J. R., Good, R. A., et al., *Lancet* **1**, 326 (1969).
25. Alper, C. A., Abramson, N., Johnston, R. B., Jr., et al., *N. Engl. J. Med.* **282**, 349 (1970).
26. Thompson, R. A., and Lachmann, P. J., *Clin. Exp. Immunol.* **27,** 23 (1977).
27. Alper, C. A., and Rosen, F. S., in *Advances in Immunology* (H. G. Kunkel and F. J. Dixon, eds.), Academic Press, New York, 1971, p. 251.
28. Alper, C. A., Abramson, N., Johnston, R. B., Jr., et al., *J. Clin. Invest.* **49**, 1975 (1970).
29. Abramson, N., Alper, C. A., Lachmann, P. J., et al., *J. Immunol.* **107**, 19 (1971).
30. Alper, C. A., Rosen, F. S., and Lachmann, P. J., *Proc. Natl. Acad. Sci.* (U.S.A.) **69**, 2910 (1972).
31. Ziegler, J. B., Alper, C. A., Rosen, F. S., et al., *J. Clin. Invest.* **55**, 668 (1975).
32. Ziegler, J. B., Rosen, F. S., Alper, C. A., et al., *J. Clin. Invest.* **56**, 761 (1975).
33. Day, N. K., Geiger, H., Stroud, R., et al., *J. Clin. Invest.* **51**, 1102 (1972).
34. Moncada, B., Day, N. K., Good, R. A., et al., *N. Engl. J. Med.* **286**, 689 (1972).
35. DeBracco, M. M. E., Windhorst, D., Stroud, R. M., et al., *Clin. Exp. Immunol.* **16**, 183 (1974).
36. Pickering, R. J., Michael, A. F., Jr., Herdman, R. C., et al., *Pediatrics* **78**, 30 (1971).
37. Hauptmann, G., Grosshans, E., Heid, E., et al., *Nouv. Presse Med.* **3**, 881 (1974).
38. Jackson, C. G., Ochs, H. D., and Wedgwood, R. J., *Fed. Proc.* **35**, 655 (abstr.) (1976).
39. Ochs, H. D., Rosenfeld, S. I., Thomas, E. D., et al., *N. Engl. J. Med.* **296**, 470 (1977).
40. Teisberg, P., Akesson, I., Olaisen, B., et al., *Nature* **264**, 253 (1976).
41. Stratton F., personal communication.
42. Glass, D., Raum, D., Gibson, D., et al., *J. Clin. Invest.* **58**, 853 (1976).
43. Alper, C. A., and Rosen, F. S., in *Advances in Human Genetics* (H. Harris and K. Hirschhorn, eds.), Plenum, New York, 1976, p. 141.
44. Agnello, V. A., *Medicine* **57,** 1 (1978).
45. Colten, H. R., *J. Clin. Invest.* **51**, 725 (1972).
46. Einstein, L. P., Alper, C. A., Bloch, K. J., et al., *N. Engl. J. Med.* **292,** 1169 (1975).
47. Klemperer, M. R., Woodworth, H. C., and Rosen, F. S., *J. Clin. Invest.* **45**, 880 (1966).
48. Alper, C. A., *J. Exp. Med.* **144**, 1111 (1976).
49. Hobart, M. J., and Lachmann, P. J., *Transplant. Rev.* **32**, 26 (1976).
50. Meo, T., Atkinson, J. P., Bernoco, M., et al., *Proc. Natl. Acad. Sci.* (U.S.A.) **74**, 1672 (1977).
51. Alper, C. A., Propp, R. P., Klemperer, M. R., et al., *J. Clin. Invest.* **48**, 553 (1969).
52. Johnston, R. B., Jr., Klemperer, M. R., Alper, C. A., et al., *J. Exp. Med.* **129**, 1275 (1969).
53. Alper, C. A., and Propp, R. P., *J. Clin. Invest.* **47**, 2181 (1968).
54. Alper, C. A., Colten, H. R., Rosen, F. S., et al., *Lancet* **2**, 1179 (1972).
55. Alper, C. A., Colten, H. R., Gear, J. S. S., et al., *J. Clin. Invest.* **57**, 222 (1976).
56. Grace, H. J., Brereton-Stiles, G. G., Vos, G. H., et al., *South Afr. Med. J.* **50**, 139 (1976).
57. Ballow, M., Shira, J. E., Harden, L., et al., *J. Clin. Invest.* **56**, 703 (1975).
58. Osofsky, S. G., Thompson, B. H., Lint, T. F., et al., *J. Pediatr.* **90**, 180 (1977).
59. Davis, A. E., III, Davis, J. S., IV, Rabson, A. R., et al., *Clin. Immunol. Immunopathol.* **8**, 543 (1977).
60. Rosenfeld, S. I., and Leddy, J. P., *J. Clin. Invest.* **53**, 67a (abstr.) (1974).
61. Rosenfeld, S. I., Kelly, M. E., and Leddy, J. P., *J. Clin. Invest.* **57**, 1626 (1976).
62. Leddy, J. P., Frank, M. M., Gaither, T., et al., *J. Clin. Invest.* **53**, 544 (1974).

63. Heusinkveld, R. S., Leddy, J. P., Klemperer, M. R., et al., *J. Clin. Invest.* **53**, 554 (1974).
64. Zimmerman, T. S., Arroyave, C. M., and Müller-Eberhard, H. J., *J. Exp. Med.* **134**, 1591 (1971).
65. Lim, D., Gewurz, A., Lint, T. F., et al., *J. Pediatr.* **89**, 42 (1976).
66. Boyer, J. T., Gall, E. P., and Norman, M. E., *J. Clin. Invest.* **56**, 905 (1975).
67. Wellek, B., and Opferkuch, W., *Clin. Exp. Immunol.* **19**, 223 (1975).
68. Petersen, B. H., Graham, J. A., and Brooks, G. F., *J. Clin. Invest,* **57**, 283 (1976).
69. Alper, C. A., Raum, D., Balavitch, D., et al., in preparation.
70. Giraldo, G., Degos, L., Beth, E., et al., *Clin. Immunol. Immunopathol.* **8**, 377 (1977).
71. Jasin, H. E., *J. Clin. Invest.* **60**, 709 (1977).
72. Granerus, G., Hallberg, L., Laurell, A. B., et al., *Acta Med. Scand.* **182**, 11 (1967).
73. Fu, S. M., Kunkel, H. G., Brusman, H. P., et al., *J. Exp. Med.* **140**, 1108 (1974).
74. Fu, S. M., Stern, R., Kunkel, H. G., et al., *J. Exp. Med.* **142**, 495 (1975).
75. Friend, P. S., Handwerger, B. S., Kim, Y., et al., *Immunogenetics* **2**, 569 (1975).
76. Raum, D., Glass, D., Carpenter, C. B., et al., *Clin. Res.* **24**, 335A (abstr.) (1976).
77. Glass, D., Gibson, D. J., Carpenter, C. B., et al., *J. Immunol.* **116**, 1734 (1976).
78. Miller, G. W., and Nussenzweig, V., *Proc. Natl. Acad. Sci.* (U.S.A.) **72**, 418 (1975).
79. Kohler, P. F., Percy, J., Campion, W. M., et al., *Am. J. Med.* **56**, 406 (1974).
80. Czop, J., and Nussenzweig, V., *J. Exp. Med.* **143,** 615 (1976).

Chapter Fifteen

Immunodeficiency Diseases

FRED S. ROSEN

Children's Hospital Medical Center and Harvard Medical School, Boston, Massachusetts

Immunity results from many interacting mechanisms, which may be specific or nonspecific; the failure of one or another specific immunity mechanism results in immunodeficiency disease. It has been known for two decades that there is a clear-cut difference between cellular and humoral immunity.

The WHO Committee on the Primary Specific Immunodeficiency Diseases recently convened in Geneva, Switzerland (November 1-7, 1977), and reclassified the primary specific immunodeficiencies (1). This classification is given in the accompanying table. As can be seen, 17 different disease entities are designated as primary specific immunodeficiencies. The phenotypic expression of each disease is given; only the functional cellular deficiency and the cellular abnormality were known. Furthermore, the table gives the presumed level of the basic cellular defect when known, as well as the pathogenetic mechanisms. When a disease happens to be genetically determined, the inheritance is listed. Also the main associated features of each of the 17 syndromes are listed. In order to clarify the terminology used in the table, reference is made to Fig. 1, which forms a basis for current knowledge of the ontogeny of human B and T lymphocytes. An attempt has been made in Table 1 to localize the cellular defect to some point in ontogeny shown in the figure. The text that follows is intended to complete the information given in the table and provide additional comments on the various disease entities listed in the table.

1. SEVERE COMBINED IMMUNODEFICIENCY

Severe combined immunodeficiency is the most profound of the cellular defects. Affected patients usually have no T or B cells; the disease is invariably fatal. It is genetically determined, and there is clear evidence of autosomal recessive and

Table 1. Classification of Primary Specific Immunodeficiencies

Designation	Usual Phenotypic Expression: Functional Deficiencies	Usual Phenotypic Expression: Cellular Abnormalities	Presumed Level of Basic Cellular Defect
1. Severe combined immunodeficiency			
a) Reticular dysgenesis	CMI, Ab, and phagocytes	↓T, B, and phagocytes	HSC
b) "Swiss type"	CMI and Ab	↓T and B	LSC
c) ADA deficiency	CMI and Ab	↓T ± B	LSC or early T
d) With B lymphocytes	CMI and Ab	↓T (B lymphocytes without or with normal isotype diversity)	Early T ± early B
e) Others (see text)		—	—
2. Thymic hypoplasia (Di-George syndrome)	CMI and impaired Ab	↓T	Thymus
3. Purine nucleoside phosphorylase deficiency	CMI ± Ab	↓T	T
4. ID with ataxia telangiectasia	CMI and Ab (partial)	↓T and plasma cells (mainly IgA, IgE ± IgG)	Early T and defective terminal differentiation of B lymphocytes
5. ID with thymoma	Ab and impaired CMI (variable)	↓Pre-B and B ±↓T	HSC
6. X-linked agamma-globulinemia	Ab	↓B	Pre-B
7. Transcobalamin II deficiency	Ab and phagocytosis	↓Plasma cells	Failure of terminal differentiation of B lymphocytes
8. Selective IgA deficiency	IgA Ab	↓IgA plasma cells ±↑B α ±↓T	Terminal differentiation of B α lymphocytes impaired

Known or Presumed Pathogenetic Mechanism	Inheritance	Main Associated Features
Unknown	AR	—
Unknown	AR	—
Metabolic effects of ADA deficiency	AR	± Chondrocyte abnormalities
Unknown	X-linked or AR	—
—	—	—
Embryopathy of 3rd and 4th pharyngeal pouch area	Usually not familial	(1) Hypoparathyroidism (2) Abnormal facies (3) Cardiovascular abnormalities
Metabolic effects of PNP deficiency	AR	Hypoplastic anemia
Unknown ? Faulty thymic epithelium ? DNA repair defect	AR	(1) Cerebellar ataxia (2) Telangiectasia (3) Ovarian dysgenesis (4) Chromosomal abnormalities
Unknown	none	(1) Thymoma (2) Eosinopenia (3) Erythroblastopenia (4) Aplastic anemia
Unknown	X-linked	—
Metabolic effects of Vitamin B_{12} deficiency	AR	(1) Pancytopenia with megaloblastic anemia (2) Intestinal villous atrophy
(1) ?↑ T_S (2) ? ↓ T_H (3) ? Intrinsic B cell defect	Unknown>AR> AD. Frequent in families of patients with varied ID	(1) Occasional 18 chromosomal deletions (2) Anti-IgA antibodies

Table 1. Classification of Primary Specific Immunodeficiencies *(continued)*

Designation	Usual Phenotypic Expression: Functional Deficiencies	Usual Phenotypic Expression: Cellular Abnormalities	Presumed Level of Basic Cellular Defect
9. Selective deficiency of one other Ig class or subclass	Ab	↓ Plasma cells ±↓ T	Unknown
10. Secretory piece deficiency	Secretory IgA Ab	↓ Intestinal IgA plasma cells	Mucosal epithelial cell
11. Ig deficiencies with increased IgM	Ab	↓ IgG and IgA plasma cells ↑ IgM plasma cells ± ↑ B lymphocytes	Failure of terminal differentiation of B δ and B α lymphocytes
12. Ig deficiencies with IgM production and without δ and α cells	Ab	Absent B δ and B α lymphocytes	Pre-B or B
13. Transient hypogammaglobulinemia of infancy	Ab	↓Plasma cells	Impaired terminal differentiation of B lymphocytes
14. Antibody deficiency with normal or hypergammaglobulinemia	Impaired Ab for some antigens (mainly primary response)	↓ B	Pre-B or early B
15. Kappa chain deficiency	Ab	↓ B_k	Pre-B
16. Wiskott-Aldrich syndrome	Ab to certain antigens (mainly polysaccharides) and CMI (progressive)	↓ T and B (progressive)	Unknown
17. Varied immunodeficiencies (common and largely unclassified)			
a) Predominant immunoglobulin deficiency	Ab ± CMI	± ↓ B	Pre-B or B in some
b) Predominant T cell deficiency	CMI ± Ab	↓ T	Early T or T helpers

Known or Presumed Pathogenetic Mechanism	Inheritance	Main Associated Features
Unknown ? ↑ TS	Unknown	—
Unknown	Unknown	—
Unknown	X-linked or AR or unknown	—
Faulty isotype diversification	AR or unknown	—
? ↓ T helper	Frequent in heterozygous individuals in families with various SCID	—
? Reduced clonal size or diversity	AR in some	—
Unknown	Unknown or familial	—
Unknown	X-linked	(1) Thrombocytopenia (2) Eczema
(1) Intrinsic B cell defect (2) Underproduction of B cells (3) ? ↑ T suppressors (4) ? ↓ T helpers (5) Autoantibodies to B cells	Unknown or familial	—
(1) Unknown (2) Autoantibodies to T cells	Unknown or familial	—

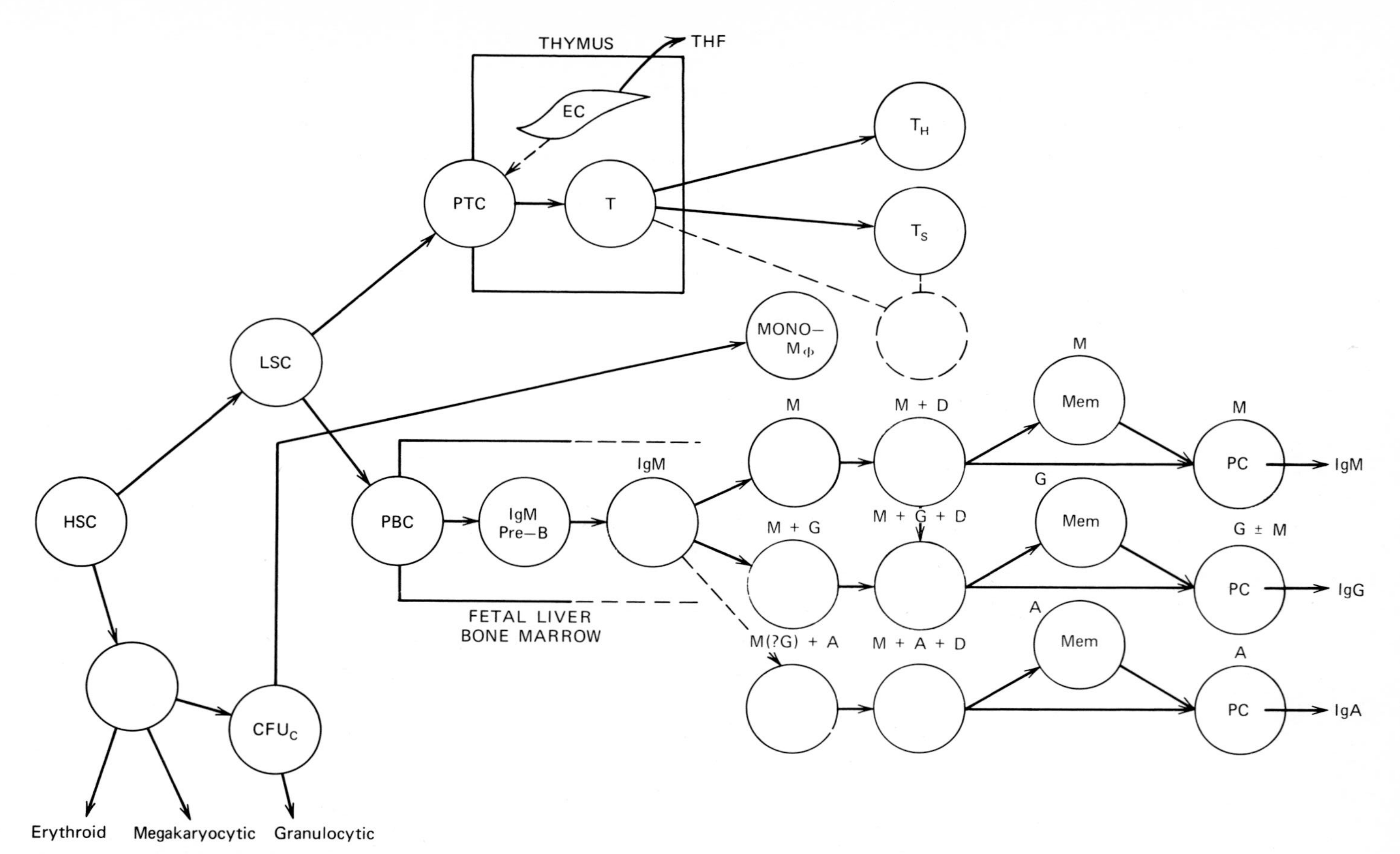

Figure 1. Cellular basis of the immune response. See text under heading "Congenital Thymic Aplasia (DiGeorge Syndrome)" for description. THF = thymic humoral factor, T = T cell, PTC = pre-T cell, EC = epithelial cell, LSC = lymphopoietic stem cell, HSC = hematopoietic stem cell, CFUc = colony-forming units in culture assay, PBC = pre-B cell, TH = thymic helper cell, TS = thymic suppressor cell, mono = monocyte, MΦ = macrophage, Mem = memory, PC = plasma cell, M = IgM, G = IgG, A = IgA, D = IgD.

X-linked recessive transmission of the disease. The clinical and laboratory findings may be quite variable from patient to patient, even among affected members of a single family.

Persistent infection of the lungs, monilial infection of the oropharynx, esophagus, and skin, chronic diarrhea, and wasting and runting begin in the early months of life and progress with monotonous regularity to a fatal termination, despite all attempts at routine therapy. Affected infants usually do not survive the first year or two of life. Examination usually reveals absence of tonsils, very small or absent lymph nodes despite chronic infection, chronic pneumonitis evidenced by a pertussis-like cough, inspiratory retractions of the chest, rales, a somewhat distended abdomen with wasting, and oral thrush.

Roentgenographic signs include pulmonary infiltration and absence of a thymic shadow. There is usually an absolute decrease in the number of circulating lymphocytes, and occasionally neutropenia. In typical cases, the immunoglobulins are markedly decreased, but variants have been described in which circulating immunoglobulins are normal or there is selective immunoglobulin deficiency. M components may be present in the circulation. Plasma cells have been found in the tissues of such patients, but antibody formation is almost always impaired or absent. Tests of delayed hypersensitivity give negative results: sensitization cannot be induced with dinitrochlorobenzene; cultured lymphocytes do not respond to phytohemagglutinin; and skin allografts are not rejected. T cells are almost always absent from the circulation, and the few lymphocytes present in the blood usually have the characteristics of B cells.

Recently, half of all infants with the autosomal recessive form of the disease have been found to lack the enzyme adenosine deaminase (ADA) from their red cells and other tissues (2). Furthermore, a mutant enzyme with abnormal electrophoretic mobility has been detected in fibroblast cultures from affected infants (3). This discovery has led to the prenatal diagnosis of the disease (4).

The metabolic consequences of ADA deficiency are interesting in that they may ultimately explain why only the lymphoid tissue is susceptible to damage by enzyme deficiency. The enzyme is ubiquitous in all mammalian tissue. Thymus contains 10 to 13 times more ADA than other tissues (5). It has been proposed that adenosine accumulation blocks orotic acid to orotodine conversion, thereby inhibiting DNA synthesis. This has not been borne out by attempts to reverse the block with uridine. It has been shown that adenosine triphosphate (ATP) is synthesized at 9 to 10 times the normal rate in ADA-deficient red cells. This effect can be mimicked in normal red cells by treatment with coformycin, an ADA inhibitor (6). Coformycin also inhibits null to T cell maturation in vitro (7). It is possible but unlikely that massive ATP accumulations cause increased cyclic AMP formation as the immunosuppressive event. Finally, the toxic metabolite may be deoxy-ATP, synthesized in excess from deoxyadenosine. All these possibilities require further exploration.

The establishment of immunologic competence with transplants of bone marrow in these infants is still experimental but successful; however, it should only be carried out in those centers with adequate manpower, clinical and laboratory experience, and physical facilities for what is an exacting ordeal.

A donor of bone marrow whose cells are HLA identical and can be shown to be histocompatible in vitro by mixed lymphocyte culture (MLC) should be identified. In practice, this almost always means a sibling. However, a successful transplant from an MLC-identical maternal uncle has been accomplished, despite HLA nonidentity between donor and recipient. An unrelated donor has been used in one instance (8). Administration of a suitable dose of bone marrow cells from the donor when the infant is as free of infection as possible is accomplished with 50×10^6 nucleated cells per kg intravenously. More cells are optimal for intraperitoneal injection, perhaps 50×10^7. Evidence that the graft has become established and that immunologic reconstitution (T cell function as shown by phytohemagglutinin responses, B cell function by immunoglobulin synthesis) has occurred usually requires three to eight weeks.

In skilled hands, patients with this hitherto fatal disease have been cured and appear normal. Nevertheless, success is not universal; there is much to learn; and the treatment is heroic. In a few cases, ADA replacement by infusion of frozen red cells has corrected the immunodeficiency (9).

2. CONGENITAL THYMIC APLASIA (DiGEORGE SYNDROME)

Congenital thymic aplasia (DiGeorge syndrome, third and fourth pharyngeal pouch syndrome) results from a failure of the normal embryogenesis of the thymus and parathyroid glands, which are derived from the third and fourth pharyngeal clefts. The syndrome is not genetically determined but appears rather to result from some intrauterine accident before the eighth week of gestation. Affected infants invariably have neonatal tetany. Anomalies of the great blood vessels are very frequently encountered, usually right-sided aortic arch, as in the tetralogy of Fallot. These cardiac complications are the cause of late death in these children. Mental subnormality also accompanies this syndrome.

The T cell defect in children with congenital thymic aplasia varies from the most profound to the barely discernible. In any case, T cell function improves in these children with age, so that by 5 years of age no T cell deficit can be ascertained. It is not clear how this grossly retarded T cell maturation occurs in the absence of a thymus gland. Some children may have a small thymic remnant, but T cell maturation may occur at sites other than the thymus.

Transplants of fetal thymus into these infants result in a rapid acquisition of T cell function (10,11).

3. PURINE NUCLEOSIDE PHOSPHORYLASE (PNP) DEFICIENCY

The deficiency of purine nucleoside phosphorylase (PNP) is inherited as an autosomal recessive defect (12). Affected infants have very poor T cell function and hypoplastic anemia. It is, of course, proof of the importance of the purine salvage pathway that defects in ADA or PNP cause profound immunodeficiency. The metabolic consequences of PNP deficiency are more obscure than the consequences of ADA deficiency. Deoxyinosine may be an important metabolite in PNP deficiency.

4. IMMUNODEFICIENCY WITH ATAXIA TELANGIECTASIA

Ataxia telangiectasia is an autosomal recessive disease in which abnormalities of the thymus have been found at postmortem examination. Gradually progressive cerebellar ataxia begins in early childhood. This is associated with increasing telangiectasia, which first becomes apparent as a rather inconspicuous dilatation of small blood vessels in the bulbar conjunctivae and ultimately is visible in the skin at about 5 years of age. Gonadal dysgenesis and failure of sexual maturation may be present in those who survive into the second decade. In late childhood, recurrent sinobronchial infections begin in many patients, often leading to bronchiectasis. There is also a tendency to the development of malignant tumors, particularly of the lymphoid system. These reflect an immunologic disturbance affecting T cell function, as shown by blunting of delayed hypersensitivity reactions, failure to reject allografts normally, and reduced response of the lymphocytes to phytohemagglutinin. At postmortem examination late in the disease, the thymus is abnormally small and has a decreased number of lymphocytes; there is a poor differentiation between cortex and medulla and decided diminution in Hassall's corpuscles. The number of circulating lymphocytes and the architecture of the lymph nodes vary considerably and do not always correlate well with the patient's history. The most consistent B cell defect is a low level or absence of IgA in the serum, which occurs in about 70% of affected persons and may precede clinical evidence of immunologic deficiency by a number of years (13).

5. THYMOMA

The features of this disease are given in the table.

6. X-LINKED AGAMMAGLOBULINEMIA

X-linked agammaglobulinemia usually manifests itself in the second year of life, although the onset of the characteristically severe, recurrent infections may occur at any age from 8 months to 3 years. The infections are those caused by the common pyogenic organisms—*Staphylococcus aureus,* pneumococci, meningococci, *Hemophilus influenzae,* and less often β-hemolytic streptococci or *Pseudomonas.* They differ from infections in normal children only in their frequency, severity, and the tendency for infection with the same organism to occur more than once. Pyoderma, purulent conjunctivitis, pharyngitis, otitis media, sinusitis, bronchitis, pneumonia, empyema, purulent arthritis, meningitis, and sepsis occur with surprising frequency and may be associated with unusually high fever and unexpected elevation or depression of the leukocyte count. A rather indolent rheumatoid-like arthritis with sterile effusion into one of the large joints develops in about one-third of patients and may be the presenting complaint. The children usually, but not always, handle most viral infections normally.

There should be a high index of suspicion about the diagnosis of X-linked agammaglobulinemia on the basis of the history of repeated severe bacterial infections. A careful family history may uncover instances of death from overwhelming infection or multiple severe infections in male siblings, maternal uncles, or male offspring of maternal aunts. Examination reveals little except the signs of infection, evidence of joint involvement if present, and unusually small, smooth tonsils. Lateral films of the pharynx fail to reveal an adenoid shadow. Lymph nodes are small but palpable; regional nodes may be swollen and tender during episodes of infection. Immunochemical assay reveals a marked diminution of IgM, IgA, and IgG globulins in the serum. It is important to remember that, because of individual variations and the low levels of immunoglobulins normally found in the early months of life, the diagnosis cannot be firmly established by immunoelectrophoresis until 6 to 8 months of age. However, failure of IgM or IgA to appear in significant concentration and a steady fall in IgG during the first 3 to 4 months of life should suggest the diagnosis, especially in the presence of a positive family history. Isohemagglutinins are usually absent or in very low titer. Injection of vaccines is not followed by an adequate antibody rise, and removal of a stimulated regional lymph node discloses absence of the expected germinal centers, secondary follicles, and plasma cells.

The thymus is normal, but lymph nodes and spleen lack the usual follicular architecture. Germinal centers are absent, and there are few if any plasma cells in the medullary cores or red pulp. Although the number of lymphocytes in the tissues appears diminished, they are present in the thymus-dependent areas of lymphoid tissue, and normal numbers are found in the blood. Plasma cells are absent from the bone marrow. However, plasma cells may be normally absent from the bone marrow in children under 5 years of age, so this is an unhelpful finding. Study of the circulating lymphocytes has revealed normal numbers of T cells but complete absence of B cells. We have found normal numbers of B cells in only one case of proved X-linked agammaglobulinemia. These B cells are abnormal in that they are unresponsive to the T cell mitogen and pokeweed mitogen and do not synthesize immunoglobulins in vitro (14).

Provided the diagnosis is made and treatment begun before repeated infections have produced serious anatomic damage (e.g., bronchiectasis, pulmonary insufficiency, middle ear deafness), the immediate prognosis for these children is excellent, and they gain and grow normally. However, in later childhood, adolescence, or early adult life, complications may develop in some of these patients. Slowly progressive neurologic disease, suggesting a "slow virus" infection, accompanies a dermatomyositis-like syndrome with brawny edema, perivascular mononuclear infiltrates, and, terminally, severe systemic symptoms and death. Thus far, no consistent cause for these complications has been found. An enterovirus was repeatedly isolated from blood, stool, and spinal fluid in the last patient to succumb with the dermatomyositis-like picture and from several other patients with this syndrome (15).

Vigorous antimicrobial therapy is indicated for individual infections, which respond to treatment as in normal individuals. Regular injections of gamma globulin, which is almost pure IgG, in doses adequate to maintain a plasma concentration of IgG globulin above 200 mg per 100 ml are essential. Maintenance therapy is initiated with a loading dose of 0.3 gm (1.8 ml) per kg of IgG globulin. This may be given in divided doses over a period of a week in order to minimize discomfort. Thereafter, an average dose of 0.1 gm (0.6 ml) per kg per month (the volume of the injection may be scaled down if injections are given every two or three weeks) is required to maintain a protective level of antibody. Intramuscular administration is necessary to avoid reactions with the standard preparation. A preparation satisfactory for intravenous administration has been shown to be effective in preventing infections in these patients and is being developed for clinical trials. Prophylaxis with gamma globulin is usually effective in preventing invasive bacterial infection and communicable disease, and its institution generally cures hydrarthrosis. It does not control localized superficial infection of skin or respiratory tract; in a few instances, antimicrobial drugs may have to be given in addition to control chronic sinusitis, most frequently due to *H. influenzae*. Infections may be prevented for considerable periods by the administration of broad-spectrum antibiotics without gamma globulin.

7. TRANSCOBALAMIN II DEFICIENCY

The features of this deficiency are given in the table.

8 and 9. SELECTIVE IMMUNOGLOBULIN DEFICIENCIES (DYSGAMMAGLOBULINEMIA)

The term "selective immunoglobulin deficiencies" is used to describe consistent deficiencies of one or more of the recognizable plasma immunoglobulins. Although often associated with the clinical manifestations of the antibody deficiency syndrome, some instances of selective immunoglobulin deficiency may be chance laboratory findings in otherwise apparently normal individuals.

Selective deficiency of IgG subclasses may occur, in which the patient is unable to synthesize one or more of the IgG subclasses and thus fails to produce antibodies in one or more of the four presently identified IgG subclasses. This results in failure to respond to particular types of antigens, in increased susceptibility to a limited spectrum of bacterial infections, and in a reduction in total serum IgG concentration proportional to the percentage of the total IgG pool accounted for by the deficient IgG subclass. Of course, a deficiency in IgG_1 is most severe, since this subclass constitutes over 70% of the IgG (16,17).

Selective IgA deficiency is observed with considerable frequency (3 to 7 per 1,000 population). In a few patients, this may portend the development of ataxia telangiectasia, but an appreciable number of such individuals remain healthy throughout life. However, a high incidence of rheumatoid arthritis, systemic lupus erythematosus, and malabsorption syndrome has been observed among this group of patients (18). A significant number of IgA-deficient individuals have circulating antibodies to IgA and have anaphylactic reactions upon receiving whole blood or plasma (19).

10. SECRETORY PIECE DEFICIENCY

Only two cases of this have been observed in a single family.

11. X-LINKED IMMUNODEFICIENCY WITH INCREASED IgM

In a few instances, patients are observed with manifestations similar to those in X-linked agammaglobulinemia, but with higher levels of immunoglobulins, which, when analyzed, turn out to reflect a marked deficiency of serum IgA and IgG but an elevation in the concentration of IgM. The congenital form of this disease seems to occur almost entirely in males and has a suggestive X-linked pattern of inheritance. Except for a greater frequency of "autoimmune" hematologic disorders (neutropenia, hemolytic anemia, thrombocytopenia), the clinical course in these patients resembles that of X-linked agammaglobulinemia. Histologically, there is disorganization of the follicular architecture of the lymphoid tissues, but PAS-positive plasmacytoid cells containing IgM are present, and even tonsillar hypertrophy due to these cells has been observed. Only B cells with IgM surface fluorescence are found. No B cells with surface IgA or IgG are present. Similar disturbances of the immunoglobulin picture associated with the antibody deficiency syndrome have been seen in adults with frequent respiratory tract infections and bronchiectasis, and in some infants with congenital rubella.

12. Ig DEFICIENCIES WITH IgM PRODUCTION AND WITHOUT γ AND α CELLS

Cases are defined as stated in the table.

13. TRANSIENT HYPOGAMMAGLOBULINEMIA OF INFANCY

Normally, the synthesis of immunoglobulins in response to infection and other antigenic stimuli begins after birth. However, if the fetus is infected in utero after the twentieth week of gestation by rubella virus, cytomegalovirus, *Toxoplasma,* or *Treponema pallidum*, he (or she) can mount an impressive antibody response to the invasive pathogen. This antibody response, consisting largely of IgM and to a lesser extent of IgA and IgG antibodies, can be helpful in the diagnosis of prenatal infection. A cord or neonatal serum level of IgM in excess of 20 mg per 100 ml is considered presumptive evidence of intrauterine infection. The level of IgG globulin, which is passively acquired by transplacental passage, falls rapidly during the first month of life, levels off during the second month, and soon begins to rise. Rarely, there is delay in the maturation of B cells and their immunologic function; the level of IgG globulins received by passive transfer from the mother continues to fall and is not adequately raised by immunoglobulins synthesized by the infant, so that within a few months the total gamma globulin level is much lower than usual for that age. The infants have overt infections, unexplained episodes of fever, and often bronchitis with wheezing. Regular injections of gamma globulin (see below) will protect them from severe, invasive infections. The injections may be discontinued when the IgG globulins begin to rise toward normal levels, usually before the age of 3 years. The cause of this transient hypogammaglobulinemia is not known. Normal numbers of B cells are present in the circulation of affected patients.

14. IMMUNODEFICIENCY WITH NORMAL OR HYPERGAMMAGLOBULINEMIA

Rare cases of immunodeficiency with normal or increased immunoglobulins have been observed, in which the classic picture of the antibody deficiency syndrome was accompanied by a normal or even increased level of immunoglobulins and the presence of plasma cells in the tissues, but a failure to form specific antibodies to a variety of antigens. These have not been sufficiently studied with modern methods to provide an adequate explanation.

15. KAPPA CHAIN DEFICIENCY

Two cases have been reported as outlined in the table.

16. IMMUNODEFICIENCY WITH THROMBOCYTOPENIA AND ECZEMA (WISKOTT-ALDRICH SYNDROME)

The Wiskott-Aldrich syndrome is an X-linked recessive disorder that is usually manifested by eczema, thrombocytopenia, and a wide variety of infections beginning late in the first year, although it may present rarely as thrombocytopenia alone. Death may occur from hemorrhage, infection, or the development of a malignant process similar to the Letterer-Siwe type of reticuloendotheliosis.

The infections may be caused by a wide variety of microorganisms, including viruses, bacteria, fungi, and *Pneumocystis carinii.* Transient episodes of arthritis have been observed.

Results of studies of the pathogenesis of the Wiskott-Aldrich syndrome are confusing. The lymphoid tissues appear normal early in the course of the disease, but as it progresses there may be a loss of lymphocytes from the thymus and paracortical areas of the lymph nodes. The peripheral lymphocyte count may decrease, and there is a variable loss of cellular immunity, resulting in increased susceptibility to viral or fungal disease. Studies of immunoglobulin production in such patients suggest normal responses to a variety of antigens. IgM values are often low, and isohemagglutinins and Forssman antibodies, normally present as "natural" antibodies, are usually lacking. The failure of these patients to respond to pneumococcal polysaccharides has led to the postulation that they have a general inability to respond to polysaccharide antigens, as opposed to normal responses to protein antigens. Whether this failure resides in the recognition system of the lymphocytes, in a deficit of the macrophages in processing such antigens, or in a qualitative deficiency of plasma cell function is not clear. Since polysaccharides are widely distributed and important constituents of bacteria and fungi, it is reasonable that such a selective immunologic deficiency might have a serious impact upon resistance (20,21).

Bone marrow transplantation has been effective in some of these patients, using histoidentical sibling donors (22).

17. VARIED UNCLASSIFIED IMMUNODEFICIENCY (ACQUIRED HYPOGAMMAGLOBULINEMIA)

Varied unclassified immunodeficiency is the most common form of immunodeficiency with serious clinical consequences and probably includes a number of entities; it occurs in either sex at any age without any known causative factor, either genetic or acquired, although a predisposition may be inherited, since its development has been reported in siblings or among relatives.

The picture is that of the antibody deficiency syndrome associated with immunoglobulin deficiency, which may be somewhat less severe than in the X-linked form of agammaglobulinemia. Pathologically, there is necrobiotic change in the follicular architecture of the lymph nodes and spleen, or lymphadenopathy and splenomegaly due to reticulum cell hyperplasia. The predominant infections are sinusitis and pneumonia, often leading to bronchiectasis unless intensively treated. Although the rheumatoid arthritis-like complications are occasionally seen, a sprue-like malabsorption syndrome and pernicious anemia are more common (23). Recent work has demonstrated that this malabsorption syndrome is often due to *Giardia lamblia,* demonstrated either in aspirates of duodenal fluid or in biopsy specimens of duodenal mucosa (24).

Management is the same as for X-linked agammaglobulinemia: substitution therapy with regular injections of large doses of immune serum globulin for prophylaxis and intensive antimicrobial therapy for acute infections. The chronic diarrhea and malabsorption due to giardiasis, which may give a picture of protein-losing enteropathy, usually respond promptly to metronidazole (Flagyl) in doses of 0.25 gm three times a day for five days.

Patients with "acquired" agammaglobulinemia may have no B cells, but, more commonly, normal numbers of B cells or even increased numbers of B cells are found. In some patients the B cells do not synthesize immunoglobulin; in others, immunoglobulin synthesis is normal, but there is no secretion of the immunoglobulin formed (25). We have studied one patient whose B cells functioned normally in vitro when cultured in normal AB+ serum, but did not in the patient's serum. Obviously, a whole spectrum of B cell maturation failure is presented by these patients. In some patients, T cell function deteriorates progressively. This is particularly true of patients who have an associated thymoma.

REFERENCES

1. WHO Committee, *Primary Immunodeficiencies,* Report of WHO Committee, in preparation.
2. Giblett, E. R., Anderson, J. E., Cohen, F., Pollara, B., and Meuwissen, H. J., *Lancet* **2**, 1067 (1972).
3. Hirschhorn, R., Beratis, N., and Rosen, F. S., *Proc. Natl. Acad. Sci.* **73**, 213 (1976).
4. Hirschhorn, R., Beratis, N., Rosen, F. S., Parkman, R., Stein, R., and Polmar, S., *Lancet* **1**, 73 (1975).
5. Hirschhorn, R., Martiniuk, F., and Rosen, F. S., *Clin. Immunol. Immunopathol.* **9**, 287 (1978).
6. Agarwal, R. P., Crabtree, G. W., Parks, R. E., Jr., Nelson, J. A., Keightley, R., Parkman, R., Rosen, F. S., Stern, R. C., and Polmar, S. H., *J. Clin. Invest.* **57**, 1025 (1976).
7. Ballet, J. J., Insel, R., Merler, E., and Rosen, F. S., *J. Exp. Med.* **143**, 1271 (1976).
8. O'Reilly, R. J., Dupont, B., Pohwa, S., Grimes, E., Smithwick, E. M., Pohwa, R., Schwartz, S.,

Hansen, J. A., Siegal, F. P., Sorell, M., Sveygaard, A., Jersild, C., Thomsen, M., Platz, P., L'Esperance, P., and Good, R. A., *N. Engl. J. Med.* **297**, 1311 (1977).
9. Polmar, S. H., Wetzler, E. M., Stern, R. C., and Hirschhorn, R., *Lancet* **2**, 743 (1975).
10. August, C., Rosen, F. S., Filler, R. M., Janeway, C. A., Markowski, B., and Kay, H. E. M., *Lancet* **2**, 1210 (1968).
11. Cleveland, W. W., Fogel, B. J., Brown, W. T., and Kay, H. E. M., *Lancet* **2**, 1211 (1968).
12. Giblett, E. L., Ammann, A. J., Nara, D. W., Sandman, R., and Diamond, L. K., *Lancet* **1**, 1010 (1975).
13. Peterson, R. D. A., Kelly, W. D., and Good, R. A., *Lancet* **1**, 1189 (1964).
14. Geha, R. S., Rosen, F. S., and Merler, E., *J. Clin. Invest.* **52**, 1726 (1973).
15. Wilfert, C. M., Buckley, R. H., Mohanakumar, T., Griffith, J. F., Katz, S. L., Whisnant, J. K., Eggleston, P. A., Moore, M., Treadwell, E., Oxman, M. N., and Rosen, F. S., *N. Engl. J. Med.* **296**, 1485 (1977).
16. Schur, P., Borel, H., Gelfand, E. W., Alper, C. A., and Rosen, F. S., *N. Engl. J. Med.* **283**, 631 (1970).
17. Yount, W. J., Hong, R., Seligmann, M., Good, R., and Kunkel, H. G., *J. Clin. Invest.* **49**, 1957 (1970).
18. Ammann, A. J., and Hong, R., *Clin. Exp. Immunol.* **7**, 833 (1970).
19. Vyas, G. N., Perkins, H. A., and Fudenberg, H. H., *Lancet* **2**, 312 (1968).
20. Cooper, M. D., Chase, H. P., Lowman, J. T., Krivit, W., and Good, R. A., *Am. J. Med.* **44**, 499 (1968).
21. Blaese, R. M., Brown, R. S., Strober, W., and Waldmann, T. A., *Lancet* **1**, 1056 (1968).
22. Parkman, R., Rappeport, J., Geha, R., Belli, J., Cassady, R., Levey, R., Nathan, D. G., and Rosen, F. S., *N. Engl. J. Med.,* **298**, 921 (1978).
23. Gelfand, E. W., Berkel, A. I., Godwin, H. A., Rocklin, R. E., David, J. R., and Rosen, F. S., *Clin. Exp. Immunol.* **11**, 187 (1972).
24. Ochs, H. D., Ament, M. E., and Davis, S. D., *N. Engl. J. Med.* **287**, 341 (1972).
25. Geha, R. S., Schneeberger, E., Gatien, J. G., Rosen, F. S., and Merler, E., *N. Engl. J. Med.* **290**, 726 (1974).

Chapter Sixteen

Mechanisms of Transplantation Immunity

RICHARD LINDQUIST
Department of Pathology, University of Connecticut Health Center, Farmington, Connecticut

Tissue and organ grafts transplanted from one animal to another will be rejected if the recipient recognizes them as alien or histoincompatible. Conversely, histocompatible grafts will survive in the new host, since they are not perceived as being foreign. Histoincompatible grafts may be either grafts exchanged between genetically dissimilar members of the same species (allografts or allogeneic grafts) or grafts exchanged between individuals of different species (xenografts or xenogeneic grafts). Allografts may also be called homografts; and xenografts, heterografts. Histocompatible grafts may be either grafts taken from and returned to a single animal (autografts or autogeneic grafts) or grafts exchanged between identical twins or highly inbred animals that are genetically identical (isografts or syngeneic grafts).

Our present understanding of graft behavior and barriers to histocompatibility (H-barriers) is based largely on studies using highly inbred animals that are genetically identical and congeneic strains that are inbred strains identical with another inbred strain except for a small chromosome segment (1). Coisogeneic strains differ only by a single locus. Using inbred strains A and B, for example, it is easy to demonstrate that syngeneic grafts exchanged between animals A_1 and A_2 and between B_1 and B_2 always survive, whereas allografts exchanged between animals A and B are always rejected. The mode of inheritance of H-barriers is demonstrated by using the F_1 hybrid of A and B, $(A \times B)F_1$, as donor. $(A \times B)F_1$ tissue is rejected by both A and B recipients, thus demonstrating that the H-barriers are inherited as codominant factors. Since $(A \times B)F_1$ cannot recognize A or B as foreign, parental grafts survive on F_1 hybrid recipients.

By using the F_2 generation as recipients for parental grafts, the number of H-barriers can be estimated (2). If there were only one H-barrier, then three out of four F_2 recipients would accept parental A target grafts because (A × B) F_1 × (A × B)F_1 matings would lead to the following offspring: (A × A), (A × B), (B × A), and (B × B). Of these only BB would recognize A grafts as foreign, and thus three-fourths of the A grafts should survive. This is not the case for most inbred strains; rather, usually only a small fraction of parental skin survives on F_2 recipients. For example, only a small number of Lewis rat skin grafts transplanted onto (Lewis × Brown Norway)F_2 recipients survive (3). By using the generalization that if there are n H-barriers between two strains, then $(3/4)^n$ of the grafts from parent to F_2 will survive. From the available data, one can calculate that 14 H-barriers exist between Lewis and Brown Norway strains.

The strengths of the different histocompatibility barriers can be determined by exchanging skin grafts between congeneic strains that differ from one another by only one H-barrier. In one study (4), the median survival times of such grafts ranged from as little as 12 days to over 300 days, with a median of about 50 days. Thus, histocompatibility barriers have a wide range of strengths. The histocompatibility barrier that produces the most rapid rejection is called the strong or major H-barrier, and the remaining H-barriers are called minor histoincompatibilities.

By comparison with our knowledge of major histocompatibility, very little is known about minor H-barriers. One reason for this is that since the major barrier is the most important barrier, most research has emphasized it. The emphasis on major histocompatibility barriers has been further justified by the fact that these barriers determine the fate of kidney grafts. Graff and Bailey waggishly suggest that weak H-barriers are overlooked because only a few investigators are "patient enough or slow thinking enough to wait 100 days for an immunologic reaction" (4a).

It should be noted that multiple minor histocompatibility barriers can act together to produce the abrupt rejection of skin. For instance, skin grafts exchanged between Lewis and Fischer inbred rats that are identical at the major H-barrier (AgB), but differ at multiple minor H-barriers, are rejected in 10–12 days, which is about the same time for graft rejection between the AgB incompatible strains, Lewis and Brown Norway (4b).

Investigation of histocompatibility barriers in many species indicates that each species has a major H-barrier. In the mouse, this major barrier is called H-2, for historical reasons which will be discussed later. In man, the major histocompatibility barrier is called HLA (formerly HL-A), for *h*uman *l*eukocyte *a*ntigen. The genetic control of these major barriers resides in the major histocompatibility gene complex (MHC).

MAJOR HISTOCOMPATIBILITY COMPLEX IN MICE

The H-2 major histocompatibility gene complex in mice is a relatively large (0.5-cM) segment on chromosome 17 located 15 cM from the centromere (5,6). It is divided into five main regions called K, I, S, G, and D. These regions are marked by the respective presence of the H-2K, Ir-1, Ss, H-2G, and H-2D genes. Although not part of the H-2 gene complex, a TL region, being about 1 cM from H-2D, is closely linked to H-2. The TLa gene marks the TL region and codes for membrane alloantigens, which can be detected on thymocytes and some leukemia cells. Of particular interest to transplantation immunology is that disparity at the TL region can lead to skin graft rejection (7).

K and D Regions

H-2K and H-2D loci code the H-2 alloantigens that have been studied by serologic techniques for many years. Serologic detection of these H antigens largely resulted from the original work of Peter Gorer, a pathologist well versed in the intricacies of human blood group antigens (8). With the aid of heterologous antisera, he found two different erythrocyte antigens, antigen I and antigen II, which occurred in different quantities in different mouse strains. Antigen II, for instance, was present on erythrocytes of A strain mice but absent from C57/Bl mice. In a series of experiments on the segregation of antigen II and susceptibility to the growth of tumors obtained from antigen II-positive mice, Gorer found that 35 out of 65 F_2 mice were antigen II-positive and susceptible to tumor growth. Of the 30 mice that resisted tumor growth, 17 were antigen II-negative. On the basis of these and similar experiments, he concluded that the fate of transplanted tumors depended on two or three genetic loci, one of which also controlled the erythrocyte antigen II. Additional experiments established that antigen II was present on tumor cells and other tissues in the antigen II-positive A strain mice.

One other very important finding that came from these studies provided direct evidence of an immune response to incompatible tumors. It was found that C57/Bl mice, which are antigen II-negative, developed alloantibodies that agglutinated antigen II-positive A strain erythrocytes after they rejected tumors of A strain origin. Antigen II was later changed to H-2 antigen to conform to Snell's H or histocompatibility factors (1).

Since the pioneering work of Gorer, a bewildering array of serologically distinct H-2 antigenic specificities has been found. Initially, specificities were symbolized by letters. The specificities quickly exceeded the number of letters in the alphabet, and numbers are now used to symbolize individual specificities, i.e., 1, 2, 3, etc. In order to indicate that the specificities are H-2 specificities rather than other minor specificities, they are written as follows: H-2.1, H-2.2, H-2.3, etc. Numerous H-2 specificities are detected on tissue of individual mice strains. For instance, DBA/2 strain mice display 13 or more H-2 specificities. These numerous H-2 specificities in an inbred strain initially suggested that the different specificities were determined, not by one H-2 genetic locus, but by a series of closely linked loci. Since alleles at H-2 are closely linked, they would be inherited as units called haplotypes. Individual haplotypes are noted by small letter superscripts, i.e., $H\text{-}2^a$, $H\text{-}2^b$, $H\text{-}2^c$, etc.

The validity of this reasoning is confirmed in recombination studies. If the different H-2 specificities are directed by closely linked loci, some back-crosses should exhibit recombination of parental H-2 specificities. These experiments have been performed, and recombinants are found with a frequency of 1.0 to 0.5%, indicating that there could be as many as 1,000 genes within the H-2 loci, or as they are now called, H-2 system or H-2 complex.

An important finding that aided in estimating the number of loci within the H-2 complex was that some H-2 antigenic specificities were not unique for a particular H-2 gene product. Rather, some specificities called *public specificities* are shared by several different H-2 gene products. *Private specificities,* on the other hand, are unique to a given H-2 gene product. Analysis of the private specificities reveals that they segregate into two series of mutually exclusive specificities. Thus, it was concluded that the H-2 complex consists of two loci called H-2K and H-2D separated by 1.0 to 0.5 cM.

Recently, it was found that the specificity H-2.7, which is unique among H-2 specificities because it is found in greater amounts on erythrocytes than on lymphocytes, segregates independently from K and D series of alloantigenic specificities (9). This specificity is assigned to the *H-2G* locus, which is located between the K and D loci but closer to the D locus than to the K locus. The H-2G locus serves as a marker for the G region of the H-2 gene complex.

I Region

The I region is marked by the immune response-1 (Ir-1) locus. It has been known for a long time that different individuals and inbred animals respond differently to the same antigenic stimulation. Since the middle 1960s considerable investigative effort has been devoted to genetic control of the immune response. Many of the early experiments were done by McDevitt and co-workers (10,11), using synthetic polypeptides as antigens. C57Bl/6 mice, they found, respond with tenfold more antibody to these antigens than do CBA mice. Since F_1 hybrids of these strains produced abundant antibody, the high response was inherited as a dominant trait. While studying the adoptive transfer of high-responder lymphocytes into irradiated low responders, in order to minimize rejection of the injected spleen cells and resulting radiation death of the recipient, these investigators examined various congeneic pairs of mice differing at H-2. In so doing, they discovered that the immune response gene was closely linked to the H-2 gene complex. By examining various H-2 recombinant strains, they found that the immune response gene, which is called Ir-1, was located within the H-2 complex between the Ss locus and the genes coding for H-2.11 and H-2.13, which in light of more recent interpretation of the H-2 complex locates Ir-1 between the H-2K and Ss loci. This region of the H-2 complex is thus called the I region. Many additional H-2-linked, as well as non-H-2-linked, immune response genes are now recognized. The immune response to more than 20 different antigens is linked to H-2, and further studies indicate that Ir-1 consists of several separate loci which subdivide the I region into the following subregions: I-A, I-B, I-J, I-E, and I-C (12).

Ir-1J is of current interest because it controls the generation of suppressor T cells. It is now clear that T lymphocytes can either help or suppress B lymphocytes' response to antigen. Debré et al. (13) examined suppressor cell activity in various inbred mice strains and found that the random copolymer of L-glutamic acid^{50}-L-tyrosine^{50} (GT) is unable to stimulate antibody production in many strains. GT complexed to methylated bovine serum albumin (GT-MBSA), on the other hand, stimulates antibody production in several of the GT nonresponder strains. Prior administration of GT to these responder strains, however, inhibits the anti-GT response following subsequent immunization with GT-MBSA. This inhibition is due to suppressor T cells, and the ability of animals to develop suppressor cells is a dominant characteristic that is closely linked to the H-2 complex and located in the I-J subregion.

Of particular interest to this discussion is the role Ir-1 plays in the immune response to H antigens (14). Ir-1 controls not only the antibody response to H-2 but also cellular immune responses to H antigens. For example, even though males of all inbred mice strains possess a Y-linked minor H antigen missing from females, females from only some strains reject male skin. Others reject male skin very slowly or not at all. Specifically, C57Bl female mice reject male C57Bl skin in 26 days, whereas C3H male skin survives indefinitely when transplanted to C3H females. Because (C57Bl × C3H)F_1 females can reject C3H male skin, the failure of C3H females to reject male skin is not because the C3H males lack the Y-linked antigen. Rather, the ability of females of various strains to reject male skin is linked to the H-2 genotype, and probably the characteristic is located in the I-A subregion.

I region incompatibilities are conveniently demonstrated in vitro by using mixed lymphocyte culture reactions (see below) rather than serologic tests. For this reason, I region H antigens are frequently called lymphocyte-defined or simply LD antigens, in contrast to the serologically defined (SD) H-2K and H-2D antigens. By using various congeneic strains of mice that differ from one another only in the I region, however, it is possible to produce antisera to I region-associated (Ia) antigens. Since at least some of these antisera interfere with mixed lymphocyte responses in vitro, it is generally concluded that at least some of the antisera are directed toward the LD antigens or antigens positioned close to the LD antigens.

About 20 Ia specificities have been described to date. It is not known yet if private and public specificities exist for Ia antigens, as they do for H-2K and D antigens; however, preliminary studies indicate that Ia3 specificity is on the same molecules as Ia8 and Ia9 specificities, which suggests that there may be private and public specificities. Some studies suggest that there may be more than one locus directing Ia antigen production. For example, genetic mapping studies have placed specificity Ia8 in the I-A subregion and workshop (W) specificity Ia-W21 in the I-C subregion. Thus, these early studies are beginning to produce a picture that resembles the classical serologically detected H-2 antigens.

S Region

The Ss locus controls the serum level of a beta-globulin in mice and marks the S region (15). Two alleles, Ss^h and Ss^l, are identified at the locus, and they determine whether the serum concentration of beta-globulin will be high or low, respectively. For example, B10.D2 mice are Ss^h and have about 17 times more Ss protein than congeneic B10K, which are Ss^l. Another locus, Slp, which is so far inseparable from the Ss locus, controls a serum protein found in male mice of some but not all strains. The dominant Slp^a allele determines the presence of this sex-limited protein (Slp), and the recessive Spl^o allele determines its absence.

Since 17 of the 26 H-2 recombinants occurred between K and Ss and 19 between Ss and D, the Ss locus must be located in the middle of the H-2 complex where it marks the S region of H-2. Because there are many unanswered questions about Ss and Slp and since Ss is inseparable from Slp and since Ss and Slp traits involve the same molecule, a revised notation based on the H-2 origin of a single Ss locus is now used. Although it was once thought that inclusion of Ss within H-2 was an accident of nature, it is now known that the S region plays a significant role in immune reactions. In mice, S region-associated genes control serum levels of the first four complement components. In man, the HLA complex codes for the classical complement components C2, C4, and C8 and for a properdin component in the alternative pathway (Bf) (16).

MAJOR HISTOCOMPATIBILITY COMPLEX IN MAN

The major histocompatibility complex in man is designated HLA (17,18). Four loci divide HLA into four regions. There are HLA-A, formerly called "La" and first locus; HLA-B, formerly called "Four" and second locus; HLA-C, formerly called AJ locus; and HLA-D. The HLA complex is found on chromosome 6. H antigens encoded by HLA-A, HLA-B, and HLA-C loci are readily detectable by serologic techniques and are analogous to H-2K, H-2D, and H-2G. Just as in the mouse, each locus has multiple alleles; 19 at the A locus and 24 at the B locus. Since these alleles account for over 95% of A and B locus genes, it is unlikely that many more alleles will be detected. This is not the case for HLA-C. Only six alleles have been so far detected, and these are found in only 50% of typed individuals.

Mixed lymphocyte reactions are used to identify D locus antigens. To date, our knowledge of HLA-D is rudimentary. Many HLA antisera contain antibodies that react with B lymphocytes, and for several reasons these antibodies appear to be reacting with antigens similar to the I region-associated (Ia) antigens in mice. The region directing the production of glycoproteins on the surfaces of B cells has been recently designated HLA-DR. Although it is too early to reach any conclusion, the probability that HLA-D is analogous to H-2I is high. Research in this area is progressing rapidly, and definite answers should be forthcoming shortly.

The HLA genes on one chromosome are called haplotypes and are inherited *en bloc* 99% of the time. An individual contains two haplotypes, one paternally derived and one maternally derived. Thus, in a mating between a father with X and Y haplotypes and a mother with Z and W haplotypes, children of four genotypes are possible: XZ, XW, YZ, and YW. Hence, among siblings there is a 25% chance of compatibility at the MHC. This probability does not take into consideration the 1% incidence of recombination within the MHC. Since HLA genes are inherited codominantly, excluding homozygosity, each individual will express eight major H antigens, two H antigens encoded by each of the A, B, C, and D loci.

The degree of H antigen polymorphism is staggering. Considering only HLA-A and B loci, there are (19 × 24) or 456 possible haplotypes and 104,196 genotypes. Adding the six alleles at the C locus, which accounts for only 50% of the C phenotypes, yields 2,736 haplotypes and 3,744,216 genotypes. Adding the alleles so far determined at the D locus yields 21,888 haplotypes and 239,553,210 genotypes! Since negative mixed lymphocyte reactions between unrelated individuals are extremely rare, many alleles are likely to exist at the D locus. Alternatively, there may be fewer alleles but more than one locus. Whatever the explanation, the polymorphism will increase by several orders of magnitude. Although this extreme degree of polymorphism poses a large obstacle to clinical transplantation, it is reassuring that we are truly individuals.

HLA typing studies of large unrelated populations have found unexpected associations between certain alleles at different HLA loci. In a large population, it is anticipated that alleles at different loci will segregate randomly. The frequency with which alleles in any combination on different loci segregate together will be the product of the frequency of each individual allele. For example, if the frequency of A1 and B8 in the population is 0.18 and 0.15, the theoretical frequency of A1 and B8 occurring together in one individual is (0.18×0.15) or 0.027. HLA typing studies, however, indicate that in reality the frequency of A1, B8 is 0.099. Thus, there is a *linkage disequilibrium* or nonrandom association between certain antigens.

CHEMICAL CHARACTERISTICS OF MAJOR H ANTIGENS

H-2K and H-2D gene products solubilized from cells with the aid of the nonionic detergent NP40 consist of two non-covalently linked polypeptide chains. The larger of the two polypeptide chains has a molecular weight of about 45,000 to 46,000 daltons, and it carries the H-2 antigenic specificities. The smaller chain has a molecular weight of about 12,000 daltons and has been identified as β_2-microglobulin. In the detergent extraction procedure, two heavy chains with their non-covalently associated light chains frequently are linked by disulfide bonds. However, if the cells are alkylated with iodoacetamide before H-2 antigens are extracted, there is no such disulfide bond linking two heavy chains. This suggests that such interchain linkage is only transitory on the cell surface. When papain is used to isolate H-2 antigens, the heavy chain is cleaved into fragments of 39,000 molecular weight which contain the amino terminus. Thus it appears that a fragment, of less than 7,000 daltons, containing the carboxy terminal region of the heavy chain is associated with the membrane.

The isolation studies clearly indicate that H-2K and H-2D private specificities are found on separate molecules; however, amino acid sequencing of the heavy chain has now been started and the preliminary results indicate that there are similarities between products of the H-2K and H-2D loci. Thus, these data support the hypothesis that these loci arose by gene reduplication.

β_2-microglobulin was originally isolated from the urine of patients with renal tubular dysfunction. It is normally present in the serum and filtered by the renal glomerulus. Normally the filtered β_2-microglobulin is reabsorbed and catabolized by renal tubular cells. One hundred amino acids make up β_2-microglobulin, and there is a single intrachain disulfide bond which forms a 57 amino acid loop. β_2-microglobulin resembles the constant domains of IgG, especially C_H3 (19,20). A single intrachain disulfide bond forms an intrachain loop in

β_2-microglobulin which is the same size and in the same locations as the loop found in IgG constant domains. Furthermore, the two molecules exhibit a 30% amino acid sequence homology. Unlike immunoglobulins, however, β_2-microglobulin is synthesized by various epithelial and mesenchymal cells, as well as by lymphocytes. The genetic material directing β_2-microglobulin synthesis is found on chromosomes different from those directing H-2 specificities and immunoglobulin. β_2-microglobulin has been found associated with major H antigens of all species so far examined. Although all major H antigens are noncovalently linked to β_2-microglobulin, not all β_2-microglobulin is linked to major H antigens. In man, for example, of 5×10^5 molecules of β_2-microglobulin molecules on the surface of a lymphocyte, only 5×10^4 are linked to an equal number of major H antigen molecules.

Attempts to isolate and characterize I region-associated (Ia) antigens are in an early stage (21). Ia antigens isolated under reducing conditions from nonionic detergent-solubilized cells contain two glycoproteins with molecular weights of about 35,000 and 25,000 daltons. The sugar moiety on both glycoproteins consists of 3,100-molecular-weight, sugar-containing mannose, galactose, glucosamine, glucose, and sialic acid, and they are the same size, charge, and composition as a carbohydrate moiety found on the heavy chains of H-2K and H-2D antigens. Biochemical studies have also been performed on Ia material isolated from serum, and these suggest that it is largely carbohydrate and almost devoid of protein. The antigenic specificity appears to reside in the carbohydrate moiety. The Ia antigenicity is destroyed by treating the material with periodate, whereas pronase does not alter its antigenicity. Furthermore, various pure sugars inhibit anti-Ia serum from interacting with their Ia antigens. In the course of these inhibition studies, the specificities for Ia.1, Ia.3, Ia.7, and Ia.15 were found to reside on *N*-acetyl-D-mannosamine, D-galactose, L-fructose, and *N*-acetyl-D-glucosamine, respectively. Thus, it appears that at least some of the Ia antigens are carbohydrate in nature and that I region genes encode glycosyl transferases which direct the assembly of oligosaccharides containing these sugars on the cell surface. Although similar oligosaccharides are found associated with H-2D and H-2K antigens, these sugars do not express antigenic specificity.

DISTRIBUTION OF H ANTIGENS

All cells of mice express H-2K and H-2D region-coded H antigens. In man, the mature erythrocyte is the exception, and it does not express H antigens. However, immature erythrocytes do express HLA-A and B antigens. During embryogenesis, H antigens are expressed early, from the time the egg is fertilized (22). At least most, if not all, H-2K and H-2D H antigens are located on the cell surface membrane. Since no new H-2 alloantibody binding sites can be demonstrated after cells are lysed, Haughton considered that no H antigens are expressed in the cell's interior (23). Cell fractionation studies, however, indicate that a small amount of H-2 alloantigens may be associated with the endoplasmic reticulum (24).

The cellular distribution of I region-associated (Ia) antigens and HLA-DR antigens is very restrictive. Only B lymphocytes have large amounts of easily detectable Ia antigens on their cell surface membranes. Macrophages, epidermal cells, and possibly endothelial cells also may express Ia antigens, but the amount is considerably less than on B lymphocytes and is not easily detectable. Some T lymphocytes also express small amounts of Ia antigens. There is some early suggestion that antigens encoded by genes located in different I subregions may have a different cellular distribution. I-J subregion, for example, may direct the expression of Ia antigens on only a subpopulation of T cells, i.e., suppressor T cells, whereas I-E region genes may be expressed only on B lymphocytes.

H ANTIGEN PARTICIPATION IN TRANSPLANTATION IMMUNITY

Much of our knowledge of H-antigen participation in transplantation immunity comes from in vitro studies using mixed lymphocyte cultures (MLC) and lymphocyte-mediated cytotoxicity (LMC).

Mixed Lymphocyte Cultures

When lymphocytes from two disparate individuals (A and C) are mixed and cultured together for several days, a clone of A lymphocytes will recognize foreign H antigens on C lymphocytes. Similarly, an H antigen-reactive clone of C lymphocytes will recognize A lymphocytes as alien. When confronted with foreign H antigens, the H antigen-reactive clones transform into blast cells, synthesize DNA, and proliferate.

Lymphocytes making up the mixed lymphocyte reactive clone are thymus-derived lymphocytes (T cells) and belong to a T cell subpopulation which in Ly 1.2-positive mouse strains contains Ly 1 antigens and lacks Ly 2,3 antigens. Because in most instances the reaction of only one individual's lymphocytes at a time is of interest, one-way MLC are studied. This is accomplished by treating stimulator lymphocytes with X-rays or mitomycin so that they are unable to react to foreign H antigens yet still provide an adequate stimulus to the responder lymphocytes. For example, if the response of A's lymphocytes to C's H antigens is of interest, C lymphocytes are irradiated with 1,500 rads and the two populations of lymphocytes (A and C x) are cultured together. When inbred animals are used for mixed lymphocyte cultures, one-way reactions can be accomplished by using lymphocytes from F_1 hybrids as stimulator lymphocytes. For example, if the response of A's lymphocytes to C's H antigens is of interest, A and $(A \times C)F_1$ lymphocytes would be cultured together. Since the F_1 lymphocytes possess both A and C H antigens, A's H antigens are not recognized as foreign. The response of A's lymphocytes to C's H antigens is followed conveniently by measuring the amount of 3H-labeled thymidine incorporated into newly synthesized DNA in responding A lymphocytes.

When F_2 hybrids and back-crosses are used as stimulator lymphocytes in mixed lymphocyte cultures, positive mixed lymphocyte responses occur only when stimulator lymphocytes contain foreign major H antigens. Stimulator lymphocytes obtained from congeneic mice indicate that maximal mixed lymphocyte responses occur when stimulator lymphocytes are disparate at the MHC's I region. Thus, I region H antigens generally provide the major stimulus for mixed lymphocyte reactions that serve as in vitro models of the initial afferent recognition phase of transplantation immunity.

Lymphocyte-Mediated Cytotoxicity

Although there are several ways to measure lymphocyte-mediated destruction of specific target cells, currently most experimenters use the release of radioactivity from ^{51}Cr-labeled target cells. Blast-transformed lymphocytes or various tumor cells conveniently serve as target cells. In this general in vitro model, cytotoxicity occurs within several hours.

Killer cells are T lymphocytes, and in Ly 1.2-positive mouse strains these killer lymphocytes are Ly 1-negative and Ly 2,3-positive, thus indicating that the mixed lymphocyte reactive cells and killer cells are two different kinds of cells.

When target cells are lymphoblasts obtained from congeneic mice, the major antigenic targets for the cytolytic T cells are encoded by K and D regions of the MHC and not by I region H antigens.

Congeneic strains of mice have proved very helpful in analyzing the participation of H antigens during the generation of specific killer cells from mixed lymphocyte reactions. In order to achieve optimal generation of killer cells from their precursors in mixed lymphocyte cultures, two H antigen-triggered signals are necessary (25). First, H antigens that are coded for by the K and/or D regions of the mouse major histocompatibility complex (MHC) directly interact with the killer cell precursor clone. Second, a helper or amplifier signal comes from the Ly 1^+, $2{,}3^-$ T cells, which are responding proliferatively to lymphocyte-defined (LD) H antigens that are encoded by the I region of the MHC. These two H antigens need not be on the same cell, and the second signal is at least in part mediated by a soluble factor. Proliferation of the Ly 1^+, Ia antigen-responsive cell is obligatory for production of the amplifying or helper signal. Both signals are necessary only for maximum production of effector cells. Disparity at only K- and/or D-coded H antigens can give rise to effector cells, but the number of effector cells generated is considerably lower than when both K and/or D regions and I region disparities exist. For instance, it has been reported that in the presence of an SD disparity, only $298/10^6$ cells were stimulated to generate effector cells, in contrast to $1{,}447/10^6$ cells when both SD and LK disparities were present.

Thus it appears that LD alloantigens provide the greatest proliferative stimulus to lymphocytes in the afferent limb of the immune response and K and D region-directed antigens are the targets for alloimmune effector lymphocytes. This distinction, however, is not absolute. K and/or D region alloantigens can provide the stimulus for proliferative responses of alloantigen-reactive lymphocytes, and alloimmune effector lymphocytes can react against LD alloantigens.

H ANTIGENS AND DISEASE

HLA typing of patients with different diseases has revealed on many occasions that one particular H antigen is associated with certain diseases, and the incidence of this association is greater than one occurring by chance only. One of the best illustrations of this association is seen with ankylosing spondylitis and HLA-B27. Although only about 6.% of the population has B27 H antigen, about 90% of patients with ankylosing spondylitis are B27-positive. The exact incidence of ankylosing spondylitis in B27-positive persons is not known. In the general population, about 5% of the B27-positive men have obvious ankylosing spondylitis. This figure, however, may be just the tip of the iceberg, because 20% of B27-positive persons who are asymptomatic show radiographic evidence of the disease.

Ankylosing spondylitis is only one of many diseases that are associated with a particular H antigen. Several theories exist to explain the association of particular H antigens with specific diseases.

1. *Linkage Hypothesis:* H antigens themselves may not be directly related to the disease; rather, it may be a nearby gene that exists in strong linkage disequilibrium with the HLA gene. Thus, the HLA gene serves as a marker of another gene that participates in the pathogenesis of the associated disease. Since many of the diseases associated with particular H antigens are immunologic in nature, MHC-linked immune response genes are logical candidates. Susceptibility to diseases produced by microbial agents may be increased in individuals who lack the relevant immune response gene. The presence of certain Ir genes also could lead to increased susceptibility. Autoimmune diseases, for example, would develop only in individuals with the relevant Ir gene. Other genes in linkage disequilibrium with HLA antigens also may play a role in disease processes. Hemochromatosis, for example, is associated with HLA-A3, and it is possible that genes producing the metabolic defect in hemochromatosis are linked to A3.
2. *Mimicry Hypothesis:* If a certain microorganism shared antigenicity with a particular HLA antigen, a person with that particular HLA antigen would be tolerant not only to the self HLA antigen but also to the cross-reacting microbial antigen. Cross-reactions between HLA antigens and M proteins of β-hemolytic streptococci have been observed. In animals, streptococcal antigens provide immunity to skin allografts. Thus, there is partial experimental support of this hypothesis.
3. *Altered Self Hypothesis:* H antigens play an important role in the immune response to some haptens, virus, tumor, and minor H antigens. For example, mouse killer cells generated in response to cells infected with lymphocytic choriomeningitis (LMC) virus only kill target cells expressing both LMC and H-2 antigens. One interpretation of this data is that the immune response is triggered by a hybrid antigen consisting of the virus and H-2 antigen, rather than just the viral antigen. Perhaps, then, only combinations of certain H antigens and viral antigens are immunogenic and lead to diseases in which immune mechanisms participate.
4. *Receptor Hypothesis:* A particular H antigen may be the actual receptor for a certain virus. If this were so, viruses would only be able to attach to cells bearing particular H antigens that serve as the receptors for the viruses.

H ANTIGEN PARTICIPATION IN CELL-CELL INTERACTIONS

Considering the economy of nature, there must be a reason why the majority of cell surface glycoproteins are H antigens. Clearly it is not to frustrate transplantation surgeons. Possibly it is to facilitate cell-cell interactions.

H antigens play an important role in the collaboration between T and B lymphocytes and between T lymphocytes and macrophages. Antibody production to most antigens requires participation of a helper T lymphocyte and an antibody-producing precursor B lymphocyte. Experiments using T cells from one mouse and B cells from another mouse indicate that optimum collaboration occurs only when both T and B cells are of the same H-2 haplotype. The use of congeneic strains indicates that B compatibility of the I-A subregion of the H-2 histocompatibility complex is required for optimum T-B lymphocyte collaboration. T lymphocyte-macrophage collaboration, at least in the guinea pig but possibly not in the mouse, also is governed by compatibility at the major histocompatibility complex.

Recent studies indicate that the major histocompatibility complex plays a prominent role in lymphocyte interaction with and destruction of cells bearing tumor, viral, and minor histocompatibility antigens. Zinkernagel and Doherty (26) discovered that cytolytic effector T cells obtained from mice infected with lymphocyte choriomeningitis (LCM) virus killed only target cells that processed *both* LCM viral antigens and H-2K- and/or H-2D-coded H antigens that were identical to the sensitizing cell. Target cells containing only LCM viral antigens were not lysed by effector cells.

Of particular interest to transplantation immunity are experiments suggesting that immunity to minor H antigens also shows H-2 restriction. For example, Bevan (27) found that lymphocyte-mediated cytolysis directed toward minor histocompatibility antigens required that sensitizing cells and target cells share H-2.

Two general hypotheses have been formed to explain this H-2 restriction: "altered self" and "intimacy" hypotheses. The "altered self" hypothesis postulates that receptors on the cytolytic T cell interact with H-2 plus "nonself" antigens. These may exist separately in a closely spaced two-antigen unit, or the "nonself" antigen may be directly attached to H-2 antigen so that a new "hybrid" antigen is produced. According to the "intimacy" hypothesis, the receptors on the cytolytic T cells react directly with the "nonself" antigen. H-2 compatibility between effector and target is necessary for the intimate, effective interaction of the two cells. Which of these hypotheses is correct or whether some other explanation exists must await further studies in the rapidly expanding area of MHC function.

The role of H antigens in other cell-cell interactions has not been studied; but it is possible that H antigens play a role in other cell-cell interactions that occur during embryogenesis and throughout life. When H-2 disparate blastular cells are mixed and implanted into foster mothers, the resulting tetraphrenic mice develop normally. In developing embryos, there is some evidence that H-2 disparity between mother and offspring is beneficial. In rodents, for example, litter size and placental weight are greater when the conceptus contains paternally derived H antigens that differ from maternal H antigens than when the conceptus contains H antigens completely syngeneic with the mother. In man, however, HLA-A and HLA-B typing have not disclosed any consistent selective survival benefit of foreign H antigens to the conceptus.

IMMUNOLOGIC MEMORY TO H ANTIGENS

Transplantation immunity, like all forms of immunity, exhibits specific immunologic memory. For instance, (BN × WF)F_1 skin grafted for the first time onto (L × Bf)F_1 is rejected in 12 days. Second grafts are rejected in accelerated fashion 6 days after grafting. Third grafts never heal onto the graft bed at all and are rejected as white grafts. Analysis of memory in transplantation immunity is complicated by the fact that antibodies that develop after the first or second graft may influence the survival of future grafts. Hyperacute rejection (see below), for example, occurs within minutes of grafting and is initiated by antibodies reacting with the graft H antigen. In order to bypass the influence of antibodies, the in vitro models of mixed lymphocyte reactions and cell-mediated cytotoxicity have been used to study immunologic memory to H antigens at the T cell level.

In most immunologic systems, memory can be explained on the basis of expanding the number of lymphocytes making up the specific antigen-reactive clone. Clonal expansion does not, however, fully explain immunologic memory to major H antigens.

It is possible to determine the number of lymphocytes that make up the clone that responds to H antigens in mixed lymphocyte cultures. Memory to H antigens is evident in time-course studies. Lymphocytes from animals specifically immunized respond more quickly than lymphocytes from animals without prior H antigen exposure. The number of cells in the H antigen-reactive clone, however, is the same in both nonimmune and immune animals. Thus, clonal expansion does not explain memory; rather, there appears to be some qualitative difference in the lymphocyte.

Immunologic memory to H antigens is also demonstrable in the generation of cytolytic T cells. Specific cytolytic T cells generated in vitro exhibit maximum killer activity five days after stimulation for the first time with disparate H antigens. It will be recalled from previous discussions that optimum generation of the killer cells requires a disparity of both H-2K and/or H-2D region-directed and H-2I region-directed alloantigens. Also, the generation of killer cells requires cellular proliferation and DNA synthesis. Killer cells that are large lymphocytes exhibit maximum cytolytic activity on day 5 when generated in vitro and thereafter become less efficient killers. Concomitantly, they become smaller, so that by day 11 in the absence of continuing H antigen stimulation, they have little cytolytic activity and are now small lymphocytes. These formerly large, formerly cytolytic lymphocytes now represent a pool of specific memory cells and are called nonlytic secondary cytolytic T cells.

When nonlytic secondary cytolytic T cells are stimulated for the second time by specific H antigen, efficient killer cell activity develops rapidly. Specific cytolytic activity is seen as early as 18 hours, and maximum activity develops on day 3. In contrast, during primary stimulation, the earliest significant cytolytic activity is seen on day 3. Unlike the primary generation of cytolytic T cells, generation of cytolytic T cells after H antigen stimulation for the second time does not require cellular proliferation or DNA synthesis. The H antigen requirement for stimulating memory cytolytic T cells also is different from that in primary stimulation. Optimum stimulation of memory cytolytic T cells requires only H-2D- and/or H-2K-directed H antigens, and subcellular fragments are suitable for stimulation.

The cytolytic activity of the secondary cytolytic cells differs from that of primary cytolytic T cells in several ways. The activity of primary cytolytic T cells is temperature-dependent. For example, no or few cytolytic T cells form effective adhesions with target cells at 5°C or 15°C, and little specific cytolytic activity is evident at 20°C. Secondary cytolytic T cells, on the other hand, form effective adhesions with target cells at 5°C and 15°C and are efficient killers at 20°C. Kinetic studies reveal that secondary cytolytic T cells also are more efficient killers at 37°C. Whereas 50% of the killing by primary cytolytic T cells occurs in 2.5 hours, secondary cytolytic T cells kill in 1.2 hours. Thus, although there is no difference in the number of cytolytic T cells generated during primary and secondary responses, there are qualitative differences in the killer cells. Secondary cytolytic T cells are more efficient than primary cells in their interaction with and lysis of specific target cells. The reason for this difference is not clear, but a reasonable speculation is that the receptors on secondary cytolytic T cells are more fully exposed and/or greater in number.

MECHANISMS OF GRAFT REJECTION

For discussion purposes, it is convenient to divide transplantation immunity into two phases: afferent and efferent. During the afferent phase the recipient recognizes the graft's alien H antigens and generates effector mechanisms. These effector mechanisms attack the graft during the efferent phase of transplantation immunity. In the next two sections the afferent and efferent phases of transplantation immunity will be discussed.

Afferent Phase of Allograft Rejection

Much of our knowledge about the afferent phase of transplantation immunity comes from studying natural or artificially produced immunologically privileged sites that allow histoincompatible grafts to survive anonymously.

Natural immunologically privileged sites include the hamster's cheek pouch, cornea, anterior chamber of the eye, brain, mammary fat pads, hair follicles, and testes. Not all of these immunologically privileged sites have been studied completely, and some of them may afford only partial protection to attack by the host's immune system.

The hamster's cheek pouch is one of the best-studied immunologically privileged sites. Histoincompatible tissue transplanted into the hamster's cheek pouch is not rejected and enjoys privileged survival. Since these animals do not develop systemic immunity to donor H antigens, the hamster's cheek pouch attains its privileged status because it prevents immunization. This conclusion also is supported by the fate of grafts within the cheek pouch in hamsters rendered immune by a conventionally placed skin graft. For example, if hamster A skin is grafted into hamster B's cheek pouch, it survives. When A skin is transplanted on B hamster's chest wall and thus renders hamster B immune to hamster A's H antigen, both the graft within the cheek pouch and the chest wall skin graft are rejected.

Because the hamster's cheek pouch lacks lymphatic drainage, it is generally concluded that an intact lymphatic drainage is necessary for the afferent, sensitizing pathway of transplantation immunity. The use of artificial immunologically privileged sites confirms this conclusion. Barker and Billingham (28) produced artificial immunologically privileged sites in guinea pigs by raising a skin flap. The skin flap is isolated from the flap's bed by a Petri dish and connected to the animal only by a vascular pedicle. As long as the vascular supply bundle connecting the skin flap to the animal is devoid of lymphatic vessels, histoincompatible skin grafted onto the skin flap survives. However, on reestablishment of the skin flap's lymphatic drainage, the skin graft is promptly rejected. Also, rejection of the graft occurs whenever the animal is systemically sensitized to donor H antigens. Thus, in regard to skin grafts, the afferent sensitizing pathway proceeds via lymphatic vessels.

In contrast to the obligatory role of lymphatic vessels in the skin grafts, in vascularized organ grafts such as kidneys, lymphatic drainage is not required for sensitizing the recipient to donor H antigens. Experimentally, this was found to be true by following the fate of transplanted histoincompatible kidneys that were deprived of their lymphatic drainage. This is most conclusively accomplished by placing the kidney in a plastic box on the recipient's back and using silicone tubing to connect the graft's artery and vein to host vessels (29). Even though these kidneys are completely deprived of lymphatic drainage, they are rejected, and rejection is as prompt as with conventionally placed kidney grafts. Thus, the afferent sensitizing phase of transplantation immunity to vascularized organ grafts does not require lymphatic drainage.

At one time there was considerable discussion as to whether the sensitization and development of effector mechanisms occurred within the graft ("peripheral sensitization") or within lymph nodes and spleen ("central sensitization"). Experiments by Strober and Gowans (30a) favored peripheral sensitization and have lessened the controversy. These authors perfused F_1 hybrid rat kidneys in vitro with lymphocyte suspensions obtained from parental rats. After the lymphocytes had circulated through the kidney, they were returned to the parental rats. Eight days later the parental rats were grafted with F_1 hybrid skin to see if they were immune. They were, and controls were not. On the basis of these experiments, the authors concluded that lymphocytes were sensitized peripherally as they circulated through the kidney. However, an alternative explanation of the results is that "sticky" H antigens are picked up by the circulating lymphocytes and carried to a central location where immunization occurs. Also, the possibility that donor "passenger" leukocytes (see below) were released from the grafts was not entirely eliminated.

Much of the early distinction between peripheral and central sensitization rested on whether a single lymphocyte could become sensitized on encountering alien H antigens or whether the microarchitecture of the lymphoid organs was an important factor in sensitization and effector cell production. We now know largely from the in vitro models of transplantation immunity that at least two and probably more cells are necessary for optimal development of transplantation immunity. Thus, development of transplantation immunity in vivo most likely occurs at any site that can accommodate the required cells. This can occur both within grafts and within lymphoid tissues.

PASSENGER LEUKOCYTES AS A SENSITIZING VEHICLE

Several years ago, in studies of the effects of antilymphocyte sera on renal allograft rejection, it was observed that kidneys obtained from donor rats pretreated with antilymphocyte sera survived better than nontreated controls (30b,c). Additional studies revealed that kidneys obtained from donors pretreated with lympholytic drugs also survived better (30d). These studies suggested that lymphoid cells within the graft (passenger leukocytes) played an important role in determining whether grafts were rejected or not.

An additional experiment by Guttmann et al. (30e) conclusively demonstrated that passenger leukocytes within kidney grafts were absolutely required for renal allograft rejection. Prospective $(A \times B)F_1$ hybrid donors were given a lethal dose of cyclophosphamide, and their bone marrow was replaced by A bone marrow cells. Several weeks after this procedure, the kidneys that consisted of $(A \times B)F_1$ parenchyma and A passenger leukocytes were transplanted into A recipients. The kidneys were not rejected. Conversely, when kidneys obtained from A donors whose bone marrow was replaced by $(A \times B)F_1$ marrow were transplanted into A recipients, there was morphologic evidence of rejection. Thus, these experiments indicated that the passenger leukocyte and not the renal parenchyma determined whether renal grafts were rejected or not.

Since it was known that renal parenchyma expressed H antigens, it was difficult to explain these results fully at the time they were performed. With our current understanding of Ia antigens (LD antigen), the explanation is obvious. Even though renal parenchyma express H antigens serologically, they do not express sufficient Ia antigen to stimulate the Ia antigen-responsive helper cells, which is necessary for generation of optimum numbers of killer lymphocytes. In vitro studies indicate that the foregoing interpretation has to be slightly altered (30f). Renal tubular cells growing in vitro without contaminating passenger leukocytes do provide the necessary stimulus to provoke blastogenesis in allogeneic lymphocytes. Therefore, it appears that renal parenchymal cells possess a sufficient amount of Ia-antigens. In vivo, however, these antigens on the tubular cells are completely encircled by basement membranes and are, therefore, sequestered from host alloantigen reactive cells. Thus the Ia-antigens cannot be presented to alloreactive lymphocytes. The passenger leukocytes, or at least the passenger B lymphocytes, on the other hand, express Ia antigen in large quantity. Therefore, the passenger leukocyte is necessary for an allograft rejection reaction.

EFFERENT PHASE OF TRANSPLANTATION IMMUNITY

Both antibody- and cell-mediated mechanisms participate in allograft rejection. Of the two kinds of mechanisms, the cellular mechanism appears to be the principal effector mechanism participating in the rejection of tissue and organ allografts transplanted into nonsensitized recipients. Early proof for this conclusion was obtained by examining skin allografts residing in specifically tolerant recipients. The adoptive transfer of specifically sensitized lymphoid cells from animals rendered immune to specific donor H antigens to the tolerant recipient bearing skin allografts is followed by rejection of the grafts. In contrast, the passive transfer of antisera directed toward donor H antigens generally is not deleterious to the well-healed-in graft. Thus, it is generally concluded that lymphoid cell-mediated effector mechanisms, not antibody-mediated mechanisms, destroy skin grafts.

Cell-Mediated Effector Mechanisms

In vitro studies have provided much information about cell-mediated effector mechanisms that participate in the destruction of histoincompatible cells. Several distinct effector mechanisms have been delineated. One major mechanism involves the ability of specifically immune cytolytic T lymphocytes to adhere to and kill cells that express the specific antigens. Because this appears to be the principal mechanism that destroys alien cells, for cytolytic T cell killing will be discussed in detail in the following paragraphs.

Nonimmune lymphoid cells also are capable of cytocidal activity if they are bound by their Fc receptors to specific antibody-coated target cells. This effector mechanism is called antibody-dependent cellular cytotoxicity (ADCC). The exact character of the cell participating in ADCC is not known.

At one time or another, almost every lymphoid cell (T, B, null, monocyte) has been identified as the effector cell. Because there is some confusion about the identity of the nonimmune effector cell that participates in ADCC, the effector cell is noncommittally called a "K" cell. Part of the confusion in identifying K cells stems from the use of different target cells. In some systems, the K cell participating in the destruction of erythrocytes is a monocyte, whereas the K cell participating in the destruction of nonerythroid cells is a lymphocyte. Even though there is still some doubt about the character of K cells (recent data suggest that K lymphocytes are null cells), one point is clear: the K cell must have a receptor for the Fc portion of immunoglobulin on its surface. It is by the Fc receptor that K cells interact with antibody-coated target cells. Not all Fc receptor-bearing cells, however, are K cells. Specific antibody in ADCC serves as a bridge molecule, bringing together the Fc receptor-bearing K cell and target cell. It is not known if the Fc receptor has an additional role in ADCC. Since the antibody must interact with the Fc receptor on the K cell, the Fc portion of the immunoglobulin must be present; Fab_2 antibody is ineffective in producing ADCC.

Activation of the complement system by ADCC antibody has been effectively ruled out by showing that ADCC proceeds with cells and serum from animals genetically deficient in C4, 5, and 6. Apart from the first interactive, recognition step, most studies find that the lethal hit step in ADCC and cytolytic T cell killing are similar. These mechanisms are discussed in the next paragraphs.

Macrophages also may participate in destruction of grafts; however, their participation is nonessential. Grafts are rejected as promptly in the absence of macrophages as in their presence. Because of the apparent trivial nature of macrophage effector mechanisms in the rejection, macrophages will not be discussed in this section. If they do participate in graft destruction, they must participate in a specific way, rather than nonspecifically, since there is good experimental evidence attesting to the extreme specificity of allograft rejection mechanisms.

Cytolytic T Lymphocytes

In 1960, Govaerts (31) demonstrated for the first time that lymphocytes obtained from the thoracic ducts of dogs rejecting a renal allograft could specifically kill cells cultured from the donor dog's other kidney. This general in vitro model using alloimmune killer cells either obtained from immune animals or generated in vitro during mixed lymphocyte reactions has been used to examine the cellular effector mechanisms participating in transplantation immunity.

Cytolytic killer cells are large lymphocytes that belong to a T cell subpopulation that in Ly 1.2 strains is Ly 2,3-positive and Ly 1-negative. This subpopulation is a minor one, comprising about 5 to 10% of T cells (32). Suppressor cells and their precursors also belong to this subpopulation; however, suppressor cells can be distinguished from effector cells by virtue of Ia antigens on the surface of suppressor cells (33). Well-differentiated effector cells, but not their precursors, possess a membrane receptor for histamine (34). It is not entirely clear if effector cells possess a surface Fc receptor or not. Recent data suggest that the effector cell precursor contains a membrane receptor for Fc but that the mature effector cell fails to express the Fc receptor (35). Recent studies indicate that killer cells also express Ly 5 and Ly 6 antigens.

The immediate precursors of alloimmune effector lymphocytes are small, T lymphocytes of subclass Ly 1^-, Ly $2,3^+$, and Ly 6^- which do not contain histamine receptors. In order to achieve optimal generation of effector cells from these precursors, in vitro studies indicate that two H antigen-triggered signals are necessary (25).

Several studies have determined the number of precursor cells that give rise to mature effector cells. Using a limiting dilution technique in which cells were cultured with nude mice lymphocytes, Teh et al. (36) found that lymph node cells obtained from RNC mice (H-2^k) contained 1 precursor cell in 480 and 1 cell in 860, which gave rise to effector cells killing H-2^d and H-2^b target cells, respectively. Lindahl and Wilson (37), using a straightforward limiting dilution assay, found that 1 in 845 H-2^b lymphocytes had the potential to become killer cells against H-2^d targets and 1 in 1,400 H-2^k lymphocytes had potential anti-H-2^d activity. Skinner and Marbrook (38) found that 1 in 1,700 H-2^a lymphocytes had the potential to develop into anti-H-2^d killer cells. Thus, several investigations have found that from 6 to 20 per 10^4 lymphocytes have the potential to develop into specific effector cells. This number is considerably smaller than the number of lymphocytes capable of responding proliferatively in mixed lymphocyte cultures to disparate major H antigens.

Several studies have attempted to determine the number of specific effector cells generated in immunized animals. Wilson (39) and Thorn and Henney (40) have made calculations that indicate that 1 to 4% of lymphocytes obtained from immunized rats and mice are specific effector cells. Since these investigators assumed that each effector could kill only one target, an assumption that is not borne out by more recent data, this percentage is probably too high. However, a recently developed plaque assay showed that between 0.05 and 2% of lymphocytes were effectors (41). Similarly, recent in vitro studies on effector cells generated in mixed lymphocyte cultures show that between 0.7 and 1% of the remaining cells are effector cells. Studies on the frequency of effector cells produced in vivo indicate that as many as 10% of spleen cells from immunized mice are specific effector cells (42). Since Teh et al. have found that the average clone developed from each precursor cell during seven days in culture contained 1,040 effector cells, these estimates on effector cell frequency appear reasonable.

Several other cell-cell interactions participate in the generation of alloimmune effector lymphocytes. Suppressor T lymphocytes that are Ly $2,3^+$/Ly 1^- may modulate the generation of effector cells, most likely by suppressing the proliferative response of the LD alloantigen-responsive Ly $1^+/2,3^-$ T cells. An additional T cell-T cell interaction is seen in the proliferative response to LD antigens. A poorly defined T cell amplifies this proliferative response (43). Cells that adhere to glass and plastic and therefore are likely to be macrophages also are required for generation of effector cells.

It is not known exactly how macrophages function in the generation of effector cells. They are, however, required for a proliferative response to foreign LD alloantigens. Since supernatants of macrophage cultures will restore mixed lymphocyte responses to macrophage-depleted cultures (44), and since 2-mercaptoethanol can substitute for macrophages (45), it is likely that macrophages provide some essential soluble factor needed by the LD alloantigen-responsive lymphocyte, rather than function to bind and present allogeneic cells to the responsive lymphocyte.

Effector lymphocytes, once generated, are short-lived. Within a few days these alloimmune effector T cells progressively differentiate into smaller T lymphocytes and concomitantly lose their alloeffector activity. On restimulation, though, these small T lymphocytes transform rapidly within 24 hours into large cells without obligatory DNA synthesis and again express efficient alloeffector activity (46). It is noteworthy that restimulation of the small T memory cells into large alloimmune effector T cells can occur independently of any collaboration with the afferent limb, i.e., LD response, and can occur without obligatory DNA synthesis. Also, isolated cellular alloantigens that are unable to stimulate the production of alloimmune effector cells in lymphocyte populations without previous exposure to the alloantigen are capable of generating alloimmune effector T cells from small memory cells (47). In vitro, over the next several days following restimulation, the number of effector cells enlarges, and this expansion is dependent on DNA synthesis.

Early in the investigations of alloimmune effector T cell destruction of specific target cells, it was thought that the actual killing process took up to two days to be effected. We know now, largely through the use of chromium labeled P-815 mastocytoma cells as targets, that this is not the case. The alloimmune effector T cell-mediated destruction can occur very rapidly, in fact, about as rapidly as antibody- and complement-mediated target cell lysis.

Recent studies have been able to separate the destruction of specific target cells by alloimmune effector T cells into at least three separate phases: (1) the recognition phase, during which effector cell and target cell establish intimate contact with one another; (2) the "hit" phase, during which the alloimmune effector T cells deliver an event or "hit" that will eventually prove fatal to the target cell; and (3) the target cell disintegration phase, during which a series of events are set in motion that lead to the actual destruction of the target cells. Each of these phases will be discussed briefly.

Recognition Phase. The interaction of alloimmune effector T cells with the appropriate target cell presumably is a manifestation of the effector cells' receptors engaging the complementary antigens on the surface of the target cell. This interaction, however, is not a passive phenomenon, for energy is required. It also requires Mg^{++}. Adherence does not take place at 5°C, and it can be abolished by cytochalasin β. This latter finding suggests that microfilaments are involved. Little is known of the alloimmune cytolytic T cell's receptor, and a discussion of the molecular nature of the elusive T cell receptor is beyond the scope of this discussion. However, the exquisite specificity of alloimmune effector T cell-mediated target cell destruction implies the existence of a receptor on the effector cell. Also suggestive are experiments that show that effector cells can be adsorbed on specific target cell monolayers and thus deplete lymphocyte populations of the specific effector cell, whereas alloeffector cells with a different specificity remain unaffected (48). Furthermore, these adherent alloeffector cells can be recovered to display their specific cytotoxicity.

Since alloantibody directed against alloantigens on target cells inhibits the cytolytic action of alloimmune effector T cells, it is generally assumed that the effector cells' receptor displays a specificity identical or very similar to the specificity of alloantibody, i.e., serologically defined alloantigens. Although it is possible that alloantibody, when reacting with its complementary antigens, sterically hinders the alloeffector cells' receptors from interacting with their distinct complementary antigens, there are some studies that suggest that the antigens reacting with alloantibody and alloeffector receptors may, in fact, be different. For instance, Edidin and Henney (49) were able to cap and internalize SD alloantigens on P-815 mastocytoma cells which are $H\text{-}2^d$. Although these "naked" targets were no longer susceptible to lysis by anti-$H\text{-}2^d$ alloantisera and complement, they could be lysed by alloimmune effector T cells. Furthermore, analysis of $H\text{-}2^b$ mutants at the K locus shows that although reciprocal immunization does not lead to alloantibody production, alloimmune effector T cells are generated and effectively destroy the reciprocal targets (50,51). Other suggestive evidence is seen in studies of human alloimmune effector T cells generated in vitro in mixed lymphocyte cultures. Sometimes these effector cells exhibit alloaggressor activity or "cross-killing" toward third-party targets that do not bear any cross-reacting serologically defined antigens (52). These studies, as I have indicated, raise the possibility that the antigens recognized by alloimmune effector T cell receptors and alloantibody may in fact be different.

Thus, there are several lines of evidence that question the usually held view that the receptors of alloimmune effector lymphocytes are directed against the serologically defined alloantigens. Since there is evidence to indicate that the H antigen targets of alloimmune cytolytic T lymphocytes differ from the SD H antigens, they are called cytolytic lymphocyte-defined H antigens or simply CLD H antigens.

The "Hit" Phase. During this phase, the adherent alloimmune effector T cells deliver a hit that eventually proves fatal to the target cell. The exact nature of the "hit" is unknown. The dynamics of this phase, though, have been investigated. By removing alloimmune effector T cells from target cells at various intervals with the aid of specific alloantisera directed at the lymphocytes, Martz (53) demonstrated that less than one hour of contact between the two cells was sufficient for the hit to be inflicted, even though actual target cell lysis required several hours. Thus, alloimmune effector T cell-dependent and T cell-independent steps in specific target cell destruction were demonstrated. In continuing these studies with the aid of ethylenediamine tetraacetic acid (EDTA) and vortexing to separate alloimmune effector T cell-target cell adhesions and adding dextran to prevent additional interactions, Martz and Benacerraf found that "hits" occurred within six minutes of alloimmune effector T cell-target cell interaction (54).

An important finding brought out by kinetic studies on cytolytic T cell killing of specific target cells is that a target cell is killed by a single hit from a single alloeffector cell and that a single alloimmune effector T cell can hit more than one target cell without loss of cytolytic efficiency (55). This conclusion is at variance with early morphologic observations that led to the conclusion that effector lymphocytes underwent "allogeneic death" while killing the specific target cell. Zagury et al. (56) have convincingly demonstrated that one alloimmune effector lymphocyte can kill several target cells. With the aid of micromanipulators, these authors were able to transfer serially a single alloimmune effector lymphocyte to several target cells and found that effector lymphocytes could each kill up to three target cells.

There is some evidence that the receptors on alloimmune effector T cells, in addition to being a recognition molecule necessary for bringing a killer cell and its target into intimate contact so that the preprogrammed killer mechanisms can be expressed, actively participate in the hit mechanism.

Kuppers and Henney (57) incubated together two populations of alloimmune effector cells, $H\text{-}2^{a}$-anti-$H\text{-}2^{d}$ and $H\text{-}2^{d}$-anti-$H\text{-}2^{b}$, and later measured remaining anti-$H\text{-}2^{d}$ and anti-$H\text{-}2^{b}$ activity. If the receptor merely serves to bring the killer cells in contact with the target cells, one would expect mutual destruction of both alloimmune effector cells in the above experiments. This was not the result. Only $H\text{-}2^{d}$-anti-$H\text{-}2^{b}$ activity was decreased. $H\text{-}2^{a}$-anti-$H\text{-}2^{d}$ activity was not decreased, even though by virtue of their own receptors they were brought into intimate contact with alloimmune effector cells, i.e., $H\text{-}2^{d}$-anti-$H\text{-}2^{b}$. Thus, the receptors appear to participate in the actual killing process, as well as serve as a recognition molecule.

Although the exact character of the "hit" remains an enigma, several possibilities exist: (1) effector lymphocytes secrete soluble cytotoxins that kill the target cell; (2) effector lymphocytes insert a protein with an ion-permeable channel into the target cell membrane; or (3) enzymes on the effector lymphocyte's membrane act on and/or destroy the target cell's membrane. Each of these possibilities will be discussed.

1. *Effector lymphocytes secrete soluble cytotoxins that kill the target cell.* Since various drugs that inhibit secretory processes by virtue of elevating cAMP and affecting microtubules and microfilaments also inhibit alloimmune effector T cell destruction of specific target cells, some investigators have concluded that secretion is necessary for the lethal hit. Electron-microscopic studies by Kalina and Berke (58) also support this view. These authors observed that alloimmune effector lymphocytes have distinctive morphologic features that separate them from other lymphocytes. They contain a well-developed golgi apparatus and contain cytoplasmic granules that the authors suggest may be secretory granules.

If secretion is necessary for target cell destruction, the most likely candidate for a soluble mediator is the nonspecific cell-toxic lymphokine called lymphotoxin. Lymphocytes stimulated by either nonspecific mitogens (59) or specific antigens (60) secrete lymphotoxin, which exhibits cytocidal activity toward nonspecific target cells. Lymphotoxin apparently consists of several groups of effector molecules (61). One group is labile with a short half-life in culture. These labile lymphotoxins are secreted shortly after in vitro stimulation with PHA and contain a subgroup with molecular weights of about 50,000. Another group is stable, is secreted after about 20 hours of culture with PHA, and has a molecular weight of about 85,000.

There are two major experimental observations that present obstacles to accepting the hypothesis that lymphotoxin-like effector molecules participate in alloimmune effector T cell-mediated cytolysis. First, lymphotoxin-like effector molecules are not found in supernatants of target cells undergoing specific destruction by alloimmune effector T cells. Second, alloimmune effector T cell-mediated target cell destruction is highly specific. Numerous studies in which alloimmune effector T cells were added to mixtures of specific and nonspecific target cells have failed to reveal nonspecific target cell killing. If lymphotoxin-like effector molecules mediate the specific target cell destruction after alloimmune effector T cells are triggered by reaction of their receptors with corresponding antigens on the target cell surface, lymphotoxins, which by demonstration and conception exhibit no specificity in terms of alloantigens, should destroy nonspecific target cells. The fact that nonspecific target cell destruction was not observed in mixtures of specific and nonspecific target cells, then, does not favor the hypothesis that lymphotoxin-like effector molecules participate in alloimmune effector T cell destruction of specific target cells.

There have been a few reports of nonspecific target cell destruction by alloimmune effector T cells, but these studies have employed target cells in monolayers rather than in suspension. In systems employing monolayer mixtures of specific and nonspecific targets, it is likely that a single alloeffector cell can by establishing simultaneous contact with both specific and nonspecific targets destroy the nonspecific target cell. Such simultaneous contact is highly unlikely in suspension cultures.

The above objections certainly are not absolute. There are possible explanations to account for these findings during alloimmune effector T cell target cell destruction mediated by lymphotoxin-like molecules. For instance, the possible lymphotoxin-like effector molecule could be extremely labile, having an extremely short life span in culture, and thus not be readily detectable in culture supernatants. Heterogeneity of the lymphotoxin secreted by PHA-stimulated lymphocytes gives some credence to this possibility. One of the groups of lymphotoxins is labile and short-lived (see above).

Another reason why lymphotoxin-like effector activity has not been found in supernatants could be that the lymphotoxin-like effector molecules are secreted onto the target cells' membranes. The evidence indicating the existence of lymphotoxin receptors on the membranes of target cells (62,63) is consistent with this interpretation. A further possibility along similar lines is that the lymphotoxin-like effector molecule is secreted or "injected" directly *into* the target cells and thus is not found free in the supernatant. This and the previous possibility coupled with antigen-specific triggering of the injection process would explain the nonspecific target cell destruction under conditions in which alloimmune effector T cells can make simultaneous contact with mixed monolayers of specific and nonspecific target cells. Support for such a view can be found in the experiments of Sellin et al. (64). These authors were able to demonstrate transfer of fluorescein from labeled immune lymphocytes to specific target cells. Their work has not been confirmed; if it were, it would indicate that mechanisms exist for the intracellular transfer of material from lymphocytes to target cell.

Exactly how transfer of fluorescein and other molecules could occur between effector lymphocyte and target cell is not known. Transfer of genetic material between bacteria is unequivocally established, and it occurs via a conjugation bridge (F. pilus). A similar transfer between macrophage and lymphocyte has been suggested, and cytoplasmic continuity between these two cells has been demonstrated by electron microscopy (65). Thus, effector lymphocytes may establish cytoplasmic bridges with target cells so that cytotoxic material can be transferred into the target cell. Sura et al. (66) have concluded on the basis of histochemical and light-microscopic observations that such cytoplasmic bridges exist between alloimmune effector lymphocytes and target, and that lymphocyte DNA and RNA are transferred into the target cell. Although such communications may exist, data more convincing than those presented by Sura et al. must be obtained to substantiate their existence.

A more likely anatomic basis of intercellular transfer may consist in specialized membrane junctions of the gap and/or septate variety. Through the former and probably the latter junctions, transfer of material with a molecular weight of about 10^3 daltons and possibly as much as 69,000 daltons has been demonstrated in a variety of nonlymphoid cells (67). McIntyre et al. (68) have identified septate-like junctions between lymphocyte clusters forming in Mishell-Dutton cultures, and there is a faint suggestion that septate junctions form between alloimmune effector lymphocytes and target cells.

Whether or not protein synthesis is necessary in the alloimmune effector T cells during the destruction of specific target cells is in dispute. The requirement for protein synthesis in the alloimmune effector T cells is of more than just peripheral interest; for if lymphotoxin-like effector molecules mediate the killing, these protein molecules have to be synthesized. If inhibitors of protein synthesis had no effect on alloimmune effector T cell destruction of specific target cells, this would be discordant with the view that the destruction is mediated by lymphotoxin-like effector molecules, unless prior synthesis and storage of the effector molecules are postulated.

Brunner and co-workers (69) found that cyclohexamide, a reversible inhibitor of protein synthesis, inhibited but did not abolish alloimmune effector T cell cytotoxicity. Using irreversible inhibitors of protein synthesis, Henney et al. (70) found that cytotoxicity of alloimmune effector T cells was completely inhibited by these inhibitors. However, in the authors' dose response studies, they found that inhibition of protein synthesis and inhibition of cytotoxicity do not necessarily go hand in hand. Pactamycin, for example, at 10^{-6} moles completely suppresses amino acid incorporation into lymphocyte proteins. This dose also inhibits 90% of migration inhibition factor (MIF) release by sensitized lymphocytes. Alloimmune effector T cell destruction of specific target cells, however, is only inhibited 20% at this concentration. It is also noteworthy that alloimmune effector T cell destruction continued undiminished for 24 hours with 10^{-6} moles pactamycin. Only at a dose of 10^{-5} moles does cytotoxicity become inhibited. Thus, this study with the aid of inhibitors of protein synthesis shows a dissociation between soluble mediator release by sensitized lymphocytes and alloimmune effector T cell destruction of specific target cells. A similar conclusion was reached after studying the effects of *Vinca* alkaloids and of agents that elevate cAMP on target cell killing and soluble mediator release.

The use of antilymphotoxin antibodies also has provided evidence that lymphotoxins do not participate in alloimmune effector lymphocyte killing mechanisms. Although addition of antilymphotoxin antibody to cultures of sensitized lymphocytes and antigens protects nonspecific target cells from destruction, antilymphotoxin has no effect on alloimmune lymphocyte-mediated destruction of specific target cells (71).

2. *Effector lymphocytes insert a protein with an ion-permeable channel into the target cell membrane.* Experiments monitoring leakage of rubidium from target cells indicate that rubidium leaks out within minutes of lymphocyte-target cell interaction; hence, it is reasoned that the lethal hit creates ion-permeable "pores" or "channels" in the target cell membrane. Henney, using dextrans of different molecular weight to see which dextran prevents further target cell destruction, found that dextrans with a minimum molecular weight of 40,000 protected target cells from disintegrating after being "hit" by alloimmune effector lymphocytes (72). On the basis of this finding, it was calculated that the hit produced a pore or channel 90 A in diameter. Similar studies performed by Ferluga and Allison (73) indicated that dextrans of 10,000 molecular weight protected target cells from disintegration.

Additional evidence favoring the view that ion-conducting channels appear in the target cell membrane comes from the studies of antibody-dependent cellular cytotoxicity (ADCC) by Henkart and Blumenthal (74). These investigators used artificial planar lipid bilayers as a target for ADCC and found a prompt increase in conductance and hence ion flow across antibody-coated lipid bilayers when lymphocytes were added. An important aspect of the work by Henkart and Blumenthal is that their antigen was DNP-lipid and that there was no protein in the membrane. Thus, the ion-conducting channels did not preexist in the membranes with the lymphocytes opening the "gate." If this conclusion holds for alloimmune effector lymphocyte-mediated destruction of specific target cells, one of the most likely possibilities is that the effector lymphocyte inserts channels into the target cell's membrane.

Although there is no experimental support for this possibility in alloimmune effector lymphocyte-mediated target cell destruction, the phenomenon of insertion into lipid bilayers with a resulting transmembrane channel is established for mellitin, a polypeptide bee venom that has hydrophobic domains which can insert and span the hydrocarbon moiety of a phospholipid bilayer. Mayer (75) has hypothesized and provided supportive evidence that in complement-mediated lysis of red cells the terminal complement components are inserted into the phospholipid bilayer of the erythrocyte membranes and create an ion-permeable transmembrane channel which impairs osmotic regulation of the cell and eventually leads to cell lysis.

Thus, it is possible that the alloimmune effector lymphocyte inserts a protein ion-permeable channel into the target cell membrane. This channel-creating protein could conceivably be lymphotoxin or another protein, or the ion-permeable channel could be created by another mechanism. If the lymphocyte-target cell junction is of the gap or septate type, it is possible that the permeable channels that develop in those junctions persist in the target cell membrane after the effector lymphocyte de-adheres and moves on to another target, as it does. Such persisting channels would lead to osmotic lysis of the target cells.

3. *Enzymes on the effector lymphocyte's membrane act on and/or destroy the target cell's membrane.* Support for this hypothesis comes from the experiments of Frye and Friore (76) and from Ferluga and Allison (77). The former investigators inhibited antibody-dependent cell-mediated cytotoxicity (ADCC) of heterologous erythrocytes by adding phospholipase A inhibitors. Thus, the authors conclude that phospholipase A located on the effector lymphocyte enzymatically converts target cell membrane phosphatidylcholine to fatty acid and lysolecithin, and the latter product, being a very potent lytic agent, actually causes target cell lysis. Whether phospholipase A participates in alloimmune lymphocyte cytotoxicity is not clear. Allison and Ferluga, however, cite unpublished experiments that indicate that the inhibitors of phospholipase A do not inhibit alloimmune effector lymphocyte-mediated cytotoxicity. Further osmotic lysis of target cells is prevented by dextrans of a molecular weight insufficient to afford protection against lysolecithin-induced lysis. Thus, ADCC and alloimmune effector lymphocyte cytotoxicity may have different mechanisms for destroying target cells.

Allison and Ferluga (78) suggest that proteolytic enzymes participate in target cell destruction. These authors find that lymphocyte membrane preparations alone are able to destroy target cells and that inhibitors of proteinases prevent the membrane-mediated destruction of targets. Morphologic supportive evidence for this hypothesis can be seen in an electron-microscopic study of Koren et al. (79). These authors conclude that in areas of contact between effector lymphocytes and target cells the target cell's membrane is damaged, whereas the lymphocyte membrane does not lose integrity. Since optimally prepared and viewed specimens were not used in this study, the evidence is only suggestive. Because recent studies by Allison have revealed that membrane preparations from nonimmune lymphocytes also can destroy target cells, there is reason to question the relevance of their work to mechanisms by which cytolytic T cells kill specific target cells.

Target Cell Disintegration Phase. Most investigators now use radioactive chromium release as an index for target cell destruction. These studies have revealed that it may be several hours, depending on effector cell:target cell ratios, after the alloimmune effector T cell's "hit" before the target cell is actually destroyed. The destructive process is temperature-dependent, and this finding has led to the reasoning that development of the "hit" into a lethal lesion is energy-dependent. This reasoning, however, has been shown to be fallacious, for antibody- and complement-induced lysis of P-815 mastocytoma cells, unlike the lysis of erythrocytes, also is temperature-dependent (80). Hence, it appears unnecessary to speculate on the energy requirements for development of the "hit" into its lethal potential. Rather, colloid osmotic lysis may be the actual mechanism of target cell destruction.

Consonant with this interpretation are the reports that target cell lysis could be prevented by extracellular high-molecular-weight polymers. The minimum molecular weight of dextran that affords this protection is 40,000 and suggests an initial alloimmune effector T cell-induced membrane "hole" of 90 Å in diameter (72). Similar studies were performed by Ferluga and Allison, but the results indicate that dextran with a molecular weight of 10,000 protected target cells from lysis (73). Further support for an initial small hit followed by colloid osmotic lysis is found in sequential studies on target membrane permeability (81,82). Following the alloimmune effector T cell hit, the target cell exhibits a gradually increasing permeability to larger and larger molecules. For instance, intracellular ATP, nicotinamide, and rubidium leak from target cells within ten minutes after specific effector cells are added to targets. Chromium that is bound to intracellular proteins and DNA leaks out only after a lag period that is directly related to the molecular size of the indicator. Thus, alloimmune effector T cells produce small holes in the target cell membrane, through which small ions freely exchange and cause disorder to osmotic regulation. The intracellular proteins, in accordance with the Gibbs-Donnan effect, produce a water influx with its attendant colloid osmotic forces, and this leads to cell swelling and hole enlargement to the point where intracellular proteins escape into the extracellular fluid.

Not all investigators agree with the above view. Sanderson (83,84), for instance, using labels of various sizes found that most are released at the same time, with no progression from small to large molecules. DNA release lags behind, but Sanderson concludes that this is because of its nuclear location rather than its large size. Time-lapse microcinematography upheld Sanderson's conclusions. Whereas in antibody- and complement-mediated lysis there was a progression of changes leading to final swelling and lysis of the cells, no such sequence was observed in target cells being killed by effector lymphocytes. Rather, these target cells underwent sudden and violent "zeiosis." Clearly, more studies are needed to clarify just how target cells undergo destruction after being lethally hit by the effector cell.

Antibody-Mediated Effector Mechanisms

It has long been recognized that specific antibodies directed against donor H antigens have a major effector function in the rejection of grafts consisting of disassociated cells such as lymphocytes. With solid grafts, however, early studies indicated that specific antibodies either played no role in graft rejection or actually prolonged graft survival. This beneficial action on graft survival was originally seen in solid tumor grafts and is called immunologic enhancement. In the case of skin grafts, antibody generally has no effect on healed grafts.

Unfortunately, in the early days of clinical transplantation, the results obtained from skin graft experiments were extrapolated to all solid grafts, and the results of this dogma based on the "tyranny of skin grafts" led to several tragedies. One of these tragedies involved a young girl (patient 30 in ref. 85a) who was to receive a transplant donated by her mother. Studies prior to transplantation revealed that the girl's serum contained cytotoxic antibodies that reacted with the mother's lymphocytes. During the transplant operation, within minutes after the vascular anastomosis was completed and the recipient's blood was allowed to circulate through the newly transplanted kidney, the kidney became cyanotic and swollen and did not make any urine. The kidney never did function, and when it was examined microscopically several days later, it was completely necrotic. Fluorescence microscopy disclosed that the vasculature was coated with immunoglobulins and complement. This form of violent rejection is called hyperacute rejection and is now recognized as being initiated by the interaction of donor preformed antigraft H antibodies with the graft.

Although presensitization initiates hyperacute rejection, the exact pathogenetic mechanisms are not fully understood. Part of the difficulty in elucidating these mechanisms has been the lack of suitable, readily available animal models; however, Guttmann has recently developed a model for hyperacute rejection of cardiac allografts in rats (85b).

This model consists of using recipients that are immunized to donor H antigens by three sequential skin grafts. For example, when (WF × BN)F_1 recipients are sensitized to (L × Bf)F_1 donor H antigens by three sequential (L × Bf)F_1 skin grafts, median survival time for donor hearts in these recipients is 62 minutes, compared to nine days in nonsensitized recipients. Thus, this is an excellent model for studying the pathogenesis of hyperacute rejection. We have used this rat model to investigate the role of complement in hyperacute rejection. Prospective sensitized recipients were given cobra venom factor, which depleted them of hemolytic complement. They then received a cardiac allograft. As long as the total hemolytic complement remains low in these recipients, hyperacute rejection is prevented. However, as soon as complement levels return toward normal, the hearts are rejected.

Although both antidonor antibody and complement are thus required for hyperacute cardiac allograft rejection in the rat model, it is not known how complement participates in hyperacute rejection. At least four not necessarily exclusive possibilities exist.

One possible mode of action of complement is that antibodies interacting with alloantigens of the graft activate the complement sequence and thereby generate chemotactic factors (C3a, C5a, and $\overline{C567}$) which attract polymorphonuclear neutrophils (PMNs). The PMNs, in turn, through their lysosomal enzymes, destroy the graft in a manner analogous to the tissue injury found in Arthus reactions. PMNs have been implicated in the pathogenesis of hyperacute rejections of kidneys on the basis of microscopic examination of organs undergoing hyperacute rejection. In the original report of hyperacute cardiac rejection in the rat by Guttmann, PMN accumulation within hyperacutely rejected hearts was observed and thus suggested the participation of PMNs in the pathogenesis of hyperacute rejection. However, further studies by Guttmann et al. (85c), using recipients depleted of PMNs, led to the conclusion that PMNs are not required for hyperacute rejection.

Since complement has been shown to promote blood coagulation by C6, another possible role for complement in hyperacute rejection is its activation of the coagulation system, with subsequent occlusion of the vasculature by clot formation and fibrin deposition. Microscopic observations of hyperacutely rejected kidneys demonstrated extensive plugging of the vasculature by the products of coagulation and suggested a role for coagulation in the pathogenesis of hyperacute rejection. This idea is supported by the studies of Boehmig et al. (85d), who found that clotting factors II, V, VIII, and IX were consumed by hyperacutely rejecting organs.

Another possible role for complement in the pathogenesis of hyperacute rejection is its direct participation in platelet aggregation. One way in which platelets of certain species, including the rat, aggregate is by the adhesion of platelets to C3b. Platelet aggregation was implicated in the pathogenesis of hyperacute rejection by Lowenhaupt, Nathan, and Menefee (85e), who presented the first evidence for platelet aggregation early in hyperacute rejection of renal allografts in presensitized dogs. They suggested that platelet blockade of vessels resulted in parenchymal damage leading to hyperacute rejection. In the rat model of hyperacute rejection of renal allografts, similar but not identical to the heart model, Forbes et al. (85f) concluded that platelets were required for hyperacute rejection because hyperacute rejection did not occur in previously sensitized recipients that were depleted of their platelets by administration of antiplatelet serum. Since the antiplatelet antibody on combining with platelet antigens probably activates the complement sequence, and since complement levels of the graft recipients were not determined after administration of the antiplatelet globulin, it is remotely possible that these investigators had in fact complement-depleted their rats, and prevented hyperacute rejection because of complement depletion rather than platelet depletion.

A final mechanism by which complement may participate in hyperacute rejection is through the lytic action of the terminal components of complement, C8 and C9. Presumably host antidonor antibody reacts with the endothelium of the graft and thus activates complement. Lysis of the endothelium would expose the blood to the thrombogenic properties of subendothelium and thus lead to coagulation within the allograft, and ultimately rejection. It is also possible that antibody reacts with H antigens on cardiac muscles and causes ion shifts that are especially hazardous to the contracting myocardium.

Which, if any, of the above possible mechanisms participates in the pathogenesis of hyperacute rejection must await the results of additional studies on the mechanisms of hyperacute rejection.

There is some evidence that antibodies may have an effector function in graft rejection during primary rejection. As mentioned, previously, although passively transferred specific antidonor serum has no effect on healed in grafts residing on tolerant mice, antibodies can adversely affect skin grafts that are recently transplanted. When specific antidonor serum is passively transferred for several days after skin grafting, the grafts are rejected more quickly than in controls (6 versus 10 days). Even in well-healed grafts, antibodies can accelerate rejection if the graft is injected with histamine. Presumably the histamine increases vascular permeability and thus facilitates antibody reacting with the graft.

Antibodies also may play a significant role in primary kidney rejection. Renal allografts performed in inbred rats provide a good model to study renal allograft rejection under controlled and partially defined H-barriers. Morphologic studies (86) of these rejecting renal allografts reveal two major alterations: most obvious is the appearance of large lymphocytes and lymphoid cells. The other major morphologic alteration is a necrotizing vasculitis involving the grafts' blood vessels. There are several reasons for believing that graft failure is a consequence of the vascular lesions and is not related to the lymphoid cell accumulation within the graft. In studies correlating renal function with the morphologic appearance of rejecting allografts, only the vascular lesions correlated in time with functional failure of the graft. Examination of renal grafts from recipients with "enhanced" grafts (87,88), and from recipients treated with azathioprine (89), emphasizes that the presence or absence of vascular lesions, and not the lymphocyte infiltrates, determines whether a graft fails or survives.

At the beginning of this section it was briefly mentioned that antibodies to donor H antigens may on occasion afford the graft protection against rejection. This phenomenon is called immunologic enhancement, and it is relatively easy to enhance the survival of renal allografts in rats either by active immunization or by passive transfer of antibodies. Microscopic examination of such enhanced renal allografts reveals that just as many or even more lymphoid cells accumulate within the interstitium of enhanced surviving grafts as within that of control nonenhanced rejecting grafts. However, the necrotizing vascular lesions are not seen in successfully enhanced grafts (87,88). Azathioprine, which is very effective in prolonging renal allograft survival in man and dogs, does not prolong the survival of rat renal allografts. Microscopic examination of the rejecting rat renal allografts in recipients treated with azathioprine reveals very few lymphoid cells within the graft. The vascular lesions, however, are present (89). Thus, these studies suggest that graft failure occurs as a result of the vascular lesions and not as a consequence of lymphoid cell accumulation within the graft.

Immunofluorescence studies indicate that the vascular lesions are initiated by antibody reacting with the vessels (90,91). As early as three days after allografts, Ig along with C3 is found on thin-walled peritubular capillaries. Thus, these findings raise the possibility that antibodies play a prominent role in the rejection of renal allografts in the rat.

REFERENCES

1. Snell, G. D., *J. Genet.* **49**, 87 (1948).
2. Little, C. C., and Tyzzer, E. E., *J. Med. Res.* **33**, 393 (1916).
3. Billingham, R. L., Hodge, B. A., and Silvers, W. K., *P.N.A.S.* **48**, 138 (1962).

4a. Graff, R. J., and Bailey, D. W., *Transplant. Rev.* **15**, 26 (1973).

4b. Mahabik, R. N., Gittmann, R. D., and Lindquist, R. R., *Transplantation* **8**, 369 (1969).

5. Klein, J., *Biology of the Mouse Histocompatibility-2 Complex,* Springer-Verlag, New York, 1975.
6. Shoeffler, D. C., and David, C. S., *Adv. Immunol.* **20**, 125 (1951).
7. Boyse, E. A., Flaherty, L., Stockert, E., and Old, L. J., *Transplantation* **13**, 431 (1972).
8. Gorer, P. A., *J. Pathol. Bacteriol.* **44**, 691 (1937).
9. David, C. S., Stimpfling, J. H., and Shreffler, D. C., *Immunogenetics* **2**, 131 (1975).
10. McDevitt, H. O., Bechtol, K. M., and Hammerling, G. T., in *Cellular Selection and Regulation in the Immune Response*, (G. M. Edelman, ed.), Raven, New York, 1975, p. 101.
11. Benacerraf, B., and McDevitt, H. D., *Science* **175**, 272 (1972).
12. Shreffer, D. C., David, C. S., Cullen, S., Frelinger, J. A., and Niederhuber, J. E., in *Quant. Biol. Cold Spring Harbor Symp.,* 1977.
13. Debré, et al., *J. Exp. Med.* **142**, 1447 (1975).
14. Gasser, D. L., and Silvers, W. K., *Adv. Immunol.* **18**, 1 (1974).
15. Shreffler, D. C., and Owen, R. D., *Genetics* **48**, 9 (1963).
16. Van Rood, J. J., Van Leeuwen, A., Termijtelen, A., and Kenning, J. J., in *The Role of Products of the Histocompatibility Gene Complex in Immune Responses* (D. H. Katz and B. Benacerraf, eds.), Academic Press, New York,
17. Snell, G. D., Dausset, J., and Nathenson, S., *Histocompatibility*, Academic Press, New York, 1976.
18. WHO-IUIS Terminology Committee, *Transplant. Proc.* **8**, 109 (1976).
19. Peterson, P. A., Cunningham, B. A., Berggard, I., and Edelman, G. M., *Proc. Natl. Acad. Sci.* (U.S.A.) **09**, 1697 (1972).
20. Smithies, D., and Poulik, M. D., *Science* **175**, 187 (1972).
21. Cullen, S. E., Freed, J. H., and Ivathenson, S. G., *Transplant. Rev.* **30**, 236 (1976).

22. Simmons, R. L., and Russell, P. S., *Ann. N.Y. Acad. Sci.* **129**, 35 (1966).
23. Haughton, G., *Transplantation* **4**, 238 (1966).
24. Ozer, J., and Wallach, D. F. H., *Transplantation* **5**, 652 (1967).
25. Bach, F. H., Segall, M., Zier, K. S., Sondel, P. M., Alter, B. J., and Bach, M. L., *Science* **180**, 403 (1973).
26. Zinkernagel, R. M., and Doherty, P. C., *Nature* **251**, 547 (1974).
27. Bevan, M. J., *J. Exp. Med.* **142**, 1349 (1975).
28. Barker, C. F., and Billingham, R. E., *J. Exp. Med.* **128**, 197 (1968).
29. Vetto, R. M., and Lawson, R. K., *Transplantation* **5**, 1537 (1967).
30a. Strober, S., and Gowans, J. L., *J. Exp. Med.* **122**, 347 (1965).
30b. Guttmann, R. D., Carpenter, C. B., Lindquist, R. R., and Merrill, J. P., *J. Exp. Med.* **126**, 1099 (1967).
30c. Guttmann, R. D., Carpenter, C. B., Lindquist, R. R., and Merrill, J. P., *Lancet* **1**, 248 (1967).
30d. Guttmann, R. D., and Lindquist, R. R., *Transplantation* **8**, 490 (1969).
30e. Guttmann, R. D., Lindquist, R. R., and Ockner, S. A., *Transplantation* **8**, 472 (1969).
30f. Cogen, R., and Lindquist, R. R., *Lab. Invest.* **22**, 494 (1970).
31. Govaerts, *J. Immunol.* (1960).
32. Cantor, H., and Boyse, E. A., *J. Exp. Med.* **141**, 1376 (1975).
33. Beverley, P. C., Woody, J., Dunlley, M., Feldmann, M., and McKenzie, I., *Nature* **262**, 495 (1976).
34. Plaut, M., *Fed. Proc.* **35**, 247 (1976).
35. Eijsuoogel, V. P., Schellekens, P. A., duBois, M. J., and Zeiglemaker, W. P., *Transplant. Rev.* **29**, 125 (1976).
36. Teh, H. S., Harley, E., Phillips, R. A., and Miller, R. G., *Immunology* **118**, 1049 (1977).
37. Lindahl, K. F., and Wilson, D. B., *J. Exp. Med.* **145**, 508 (1977).
38. Skinner, M. A., and Marbrook V., *J. Exp. Med.* **143**, 1562 (1976).
39. Wilson, D. B., *J. Exp. Med.* **122**, 143 (1965).
40. Thorn, R. M., and Henney, C. S., *J. Immunol.* **117**, 2213 (1976).
41. Bonavida, B., Ikejiri, B., and Kedar, E., *Nature* **263**, 769 (1976).
42. Berke, G., Gabison, D., and Feldman, M., *Eur. J. Immunol.* **5**, 813 (1975).
43. Plate, J. M. D., *Cell. Immunol.* **21**, 121 (1976).
44. Alter, B. J., and Bach, F. H. *Cell. Immunol.* **1**, 207 (1970).
45. Heber-Katz, E., and Glick, R. E., *Cell. Immunol.* **5**, 410 (1972).
46. MacDonald, H. R., Sordat, B., Cerottini, J.-C., and Brunner, K. T., *J. Exp. Med.* **142**, 622 (1975).
47. Engers, H. D., Thomas, K., Cerottini, J.-C., and Brunner, K. T., *J. Immunol.* **115**, 350 (1975).
48. Brondz, B. D., and Goldberg, N. E., *Folia Biol.* **16**, 20 (1970).
49. Edidin, M., and Henney, C. S., *Nature (New Biol.)* **240**, 47 (1973).
50. Forman, J., and Klein, J. *Immunogenetics* **1**, 469 (1975).
51. Nabholz, M., Young, H., Meo, T., Miggiano, Rijnbeek, A., and Shreffler, D. C., *Immunogenetics* **1**, 457 (1975).
52. Sondel, P. M., and Bach, F. H., *J. Exp. Med.* **142**, 1339 (1975).
53. Martz, E., *J. Immunol.* **115**, 261 (1975).
54. Martz, E., and Benacerraf, B. J., *J. Immunol.* **111**, 1538 (1973).
55. Brunner, K. T., Mauel, J., Rudolf, H., and Chapuis, B., *Immunology* **18**, 501 (1970).
56. Zagury, D., Bernard, J., Thierness, N., Feldman, M., and Berke, G., *Eur. J. Immunol.* **5**, 818 (1975).
57. Kuppers, R. C., and Henney, C. S., *Fed. Proc.* **35**, 247 (1976).
58. Kalina, M., and Berke, G., *Cell. Immunol.* **25**, 41 (1976).
59. Granger, G. A., and Williams, T. W., *Nature* **218**, 1253 (1968).
60. Ruddle, N. H., and Waksman, B. H., *J. Exp. Med.* **128**, 1267 (1968).
61. Walker, S. M., Lee, S. C., and Lucas, Z. J., *J. Immunol.* **116**, 807 (1976).
62. Hessinger, D. A., Daynes, R. A., and Granger, G. A., *P.N.A.S.* **70**, 3082 (1972).
63. Tsoukas, C. D., Rosenau, W., and Baxter, J. D., *J. Immunol.* **116**, 184 (1976).
64. Sellin, D., Wallach, D. F. H., and Fischer, H., *Eur. J. Immunol.* **1**, 453 (1971).
65. Lindquist, R. R., Guttmann, R. D., and Merrill, J. P., *Transplantation* **12**, 1 (1971).
66. Sura, S. N., Chernyakbovskaya, I. Yu, Kadaghidze, Z. G., Fuks, B. B., and Svet-Moldavsky, G. J., *Exp. Cell Res.* **48**, 556 (1967).

67. Lowenstein, W. R., *Ann. N.Y. Acad. Sci.* **137**, 441 (1966).
68. McIntyre, J. A., Pierce, C. W., and Karnovsky, M. J., *J. Immunol.* **116**, 1582 (1976).
69. Brunner, K. T., March, J., Cerottini, J.-C., and Chapuis, G., *Immunology* **14**, 181 (1968).
70. Henney, C. S., Graffney, J., and Bloom, B. R., *J. Exp. Med.* **140**, 837 (1974).
71. Gately, M. K., Mayer, M. M., and Henney, C. S., *Cell. Immunol.* **27**, 82 (1976).
72. Henney, C. S., *Nature* **249**, 456 (1974).
73. Ferluga, J., and Allison, A. C., *Nature* **250**, 673 (1974).
74. Henkart, P., and Blumenthal, R., *Proc. Natl. Acad. Sci.* **72**, 2789 (1975).
75. Mayer, M., *Proc. Natl. Acad. Sci.* **69**, 2954 (1972).
76. Frye, L. D., and Friore, G. J., *Nature* **258**, 333 (1975).
77. Ferluga, J., and Allison, A. C., *Nature* **255**, 708 (1975).
78. Allison, A. C., and Ferluga, J., *N. Engl. J. Med.* **295**, 165 (1976).
79. Koren, H. S., Ax, W., and Freud-Moelbert, E., *Eur. J. Immunol.* **3**, 32 (1973).
80. Martz, E., and Benacerraf, B., *Cell. Immunol.* **20**, 81 (1975).
81. Henney, C. S. J., *J. Immunol.* **110**, 73 (1973).
82. Martz, E., Burakoff, S. J., and Benacerraf, B., *P.N.A.S.* **91**, 177 (1974).
83. Sanderson, C. J., *Proc. R. Soc. Lond. B* **192**, 221 (1976).
84. Sanderson, C. J., *Proc. R. Soc. Lond. B* **192**, 241 (1976).
85a. Lindquist, R. R., Guttmann, R. D., Merrill, J. P., and Dammin, G. J., *Am. J. Pathol.* **53**, 851 (1968).
85b. Guttmann, R. D., *Transplantation* **17**, 383 (1974).
85c. Forbes, R. D. C., Kuramochi, T., Guttmann, R. D., Klassin, V., and Knauck, J., *Lab Invest.* **33**, 280 (1976).
85d. Boehmig, H. J., Giles, C. R., Amemiga, H., *Transplant. Proc.* **3**, 1105 (1971).
85e. Lowenhaupt, R. W., Nathan, P., Menefee, M. G., *Transplant. Proc.* **3**, 453 (1971).
85f. Forbes, R. D. C., Guttmann, R. D., Kurgmuehi, T., Klassin, J., and Knauck, J., *Lab. Invest.* **34**, 229 (1976).
86. Guttmann, R. D., Lindquist, R. R., Parker, R. M., Carpenter, C. B., and Merrill, J. P., *Transplantation* **5**, 668 (1967).
87. Ockner, S. A., Guttmann, R. D., and Lindquist, R. R., *Transplantation* **9**, 30 (1970).
88. Ockner, S. A., Guttmann, R. D., and Lindquist, R. R., *Transplantation* **9**, 39 (1970).
89. Shehadeh, I. H., Guttmann, R. D., and Lindquist, R. R., *Transplantation* **10**, 66 (1970).
90. Lindquist, R. R., Guttmann, R. D., and Merrill, J. P., *Am. J. Pathol.* **52**, 531 (1968).
91. Lindquist, R. R., Guttmann, R. D., and Merrill, J. P., in *Advances in Transplantation* (J. Dausset, J. Hamburger, and G. Mathe, eds.), Munksgaard, Copenhagen, 1968, p. 225.

Index

Adenosine deaminase, 313
Adjuvant, 52
Agammaglobulinemia, X-linked, 315
Aging, 92, 93, 97, 102
  general aspects, 92
  humoral immune responses, 97
  immunogenetics of, 103
  immunologic theory, 93
Aleutian mink disease, 100
Allograft rejection, 336, 339, 348
  afferent phase, 336
  antibody-mediated mechanisms, 348
  cell-mediated mechanisms, 339
Alport's syndrome, 199
Altered self hypothesis, 333
Anaphylaxis, 20, 21, 69
  bradykinin, 21
  ECF – A, 21
  histamine, 20
  SRS–A, 21
Anemia, hemolytic, 158, 318
Anergy, 54
Angiodema, 291
Ankylosing spondylitis, 333
Antibodies, 14, 39, 40, 63, 69, 127, 130, 133, 181, 346
  anti-basement membrane, 181
  anti-idiotypic, 133
  anti-kidney nephrotoxic, 181
  anti-lymphokine, 63
  anti-lymphotoxin, 346
  anti-neutrophil, 39, 40
  anty-thymocyte, 127
  cyclic production of, 130
  homocytotropic, 69
  reaginic, 14
Antibody, 14, 18, 165
  blocking, 18
  cytotoxic, 165
  IgE, 14, 18
Anticoagulants, 64, 65
Antigen, 161
Antigen-binding cells, 167
Antigen-reactive cells, 118
Arthus reaction, 31, 39, 40
Ataxia telangiectasia, 315
Autoantibodies, 148
  platelets, 148
  red blood cells, 148
  white blood cells, 148
Autoantigens, Kidd-Friedewald type, 149
Autoimmune disease, 143, 150, 157, 160
  classification of, 157
  general aspects, 143
  human, 160
  induction of, 150
Autoimmune hemolytic anemia, 153
Autoimmune responses, genetic control, 152
Autoimmunity, 99

Bactericidal function, 285
Basophils, 70
B cells, 58, 146, 251, 307, 331
Berger's disease, 238
Blast transformation, 74
Blood groups, 148
Blood vessels, integrity of, 44
β2-microglobulin, 329
Bradykinin, 4
Bursectomy, 152

Carcinoma, oat-cell, 233
Cardiac allograft, 349
Cardinoembryonic antigen, 233
Cardiolipin, 149
Carrier specificity, 52
C1r deficiency, 294
C3 deficiency, 296
C3b deficiency, inactivator, 293
C4 deficiency, 295
C5 deficiency, 298
C6 deficiency, 299
C7 deficiency, 299
C8 deficiency, 299
Cell aggregation, 2
Chediak-Higashi syndrome, 277

Chemotactic factors, 2, 5, 9, 43, 75, 81, 84, 276, 349
basophils, 75
effects of, 2
eosinophils, 5, 9, 81
neutrophils, 2, 84
Cirrhosis, hepatic, 11
Clonal deletion theory, 113
Clonal selection theory, 93, 145
Cobra venum factor, 297, 349
Cold hemagglutinins, 148
Collagen vascular disease, and complement deficiency, 301
Collie dog, gray, 273
Complement, 6, 7, 8, 209, 255, 350
alternate pathway, 255
C3, 7
C5a, 8
hyperacute rejection, 350
and immune complexes, 209
in rheumatoid synovial fluids, 255
phlogistic mediator, 7
Complement deficiency states, biological significance, 300
Cryoglobulins, 208, 261
Cryoprecipitates, 225, 233
Cutaneous basophil hypersensitivity, 51, 71, 75, 76, 80. *See also* Hypersensitivity, cutaneous basophil
basophil degranulation of, 76
eosinophils, 80
histologic manifestations, 71
passive transfer, 75, 76
Cyclic AMP, 22
Cytokines, 59
Cytotoxicity, lymphocyte-mediated, 332
Cytotoxic reactions, 339
Cytotoxins, 343

Delayed hypersensitivity, 49, 51, 54, 79, 82, 165
contact sensitivity, 51
eosinophils, 79
fibrin, 51
induction, 51
participation of neutrophils, 82
passive transfer, 54
to thyroid autoantigens, 165
Desensitization, 53
DiGeorge syndrome, 314

Encephalomyelitis, experimental allergic, 127
Endocarditis, infective, 222
Eosinophils, 51, 78
Equine infectious anemia, 100
Erythroblastosis fetalis, 262

Fibroblast activating factors, 6

Germinal centers, 316
Giardia lamblia, 320
Glomerular disease, autologous immune complex-mediated, 235
Glomerular lesions, anti-GBM antibody, 182-187
Glomerulonephritis, 33, 36, 218, 221, 232, 237, 238
acute poststreptococcal, 218
focal, 238
idiopathic membranous, 237
membranous, 232
rapidly progressive, 238
syphilitic, 221
Glomerulonephritis and dense deposit disease, 237
Goodpasture's syndrome, 190
Grave's disease, 164

H antigens, 329, 330, 332, 333, 334, 335
chemical characteristics, 329
and disease, 332
distribution, 330
immunologic memory, 334, 335
participation in cell-cell interactions, 333
Helper T cells, 110, 114
Hemolytic anemia, 158, 318
Hemosiderosis, idiopathic pulmonary, 190
Hepatitis, 225, 263
immune complexes, 225
Histamine, 291
Histocompatibility barriers, 323
Histocompatibility complex, 147
Hodgkin's disease, 11
Horror autotoxicus, 158
Human complement, 290
Hyperacute rejection, 349
Hypersensitivity, cutaneous basophil, 51, 71, 75, 76, 80
basophil degranulation of, 76
eosinophils, 80
histologic manifestations, 71
passive transfer, 75, 76
Hypogammaglobulinemia of infancy, transient, 318

Idiopathic thrombocytopenia, 153
Immune complexes, 29, 30, 31, 153, 203, 204, 206, 208, 233
biologic assays, 206
detection of, 206
physiochemical techniques, 208
properties of, 29, 30, 31
radioimmunoassay, 206
and therapeutic agents, 233
Immunoconglutinin, 149
Immunodeficiency, 307
Immunologic memory, 334, 335
Immunotherapy, 25
Inactivator, 10
anaphylatoxin, 10
C36, 10
chemotactic factor, 10

Inflammatory mediators, control of, 10, 11

Kappa chain deficiency, 319
K cells, 339
Kinins, 3

Leishmaniasis, 263
Leprosy, 11, 263
Leukokinins, 4
Leukopenias, 148
Linkage hypothesis, 333
Lupus erythematosus, 228, 229
Lymphocytes, 73
Lymphokines, 56, 57, 58, 60, 61, 62, 64, 65, 84, 166, 258
  activities of, 56
  biologic significance of, 64, 65
  chemotactic factor, 57
  chemotaxis, 56, 57
  eosinophil chemotactic factor, 57
  helper factor, 56
  inhibition of production, 58
    migration inhibition factor, 55
  in vivo activity of, 60
  leukocyte inhibitory factor, 84, 166
  lymphotoxin, 56
  macrophage, 56, 57
  macrophage activating factor, 56, 57
  macrophage chemotactic factor, 56, 57
  migration enhancement factor, 84
  migration inhibitory factor, 56, 57
  mitogenic factors, 56
  neutrophil chemotactic factor, 84
  production of, 58
    B cells, 58
    T cells, 58
  serum activity, 62
  skin reaction sites, 61
  skin reactive factor, 60
  suppressor factors, 56
Lymphotoxins, 344

Macrophage disappearance reaction, 60
Major histocompatibility complex in mice, 324-327
  I region, 326
  K and D region, 325
  S region, 327
Major histocompatibility in man, 328
Masugi nephritis, 182
Migration inhibitory factors, 55
Mimicry hypothesis, 333
Mixed leukocyte cultures, 250
Mixed lymphocyte cultures, 331
Monocyte, 273
Mononuclear cells, 50
  accumulation of, 50
  delayed reactions, 50
Mononucleosis, 263
Mother factors, 56
Myeloperoxidase deficiency, 285

Neonatal thymectomy, 152
Nephritis, 45, 190, 197
  nephrotoxic, 45
  rapidly progressive, 190
  tubulointerstitial, 190, 197
    methicillin-associated, 197
Nephropathy, Quartan malarial, 221
Neutropenia, 273, 275
  clinical and pathologic consequences, 275
  cyclic, 273
Neutrophils, 41, 42, 43, 45, 82, 272, 280, 282, 349
  accumulation of, 43
  actin dysfunction, 280
  adhesiveness, 282
  complement and, 43
  constituents of, 45
  corticosteroid therapy and, 282
  locomotion defects, 280
  migration, 282
Null cells, 339

Pancreas, 149
Panphagocytopenia, 275
Passenger leukocytes, 337, 338
Phagocyte, 271
Phagocyte paralysis syndromes, 287
Phospholipase A, 347
Plasmapheresis, 196
Platelet aggregation, 212
Primary specific immunodeficiencies, coassification of, 308
Prostaglandins, 2
Proteins, cold-precipitable, 257
Proteinuria, 42

Radioimmunoassay, 193
Raji cell, 211
RAST techniques, 15, 16
Renal tubular lesions, antibody-induced, 187, 188
Retest reaction, 51, 81
Rheumatic fever, 33
Rheumatoid arthritis, 9, 247, 252, 254, 258, 259, 260
  articular cavity, 254
  cartilage, 258
  extra-articular manifestations, 259, 260
  immunologic status, 247
  joint, 252
  synovial fluid, 254
  synovial membrane, 252
Rheumatoid factors, 149, 210, 261

Sarcoidosis, 263
Schistosomiasis, 263
Secretory piece deficiency, 317

Self-recognition, 144
Serum sickness, 29-33
Shunt nephritis, 224
Sjögren's syndrome, 263
Slow-reaching substance, 5
Slow virus infection, 99
Suppressor T cells, 110
Syphilis, 263

T cells, 58, 95, 146, 248, 249, 307, 331
  immune function of, 95
Thrombocytopenias, 148, 318
Thymoma, 315
Thymus, 147, 314, 316
  transplants, 314
Thyroglobulin, 145, 161, 162, 163
  antibodies, 162, 163
    radioimmunoassay, 163
Thyroiditis, 57, 78, 122, 161, 164, 167, 168, 169, 172, 173, 174
  antigen-binding cells, 167
  autoimmune, 57, 78, 161, 172, 173, 174
  chronic lymphocytic, 161
  cytotoxic reactions in, 167
  etiology, 174
  Hashimoto's, 122, 161, 164
  histopathology, 168, 169
  immunogenetic, 172
  lymphadenoid goiter, 161
  pathogenesis, 173
  struma lymphomatosa, 161
Tissue injury, 39, 40
  immune complexes, 39, 40
    neutrophils, 39, 40
Tolerance, 107, 108, 110
  mechanism of, 108, 110
    effector cell blockade, 108
    suppressor T cells, 110
Tolerogen, dosage, 115
Transcobalamin II deficiency, 317
Transplant recipients, anti-TBM antibodies, 199
Trypanosomiasis, 263
Tuberculosis, 263
Tumor angiogenesis factor, 5

Unresponsive state, 117, 120
  duration of, 117
  termination of, 120

Vasculitis, 39, 40, 262, 351
  necrotizing lesions, 351
  in rheumatoid arthritis, 262
Vasoactive amines, 5, 20
  histomine, 5, 20
  serotonin, 20

Wiskott-Aldrich syndrome, 319